NO ASYLUM

Also by Theresa C. Smith

SECURITY vs SURVIVAL: The Nuclear Arms Race (*editor with Indu B. Singh*)
TROJAN PEACE: Some Deterrence Propositions Tested

Also by Thomas A. Oleszczuk

POLITICAL JUSTICE IN THE USSR: Lithuania

No Asylum

State Psychiatric Repression in the Former USSR

Theresa C. Smith
Mankato-Minnesota State University

in collaboration with

Thomas A. Oleszczuk
Stern School of Business
New York University

NEW YORK UNIVERSITY PRESS
Washington Square, New York

First published in the U.S.A. in 1996 by
NEW YORK UNIVERSITY PRESS
Washington Square
New York, N.Y. 10003

Library of Congress Cataloging-in-Publication Data
Smith, Theresa C.
No asylum : state psychiatric repression in the former USSR /
Theresa C. Smith ; in collaboration with Thomas A. Oleszczuk.
p. cm.
Includes bibliographical references and index.
ISBN 0–8147–8061–X
1. Political prisoners—Soviet Union. 2. Psychiatric hospitals–
–Soviet Union. 3. Dissenters—Soviet Union. 4. Psychiatry—Soviet
Union. I. Oleszczuk, Thomas A. II. Title.
HV9713.S59 1996
365'.46'0947—dc20 96–16533
CIP

Printed in Great Britain

To all the ships at sea. . . .and one capsized sailboat

Since then [1971], the Western press has carried one report after another about the use in the USSR of 'psychiatric terror against dissidents,' and various made-up numbers and new names – Plyushch, Vaikhanskaya, Fainberg and many others – have kept on surfacing.

M. Ye. Vartanyan, quoted in A. Novikov, 1987

Contents

List of Figures

List of Tables

Acknowledgements

The author and her collaborator gratefully acknowledge the research support of the International Studies Program at City College of New York, and grants from the Graduate College and the College of Social and Behavioral Sciences at Mankato-Minnesota State University System. We also appreciate the resources and talents made available to us by Sandra Stump at the Albright College Library in Reading, Pennsylvania; Kellian Clink at the Memorial Library at Mankato, Minnesota; and by the staff of the Government Documents Center at the University of Minnesota Wilson Library.

We have benefited from the advice and assistance of our many colleagues, including Professor John E. Turner, Regents Professor at the University of Minnesota; Professor Scott Shrewsbury of the Department of Political Science at Mankato in the Minnesota State University System, Professor Niel Brasher of Shippensburg State University in Pennsylvania, and Dr Scott Bodfish, Director of Institutional Research at Wilkes University, Pennsylvania. We would also like to thank Professor George Ginsbergs for permitting us to consult his materials at the Rutgers Camden University Library during the initial data-gathering.

Since we undertook the Soviet Repressed Dissident Project in 1980, several of our graduate students have made substantial contributions to coding and verifying our data. Chief among them is Thomas Klobucar, who coded the Mercer and Koppers data as well as producing a new draft of the project codebook. Kehai Su and Amy Grau also made notable additions.

Undergraduates including Cyndi Beaver Hughes, Neal Knudson and, Kevin Lau have provided valuable and much-appreciated computer skills, coding and bibliographic assistance.

These investigations have profited from the dedication and shared insights of myriad human rights advocates and researchers, including Michael Bourdeaux and Michael Rowe of Keston College, Kent; Kathy Cosman at CSCE; Barbara Futterman of Freedom House; the staff of the Lithuanian Information Center in Brooklyn, NY.

We are most especially indebted to other researchers E.J. Driessen, S.P. de Boer, H.L. Verhaar, Ellen Mercer, and Andre Koppers for their kind permission to consult their data to corroborate, enrich and extend our own, and of course to the defining scholars in this field, Peter Reddaway and Sidney Bloch, not only for the privilege of consulting their own studies but also for permission to reprint names from their data.

The author extends her thanks to Jo L. Sotheran for the many original contributions to this project, including lengthy efforts formalizing the first codebook. The author remains perpetually indebted to Bruce E. Auerbach, for much else besides his theoretical cast of mind.

Any surviving errors, are, of course, our own.

Special gratitude is due to Dean Barbara Keating at Mankato for facilitating the academic leave during which this book was written.

1 Political Hospitalization: Conception, Conceptualization and Conduct

> It's no secret to anyone that you can have schizophrenia without schizophrenia.
>
> Attributed to V.M. Morozov, in Koppers, 1990:36

> You are not a schizophrenic, but we will not annul the diagnosis. You earned it at the KGB.
>
> Dr Igor Goncharenko to A.M. Ilchenko, in Mercer, 1991:8

Leonid F. Dobrov: After petitioning the Supreme Soviet in 1985 for schools, newspapers, radio, and television in his native Gagauz language, L.F. Dobrov was whisked off the Moscow streets and transported to a psychiatric hospital. He spent three years in psychiatric hospitals before escaping and was still in hiding in 1991. (Mercer, 1991b)

Mikhail V. Ivankov-Nikolov: In 1956, while in Taiwan, the crew of his ship, the Soviet tanker *Tuapse*, requested asylum in the US. Ivankov-Nikolov, a radio operator, returned to the USSR, assured by Soviet embassy staff that there would be no retaliation. On arrival he was promptly arrested and spent over a decade in psychiatric detention. (Koppers, 1990)

Annasoltan Kekilova: A nonconformist Turkmeni poet, Kekilova found herself unable to publish in Turkmenistan, and migrated to Moscow. Contemplating leaving the country, she returned to Turkmenistan to gather her documents. There she was arrested and forcibly confined for several years to a psychiatric hospital, where she died. (Shchipakhina, 1988)

Aleksei Vasilievich Nikitin: A Communist engineer expelled from the Party for agitating for mine workers' safety and bonuses, Nikitin fell under KGB surveillance after a mine explosion he had feared took place, killing several. After repeated arrests, failed attempts to find work or to emigrate, and a meeting with Western journalists, Nikitin was forcibly detained in 1980.

He died of a drug overdose in 1984 in Talgar Special Psychiatric Hospital. (Amnesty International, Koppers, 1990)

INTRODUCTION

Many states confront episodic phenomena of political, national, ethnic and religious dissidents who defy societal norms. The Soviet experience with dissident movements was unprecedented for its duration, intensity, mass recruiting base, and its significance in the erosion and collapse of the Union. The Soviet experience was unique in both the size and degree of organization of nonconformist informal groups. The dissident movements at their apex comprised perhaps a quarter of a million or more diverse individuals (Hubner, 1980:84), of whom hundreds, possibly thousands, of the more vocal or irritating nonconformists were confined to psychiatric hospitals for extended periods. Even pariah states, such as South Africa at the height of its defence of apartheid, did not resort systematically to this measure to inhibit political upheaval.

This book presents a quantitative assessment of the incidence of state repression via the peculiar institution of forced psychiatric internment of evidently healthy individuals in the Soviet state. It considers who is targeted, and what political, economic, religious and other causes catalyze psychiatric repression. The analyses document patterns in extent, severity, timing and location of psychiatric detention. The possible roles of political cultural predisposition, professional socialization and training, and intergenerational conflict in explaining political use of mental hospitalization are examined. As we will show, our evidence is most coherent with the hypothesis of instrumental state use of psychiatric medicine to manipulate, deflect, defuse, discredit or disperse the multifaceted dissident and nonconformist movements.

HISTORY OF POLITICAL INTERNMENT

The early notion that demonic possession caused mental illness implied religion might be the only prophylaxis. Under Prince Vladimir in the tenth century, monks were ordered to aid the mentally ill. In 1551 Ivan Grozni (the Terrible) similarly instructed the Church to attend to those of unsound mind. Pyotr Veliki (Peter the Great), under a different cosmology, ordered that care be provided in psychiatric hospitals rather than monasteries in

1723. In 1762 Pyotr III again decreed separate non-Church facilities for the mentally ill (Miller, 1985:14, Babayan, 1985:2), but these instructions remained dead letter until the rule of Catherine the Great.

Thus the Tsars and a Tsarina laid the foundation for a dual system of mental health care, begun as early as the tenth and the eleventh centuries in the Russian Orthodox monasteries of Kievan Rus and diversified with the edict on non-Church hospitals in 1762. They also formalized the practice of detaining obstreperous critics of the regime on grounds of mental imbalance, and advanced the concept of 'litigious insanity' (Gluzman, 1989:36), establishing a politically useful diagnosis and the historical precedent of ordering hospitalization of dissenters and religious nonconformists.

Though sporadic use of internment had been made previously,[1] the first prominent case of punitive psychiatric detention, Chaadaev's, dates from 1836. Tsar Nicholas I declared the eminent literary figure Pyotr Y. Chaadaev insane following circulation of Chaadaev's article denouncing Tsarism, and ordered him held under house arrest – benevolently, of course – for a year (Tempest, 1986). However, the Tsarist practice of imprisoning political deviants was neither widespread nor systematic (Reddaway, 1972:231–2). Though our data show previous instances, methodical political use of psychiatric hospitals as prisons did not begin until well into the Soviet period, 1936 to 1938, when Andrei Vyshinsky initiated psychiatric detention at the behest of Stalin's Chief of Secret Police, the 'nation's favourite son' and Minister of Internal Affairs Nikolai Yezhov. Alexander Podrabinek suggests that after Stalin's death in 1953 the practice of punitive medicine to deter dissent intensified dramatically (1980:58, 70), apparently cresting during the years 1960–81[2] in the period during which our original demographic and quantitative data were the richest and most detailed, with intervals of heightened repression including the late sixties and 1977–78. Boris M. Segal, former director of the Department of Clinical Psychology and Psychotherapy at the Moscow Institute of Psychiatry, saw the overtly political trials of 1966–68 as the beginning of notable abuse of psychiatry for political purposes (Segal, 1976:274). After Leonid Ilyich Brezhnev's death in 1982, the brief administrations of Yuri Vladimirovich Andropov and Konstantin Ustinovich Chernenko were characterized by a reduction in the number of political detainees, as though the state began to abandon this tactic.

Under Gorbachev and glasnost, the number of activists involuntarily hospitalized remained low, and the geographical pattern of commitments may have shifted. Political arrests in general declined after 1986, early in the administration of Mikhail Sergeyevich Gorbachev, according to Amnesty International and other sources. The number of critics known to be detained in psychiatric hospitals also fell precipitously through the late 1980s (Amnesty International, 1989) to singularly few in the early 1990s.[3]

While there is evidence that psychiatric detention declined in this era, it did not disappear entirely. The March 1991 cancellation by Soviet Health Ministry authorities of a 16-person World Psychiatric Association delegation visit to Soviet mental hospitals, on the pretext that the Ministry lacked foreign currency adequate to extend hospitality, reinforced the Association's concerns that in early 1991 'abuse of psychiatry is still widespread in the Soviet Union',[4] a concern not quelled by the rescheduled visit which took place in June 1991. However apparently no well-known political detainees remained by 1995, even though those lesser known and 'complainers' might still be hospitalized, and the Russian government was not immune from attempts to co-opt psychiatry for political purposes.

Open sources of information proliferated in the late 1980s, only to wither under Boris Nikolayevich Yeltsin as the economy spiralled steeply downward. In the wake of the collapse of the ruble,[5] at least one Soviet psychiatric hospital, Kashchenko, Moscow's largest, turned to church volunteers and contributors to allow it to survive (*Ogonek*, 1990, in Reddaway, 1991:47). Television news broadcast in 1994 alleged St Petersburg hospitals were releasing their patients for lack of food.

DISTINCTIVE FEATURES OF THE SOVIET EXPERIENCE

What is extraordinary about the Soviet case is not that the USSR jailed political dissidents. All societies define conformity and penalize nonconformists. Therefore we dispense with the argument that other societies do not hold political prisoners (for example, Jacobo Timerman in Argentina, Steve Biko in South Africa, Leonard Peltier in the US, according to some analyses), whether in stadiums, psychiatric hospitals and clinics, or elsewhere, since nation-states do define and prosecute crimes against the state.

Instead, the distinctive characteristic of the Soviet case is the unprecedented *number* of political hospitalizations, resulting from the scale and conspicuousness of the Soviet dissident movement and consequent dramatic accumulation of political prisoners. Extraordinary too are the organizational networks which garnered information on internees and made it known in the West under conditions of great uncertainty, deprivation and high risk. Although new evidence may document similar phenomena in central Europe, Cuba, and elsewhere,[6] political use of mental hospitals emerges as an exceptional and costly strategy for coping with regime critics, and one which is usefully explained within a larger theory of regime response to dissidence, state terror, and political opposition in general (Stohl and Lopez, 1984). The question of regime response to resistance assumed a new urgency globally in the 1980s and 1990s as more governments resorted to 'disappearing' the political nuisances among them rather than engaging in the complex, lengthy and rule-bound procedures of arrest, trial and hospitalization or imprisonment.

Charges defining political crimes are characterized by their vagueness, and permissiveness with respect to enforcement decisions (Turk, 1982:54), though provisions of the ordinary civil and criminal codes can also be used for political purposes. In the US explicitly political crimes include espionage, altering election returns, civil (human) rights violations, selective service-related charges, passport and visa crimes, and racketeering.[7] In contrast to the USSR, US political crimes usually do not result in large numbers of arrests, nor in the creation of an extensive network of informal activist groups supporting those arrested. (The anti-slavery and anti-war movements are exceptions, if political crime is defined more broadly.) The probability of conviction for essentially political charges as narrowly defined not to include economic crimes is low historically in the US (Turk, 1969:137), and occasionally undependable in the USSR. Failure of the courts to convict universally and conveniently, despite the educational value of occasionally disbarring attorneys who defended dissidents, may be one reason for Soviet resort to political use of psychiatric commitments.

Salient aspects in the practice and structure of Soviet psychiatry which distinguished Soviet practice from that of most other countries outside Eastern Europe and perhaps Cuba and the PRC include:

1. An unusually ambiguous definition of mental disease.
2. Structural features of medicine and politics which facilitated regime influence on psychiatrists and their practice of medicine. Communist Party and KGB/MVD influence on arrests and detentions, and in management of special regime hospitals, as well as state connections to the structure of academic psychiatry, compromised the neutrality and independence of diagnosticians.
3. Inconsistent and inappropriate application of criteria for competence to face trial ('imputability' in Soviet terms).
4. Structural features of the law and legal practice which maximized the probability of insanity findings and the risks of use of hospitalization as retribution.
5. Reports of punitive transfer between mental institutions.
6. Punitive use of pharmaceuticals, and of industrial chemicals not suited for any medical use on humans.

These features, because they made possible though not inevitable systematic violation of fundamental human rights of religious activists, organizers of unofficial groups and nascent political parties, and other political and religious nonconformists, constitute essential elements of an explanation of psychiatric repression and so merit further exploration.

DISTINCTIVE ASPECTS OF SOVIET PSYCHIATRY: PRACTICE

1. Ambiguous Definition of Mental Disease, Leading to Hospitalization of the Healthy

The Soviet Union hospitalized individuals with no discernible mental illness, or with minor mental aberrations not requiring confinement. In particular, dissidents designated 'socially dangerous' in the sense of undermining discretionarily defined socialist values were committed when appropriate medical criteria as these would be interpreted in the West, such as posing a *physical* danger to themselves or others, were not met. A broad, inappropriately ambiguous definition of dangerousness, or even failure to compose any definition, and a diffuse operational definition of mental disease not sustainable in other societies facilitated these detentions (Merskey and Shafran, 1986:247–50).

Culture-bound low threshold definitions of mental illness in conformist societies may imply more diagnoses of mental illness there in general. This predisposition was exacerbated in the USSR where dissident attitudes could be defined as maladjusted and morbid, even in adolescents where they might otherwise or elsewhere be considered experimental, temporary, or even normal.[8]

Historical Development of a Broad Definition of Mental Disorder and Corresponding Diagnostic Criteria

Soviet practice employed a broader definition of mental illness than is generally employed in Western countries, despite the American Psychiatric Association's *Diagnostic and Statistical Manual of Mental Disorders'* (DSM-IV) forthright comment on Western diagnoses: '. . . it must be admitted that no definition adequately specifies precise boundaries for the concept of "mental disorder" ' (*DSM-IV*, 1994:xxi). The *DSM-IV* does succeed in specifying the symptoms and, most importantly, time parameters characterizing syndromes defined in the *Manual*. Schizophrenia is defined as 'a disturbance that lasts for at least six months and includes at least one month of active-phase symptoms (. . . delusions, hallucinations, disorganized speech, grossly disorganized or catatonic behavior, negative symptoms)' (ibid.:273). By contrast, the Soviet operational definition of schizophrenia has been so diffuse as to include conditions which would either be diagnosed as other mental disorders elsewhere, or would not be diagnosed as pathological at all. A broad, asymptomatic definition of psychopathy was also widely used in the Soviet Union.[9] This definitional latitude is meaningful since asymptomatic schizophrenia and 'psychopathy' rather than paranoia or other serious disturbances have been alleged as the reasons for hospitalizing many apparently healthy nonconformists.

It can be argued that psychiatry in general and great power psychiatry in particular failed to define schizophrenic states unambiguously (Scheflen, 1981; American Psychiatric Association, 1994). A 1973 World Health Organization crossnational study found the greatest latitude in the application of this term in Washington, DC and in Moscow (WHO, 1973; Bloch and Reddaway, 1977:245–6). However, in the Soviet case, particular psychiatrists expanded upon even these already insupportably general criteria.

In the West, serious mental dysfunction tends to be attributed to physiological, chromosomal, chemical or other material causes, while Soviets often favoured class-based and environmental explanations for neurotic behaviour.[10] In an exception to this general approach, prevalent Soviet views of schizophrenia hypothesized a genetic origin for the condition, with a consequent presumption of incurability which has had deleterious human rights consequences irrespective of the accuracy of the hypothesis.

During the 1920s and 1930s the Soviet child psychiatrist G.E. Sukhareva elaborated a classification of schizophrenia by type of onset and evolution.[11] Her classification[12] was adapted for adults and attributed to Academician Andrei Vladimirovich Snezhnevsky, the single most influential Soviet psychiatrist even perhaps beyond his death in 1987. This typology rendered Soviet psychiatry vulnerable to charges of non-scientific, non-falsifiable, diagnoses, not based on manifestations of disease but on hypothetical future states:[13]

1. sluggish or chronic
2. acute
3. shift-like mixed form.

A.V. Snezhnevsky renamed the first two of these phases of schizophrenia 'continuous' and 'periodic', although the term 'sluggish' persisted in diagnostic use. Snezhnevsky explicitly presumed genetic risk factors catalyzed by environment (Miller, 1985:16). Because of Snezhnevsky's dominance of the authoritative Serbsky Central Scientific Research Institute of General and Forensic Psychiatry (Serbsky) in Moscow, and his influence on the major journal, the *Korsakov Journal of Neuropathology and Psychiatry*, this interpretation of serious mental disorder acquired the most authority and prestige across the Soviet Union. A.V. Snezhnevsky's views were propagated among generations of Soviet psychiatrists through his role as Director of the Institute of Psychiatry at the Academy of Medical Sciences. In this capacity, he also advised the Ministry of Health on psychiatric medicine policy, advanced education, and research. Subsequently the focus of research and diagnosis shifted to the genetics of schizophrenia and the expectation of discovering a hypothesized 'biological structure of the schizophrenic genotype'(Babayan, 1985:43), hinted at in 1995 Western studies on human chromosome six.

The implications for dissidents of this typology and the presumption of genetic origin of mental disease were dire. Politically suspect individuals, after an initial authoritative labelling as schizophrenic, which could be had briskly and on an emergency basis *post hoc ergo propter hoc*, could only be found mentally sound with great difficulty. They might be subject to long-term hospitalization or psychiatric clinic surveillance. The absence of observable symptoms, rather than undermining the diagnosis of grave illness, merely resulted in a classification of intermittent disease.

Further, since genetic etiology was advanced as the main or only cause, allegations of mental illness could result in clinical supervision or insanity diagnoses of whole families.[14] Illustrating the wide possibilities of abuse following from the assumption of a schizophrenic or other psychotic genotype, Boris Vinokurov, of Gostelradio, was found insane *along with his wife and daughter* after he called a little prematurely for a 'bipartisan' economy and communication system (Antebi, 1977:192), much less radical than those later proposed under Gorbachev.

Dr Georgi Vasilievich Morozov (a Director at Serbsky,[15] 1957–85), extending the sluggish, acute and mixed-form typology from schizophrenia to paranoia, expanded further the scope of politically expedient diagnoses. 'Particularly in the case of paranoiac delusions . . . these activities are frequently accompanied by outwardly well-ordered behaviour . . . The main feature of such patients is their dissimulation . . .' (1974:40); that is, they appear *healthy*. A further extension of irrefutable, hence politically expedient, diagnoses has been made in the definition of 'zealotry delirium', an obsession with one particular subject such as press freedom (but not ballet or the cello) in an otherwise admittedly healthy individual (Vartanyan in Novikov, 1987). 'Resistance to therapy' (Babayan, 1985:68) via insistence that one is of sound mind might also be interpreted as a sign of illness, a ploy not unknown to Western psychiatrists.

This classification of schizophrenic and paranoiac conditions which defined an asymptomatic state in the course of the disease not only did not require empirical evidence for support but could not contemplate any contradictory empirical evidence of *sanity* except as brief remission in a relentless decline. Thus such diagnoses could not be refuted.[16] The typology was therefore inherently vulnerable to systematic discretionary instrumental misuse as well as to accidental misdiagnosis and benevolent misclassification. Via this classification system, healthy but obstreperous people might be hospitalized on claims of sluggish or dispositional mental disorders characterized by the absence of discernible symptoms.[17] Not coincidentally many hospitalized dissidents were classified as suffering from 'sluggish' or 'creeping' schizophrenia, implying both irrefutable diagnoses and incurable disease, with 'reformist delusions', a diagnosis found at least into the mid- and late 1980s.[18]

The cases of Leonid Plyushch (Bloch and Reddaway, 1977; Koppers, 1990:138–9 and Sapiets *et al.*, 1976:x, 83–5), and Zhores A. Medvedev (Koppers, 1990:125) provide two of the more spectacular examples of dissidents found asymptomatically insane because of their human rights activity. Zhores Aleksandrovich Medvedev, a gerontologist, was arrested and hospitalized in 1970 for his samizdat[19] publications, including *The Fall and Rise of T.D. Lysenko*. Found to be suffering from 'sluggish schizophrenia . . . paranoid delusions of reform', he spent much of 1970 confined to psychiatric institutions. The Ukrainian mathematician Leonid Ivanovich Plyushch, who lost his job as a result of samizdat work, was arrested in 1972. He too was diagnosed schizophrenic with messianic and reformist delusions, after helping to found the Action Group for the Defence of Human Rights and relaying information to the Group from Ukraine. Plyushch spent nearly four years in psychiatric detention, where he survived massive doses of drugs, and lived to emigrate in 1976.

Over-use of schizophrenia diagnoses remained evident as late as 1991. In that year the World Psychiatric Association interviewed ten formerly or currently hospitalized dissidents in the USSR, all of whom had been diagnosed as schizophrenic, but the WPA team could confirm the schizophrenia finding in only *one* instance (WPA, 1991:9).

Hospitalization of Healthy Individuals: Allegations and Evidence

Undeniably, in the Soviet Union healthy individuals were hospitalized involuntarily, or 'voluntarily' by relatives and others, for reasons of political activity or religious observance. Good faith estimates of the total number detained vary over time and by observer from 200 to 2000 (V. Bukovsky's

1970 estimate, in US Senate, 1973:32) or even 7000 (Dr Norman Hirt's estimate, ibid.:28). Bloch and Reddaway's estimate of 'several hundred' or perhaps approximately 350 at any one time appears to us most accurate (Bloch and Reddaway, 1977:260–1). Since co-workers and trade union representatives, as well as physicians at clinics or neuropsychiatric dispensaries and others could initiate 'voluntary' hospitalization (Salvendry, 1975:234), and the records of those involuntarily committed might be altered to reflect voluntary admission, entailing fewer reviews, both purportedly voluntary and involuntary commitment procedures presented a risk of political abuse.

Western psychiatrists repeatedly have found no basis for the hospitalization of many or all of those dissident individuals they examined in the USSR, and they have been joined in this assessment by Soviet colleagues on notable occasions. The Soviet psychiatrist Dr Anatoly Ivanovich Koryagin[20] found that *none* of the 15 nonconformists he interviewed required hospitalization (Koryagin, 1981). Dr Semyon Gluzman similarly found a pattern of forced hospitalization of sane people, and in particular opposed the finding of insanity in Gen. P.G. Grigorenko's case. Frequently, detained individuals have been found sane or not in need of treatment by *both* Soviet as well as Western psychiatrists (see Table 1.1).

Beyond doubt unnecessary hospitalizations continued into the 90s, as indicated in our data, other studies, and in Soviet public perceptions. A 1990 public opinion poll taken in Moscow and a small town shows that roughly an eighth to a third of respondents admitted to personal knowledge of a 'recent' case of psychiatric abuse.[21] According to one *Izvestia* account[22] in late December 1990, nearly 200 of the 600 prisoners still held in the special psychiatric hospital (SPH – later called strict supervision or strict observation hospitals) at Dvoryanskoye in Volgograd Oblast were being held without medical justification, including the political detainee Vladimir Novikov. Roy Alexandrovich Medvedev, Zhores' brother, also indicated ongoing abuse of psychiatry in 1990, even though the special psychiatric hospitals had purportedly already been transferred to the Ministry of Health and relevant units of the KGB[23] had been shut down. Medvedev saw this continuation of punitive psychiatry as a function of local political needs rather than a pattern of national suppression. In an interview with Tatyana Kuropayeva,[24] Medvedev is quoted as asserting '. . . I receive letters from people who are clearly absolutely healthy, but who got drawn into this psychiatric machine and have still not managed to extricate themselves from it.'

Medvedev's understanding that psychiatric repression had resolved itself into a local phenomenon may reflect the establishment in 1988 of new posts for chief psychiatrists of cities, districts and regions. These posts existed outside the mental hospital administration and would therefore have been vulnerable at least in principle to local political manipulation.

Reddaway indicated (1991:47–8) that the strict observation hospitals still retained 'many' unjustifiably as late as 1991, among whom were political and religious detainees. Cronid Lubarsky's *Vesti iz SSSR/USSR News Brief* list for October 1991, as the Union crumbled, included 11 confirmable political prisoners still held in psychiatric hospitals.

By January 1993 the Council on Security and Cooperation in Europe (CSCE), an intergovernmental agency with human rights interests, knew of no new cases of post-Soviet punitive psychiatry, and reliable sources indicated this was no longer an ongoing concern, but the CSCE hazarded that some cases might have taken place in outlying areas (CSCE, 1993:32).

These reports constitute more than sporadic and unsupported allegations. They clearly amount to evidence over time of hospitalization of healthy individuals.

Hospitalization of Healthy Individuals: Methodical and Large-Scale

The Soviet experience with punitive hospitalization differed from that of other countries in that healthy people were not detained idiosyncratically or occasionally but systematically at predictable times. Detentions followed behaviour critical of the government, religious observances, and actions advocating prohibited causes. Forced hospitalizations took place on a scale corresponding to the activity level of the dissident movement.

Zoya Serebryakova, then Chief Psychiatrist of the Soviet Ministry of Health, publicly announced in a Congress in Moscow in May 1981 that in a particular Moscow mental hospital 1.2 per cent of the inmates were incarcerated for complaints against the government (Amnesty International, 1983:9). This announcement is particularly remarkable considering that Serebryakova had been an advisor to the Ministry of Health for many years and must have been aware of – if she did not in fact help devise – practices facilitating hospitalization of dissidents and 'complainers'. Further, a number of other Soviet psychiatrists (Gluzman, Koryagin, Papiashvili) and at least one feldsher/ambulance service worker[25] (Podrabinek) openly identified a methodical practice of hospitalization of individuals noted for their political or religious behaviour. A director of the Serbsky Institute after Snezhnevsky, T. Dmitriyeva, herself acknowledged 'decades' of such abuses.[26]

However, this evidence must be understood within a larger comparative perspective. Hospitalization of some individuals without mental illness is not unique to the Soviet state. An extreme example is found in Bloch and Reddaway's account of two women forcibly interned in England for 50 years simply because they each had borne a natural child (1977:29).[27] The United States National Institute of Health reports psychiatric confinement of individuals in US hospitals, in categories not clearly requiring hospitalization, including retardation, transient disturbances, undiagnosed mental illness, and *no* mental disorder[28] (Atay, 1993; US Department of Health, 1963; Turk, 1969:142–3, 169). For 1990, Atay *et al.* showed that approximately two per cent of all additions to resident mental hospitals and about one per cent of all residents in US mental institutions exhibited *no* mental disorder whatsoever, in US residential state and county hospitals (Atay *et al.*, 1993).[29]

The implication of the US reports is that some nonconforming individuals in the US who are presumed sane become mental hospital residents as a result of family complaints, persuadable judges, psychiatrists' and other physicians' decisions, and idiosyncratic factors. Although these hospitalizations may be needless and therefore harmful, they are not necessarily systematically related to policies of state repression.

Diagnostic Variability as an 'Innocent' Cause of Hospitalization of Healthy Activists

Healthy people might be hospitalized by mistake, benevolently as a means of draft avoidance[30] or evasion of a prison camp term, or for other reasons. Marginal cases might be hospitalized because of conflicts in their doctors' academic training. Non-marginal cases might be hospitalized simply through poor practice of psychiatry, a question of quality rather than perspective in academic training. In the West, Baldessarini (1970:59) asserted that variations in diagnostic criteria – for example, variations resulting from instruction in different schools – might account for an individual's being found schizophrenic in New York and found to be suffering mainly from affective disorders in London. Diagnostic variability can be documented not only across regions, but also in the same place, simultaneously and over time. Such divergences can even be found when people are admitted to a second hospital in the same Western city at about the same time. Perhaps it is not surprising, then, that findings of schizophrenia could be six times more common in Moscow than in Leningrad; seven times as frequent in the Tadzhik SSR as in Georgia (US Senate, 1973:26). Because diagnostic variability is real, not all inconsistencies and variations in reclassification can be attributed to regime preference in the Soviet case, and thus to punitive use of psychiatry, although some anomalies are more suspect than others. The fact that Gen. P.G. Grigorenko was found healthy in Tashkent and paranoid on transfer to the Serbsky Institute in Moscow (Rubenstein, 1980, 1985:140) reflected a suspect reclassification because of the prominence of the individual concerned, the vagueness of evidence relied upon, and the interests apparently served by his reclassification, as well as the known proclivities of classification which inhered in the Serbsky Institute, a reliable source of a schizophrenia finding.

Diagnostic variability naturally arose in the Soviet case since Soviet psychiatry was no more monolithic than the Soviet government. Schools which competed with the dominant and schizophrenia-obsessed Snezhnevsky School (Serbsky Central Scientific Research Institute of General and Forensic Psychiatry) for academic standing and for political power did and still do exist outside Moscow, in Leningrad/St Petersburg, Tbilisi, Riga, Kiev and elsewhere. The Bekhterev Institute in St Petersburg advocates an interpretation of serious mental disease which contrasts sharply with that of the Moscow school in that it views environmental factors as the more powerful inducers of schizophrenia, and relies on psychotherapy, psychophysiological therapy, and behaviour modification treatments rather than chemicals. The St Petersburg school criticizes Snezhnevsky for over- and mis-diagnosing schizophrenia and for the '". . . labelling impact" [of] imposing an *unsubstantiated* diagnosis . . . which will itself have negative consequences' (Miller, 1985:20, citing Kazanetz, 1979; Reddaway, 1991:46–8), especially if the genetic or permanent basis for mental disease is accepted.

Diagnostic variability enhances the opportunity for political use of psychiatry. Since individuals could be sent for examination to a location likely to yield the preferred diagnosis, those with the authority to order the evaluation could select a convenient institution. Not only procurators, prison administrators and chief psychiatrists wielded the authority to request psychiatric examinations. Even one doctor in general practice could order an examination for a civil commitment. Those with *de facto* power to order an examination of an unwilling person by forcing individuals to be committed at least for short periods, included KGB officers working with ambulance attendants, military registration offices, governing committees of the district soviets, city Party Committees, town councils, Party Raykoms (District Party Committees), police, and even offices of the State Motor Vehicle Inspectorate (cf. Koryagin in van Voren, 1987:45), as well as employers, and local clinics.

Evidence of Needless Hospitalizations from Selected International Visits, and Soviet Reassessments

Because Soviet authorities for many years insisted that dissident psychoprisoners were genuinely mentally ill, it is necessary at the outset of this inquiry to establish that empirical evidence supports allegations of medically unnecessary and therefore potentially political hospitalizations. In a subsequent chapter data are discussed in greater detail.

Médecins Sans Frontières (MSF) member Dr Bernard Granger indicated that of 150 apparent victims of psychiatric abuse evaluated by MSF from 1987 to 1989 the vast majority 'displayed no illnesses adequate to warrant the treatment they received in the USSR' (IAPUP, 1990, No. 23:5). A similar conclusion was reached by the Independent Psychiatric Association (IPA), which from April to June 1989 met with and evaluated 44 Soviets who alleged they were victims of psychiatric abuse. In the IPA's opinion, only 25 per cent were unambiguously mentally ill; the majority (54.5 per cent or 24) were sound or else exhibited minor 'character or personality' disorders (IAPUP, 1989, No. 22:32).

Subsequently the most rigorous independent professional psychiatric evidence of needless hospitalization of Soviet political dissidents[31] was derived from the visits of a US Delegation to the USSR, invited by the Soviets and sent under the auspices of the US Department of State, and from a later visit by representatives of the World Psychiatric Association (WPA). In both cases carefully structured and documented interviews were held with hospitalized or recently released Soviets in the USSR, over the period 26 February–12 March 1989 by the US Department of State-sponsored American Psychiatric Association mental health professionals and other interested experts, and over 9–29 June 1991 by the WPA team. Some of their sanity findings are summarized in Table 1.1 below.

During the 1989 visit, the delegation interviewed 27 of an initial list of 48 individuals thought by the Helsinki Commission and others to be political detainees. Of the 27, 15 remained hospitalized and 12 had been released.[32] From the delegation's description of pre-arrest behaviour, at least nine of the 15 still hospitalized in 1989 would qualify as political detainees in our definition, as would at least 11 of the 12 recent releases. Thus at least 20/27 or about three-quarters of those seen formally were undeniably political detainees whose mental status is relevant to this study. Of the 12 recent releases the delegation found that nine (75 per cent) had *no* mental illness, and three had mild conditions not indicating hospitalization. Among those 15 still hospitalized, nine were diagnosed as seriously ill, and six (40 per cent) were seen as unjustifiably interned according to the American Psychiatric Association's *Diagnostic and Statistical Manual (of Mental Disorders)-III-R* or the World Health Organization's *International Classification of Diseases-10* draft. Those held without cause included one, recently rehospitalized after human rights activity, labelled 'schizophrenic'.

The most conservative interpretation of these numbers is that nine of the 15 (60 per cent) still hospitalized were in need of some treatment. Equally, a slight majority of 52 per cent of the whole group (14/27 in 1989:17 for their Table 2 comparing Soviet and US diagnoses) had been hospitalized with *no* mental illness whatsoever. Nine of 27 interviewed or only one-third of those diagnosed by Westerners were correctly hospitalized according to intersubjectively accepted international standards. Two-thirds were not. Considering that of the initial 48 the Delegation requested to see, perhaps 30 had been discharged prior to the arrival of the US experts (one emigrated, one was in prison, 26 were reported released and at least two more discharges took place), conjecturally the 30 releases also represent unnecessary hospitalizations, though in principle some could be remissions or cures. The delegation met with 12 such released individuals. If there were 18 more, and they are interpreted as releases occasioned by the imminent arrival of sceptical observers, then the internationally valid Soviet diagnosis rate from the evidence of the 1989 visit may be as low as 9/45 [9/(27 + 18)], or 20 per cent. This figure is a damning one because ample time had elapsed since large-scale releases began to reduce the mental hospital resident population to a core of those intersubjectively recognizable as gravely ill, assuming central direction and control of the hospitalization process. Releases from mental hospitals date at least to 1983; large-scale releases from the USSR's mental hospitals had begun in 1987, continuing in 1988 and early 1989.

The US delegation's own assessment was that among those they interviewed, 20/27 or 74 per cent of the patients' 'placement and treatment were questionable' (1989:7). Those seen in strict observation (SPH) hospitals in Kazan, Chernyakhovsk and elsewhere as a rule did not require such stark conditions. Diagnoses of schizophrenia were overused (24/27 [89 per cent] or 13/15 of those hospitalized [87 per cent] and 11/12 of those released [92 per cent]), while the US delegation could corroborate only four cases of schizophrenia among the hospitalized and none among the recent releases, or about 15 per cent overall, compared to the 89 per cent prevalence claimed.

In its June 1991 visit to Soviet mental hospitals, the WPA team found itself in the centre of international and domestic upheaval in what was soon to cease being the USSR. Conservative forces in Soviet psychiatry appeared dominant. Despite the fact that the WPA visit was a mutually agreed condition to readmission of the Soviet All-Union Society of Neurologists and Psychiatrists (AUSNP, later All-Union Society of Soviet Psychiatrists and Narcologists) to the WPA, much of the WPA's prearranged investigation was obstructed. Nevertheless the WPA team did interview ten people, seven from a list of 15 initially suggested to the AUSNP, and three from a list proposed by Dr Yuri Savenko, of the Independent Psychiatric Association, a WPA member. The WPA team, over objections, was also allowed eventually to interview inmates at Serbsky. No access was allowed to alcohol and drug treatment/detention centres, which remained under the control of the Ministry of the Interior.

By the WPA's narrow definition, at least four of those interviewed were undeniably political detainees. The WPA study provided adequate information in its case studies to argue that at least eight or nine of the individuals hospitalized should be considered political or religious dissenters by our definition, for activities varying from petitioning, demonstrating, advancing anti-Soviet or emphatically religious views, or repeatedly advancing environmental, work and industrial safety complaints.[33] Thus these figures, like those of the US delegation in 1989, can reveal the extent of diagnostic error of psychiatrically imprisoned dissidents.

The WPA group found an over-reliance on schizophrenia diagnoses, as had the APA group previously. All ten of those they interviewed had been categorized as schizophrenic, but only one correctly so in the WPA psychiatrists' view. Even in that case some question arose whether it was instead a schizoid personality disorder rather than schizophrenia. The other nine were not found to have been schizophrenic. At least five were never mentally ill, and six never previously ill, though three of those persistently healthy political detainees had been confined to strict observation hospitals. No more than two or possibly three were interpreted as still ill in 1991, though eight remained on the register with local or republic psychiatric clinics as needing follow-up care. This evidence substantiates a high rate of intersubjectively invalid diagnoses ranging from 9/10 incorrect schizophrenia diagnoses to 5/10 incorrect identifications of mental illness, overhospitalization, and excessive use of the psychiatric register.

Given the behaviour that precipitated the detentions of those hospitalized, these results clearly show political abuse and possibly incompetence in a structured sample over whom the Soviet authorities exerted considerable control, suggesting that the true rates of political diagnosis could have been even higher than those voluntarily revealed to outside observers.

In 1989 the AUSNP in conjunction with the USSR Ministry of Health composed a Medical Ethical Examining Commission of the AUSNP, to be responsible for reviewing appeals of hospitalization. The Commission, chaired by Dr B.P. Belov, had re-evaluated 112 cases of the 506 reaching it by 12 June 1991. Though the Commission had confirmed the diagnosis in 66 instances (59 per cent), it had also stated that 25 of the 112 (22 per cent) were mentally healthy. Twenty of the 25 so reclassified (80 per cent) had previously been held to be schizophrenic. Without specification, the Commission also reported a pattern of unwarranted hospitalization.

The extent of purely political variability in diagnosis – that is, a measure of instrumental use of psychiatry – can be seen in these Belov Commission statistics in the WPA report. When Soviet experts re-examined the same patients under a changed All-Union political climate, still relying on the same Soviet training and Soviet diagnostic criteria, they also detected overuse of schizophrenia labelling, and they found legally competent some (8) who had been confined as well as determining that others (55) did not need to be on the register. If a count of those held legally competent (8), not requiring follow-up care via the registry though forced onto the registry (55), and/or mentally healthy (25) together comprise a measure of overdiagnosis of serious mental illness which required hospitalization, in these first 112 reviews 88 significant errors took place which affected at a minimum 55 unwilling patients (A.G. Vigon, 1991). A misdiagnosis rate of 55/112 people=49 per cent follows, which can be viewed as a rough approximation of the overdiagnosis rate attributable to political climate change. Professor Lukacher (*Meditsinskaya Gazeta* 14 June 1991, reprinted in WPA, 1991:44, Appendix 9:1) conservatively found a 20 per cent error rate, finding illness where there was none, in 104 appeals to the Belov Commission.[34]

The cases of individuals making their complaints heard in the Belov Commission are not a random sample of all compulsorily hospitalized dissidents and probably also do not constitute a systematic or representative sample, but instead represent those protestors most astute politically, best connected, and best able to make their claims known. As other lesser known cases are reviewed, the numbers found 'practically healthy', competent, or not in need of follow-up psychiatric care might decline, at least on the presumption that those most likely to be coherent and sane as well as vocal, hence best able to publicize their cases, had already been heard by 1991. Thus the misdiagnosis rate could be overestimated in these figures.

On the other hand it might remain high, or could even be underestimated. Professor V.P. Belov's letter from the Commission (WPA, 1991:42, Appendix 6:2) indicated that many requests for reconsideration originated from individuals whose diagnosis originally ensued from an 'industrial dispute' rather than any clear mental condition, implying that these are not 'political' cases. However, because workplace health and safety concerns are correctly perceived as related to nationality, class or stratum, and other demographic and socioeconomic characteristics of those affected, many 'industrial disputes' can and should also be conceptualized as human rights concerns. It is not a coincidence, for example, that employment in mining radioactive materials and exposure to nuclear waste contamination has been distributed mainly among indigenous peoples, prisoners and other national minorities in countries mining uranium. Nationality patterns in recruitment of emergency workers to contain the Chernobyl meltdown were partly responsible for the pyrotechnic political consequences of the reactor accident (Feshbach and Friendly, 1992). Since industrial risks, contamination and ecological incidents were widespread across the Union, and catalyzed some Green Movements (including the international anti-nuclear weapons group named for Kazakhstan, Nevada and Mururoa), as well as nascent political parties, industrial disputes might account for a significant proportion of forced hospitalization cases under review, which would definitely expand the statistics on unjustified hospitalizations. The proportion of cases found competent or virtually healthy on review would continue to be substantial irrespective of other more narrowly political or religious concerns. The WPA report concluded that those reviewed up to the 1991 visit may represent the 'tip of a very large iceberg'.

The Meaning of Hospitalization of Healthy Individuals

The evidence of hospitalization of healthy political and religious nonconformists in the USSR is incontrovertible. It derives from multiple sources, is verified by observers of several nationalities, has been acknowledged by highly placed Ministry of Health officials, and has come to the attention of international professional and governmental agencies including but not limited to the World Psychiatric Association, the World Health Organization, and the United Nations Economic and Social Council Commission on Human Rights. The All Union Society of Psychiatrists and Neurologists itself made a public concession on this point on 17 October 1989 at the General Assembly of the WPA in Athens, as part of a set of conditions for its qualified readmission to the WPA, though neither the admission of abuse nor the conditions were aired until much later within the USSR. What remains to be clarified are the scale and meaning of this phenomenon.

Table 1.1 summarizes not only Western but also Soviet findings of sanity for many hospitalized dissidents. As Table 1.1 reflects, the US Helsinki Watch Committee indicated that among their records only one of all dissidents who emigrated, Nikolai Baranov, was involuntarily hospitalized in the West (Committee *Report on Abuse of Psychiatry for Political Purposes*, 1987). Mercer lists only two detainees (A. Chekanavichius, Y.V. Glukhov) believed to be mentally ill, found as a result of detailed interviews and visits to Soviet psychiatric hospitals in 1989. We share Mercer's concern for caution in interpreting this information, since the true state of mind of dissident detainees cannot be known with certainty, especially from secondary sources. And the conditions in SPHs might have induced mental illness or exacerbated existing conditions.[35] Forcible confinement,

Table 1.1 Soviet and Western Views: Mental State of Selected Hospitalized Dissidents according to Psychiatrists and Other Mental Health Professionals

West: Ill	*West: Sane*	*Soviet: Sane*
	N.Sh. Akhmetov	
N. Baranov		
		S.I. Belov
		S.P. Belov
	Yu. S. Belov	Yu. S. Belov
		V. Borisov
	V.K. Bukovsky	V.K. Bukovsky
		O. Bykov
A. Cehanavicius		
	V.V. Davydov (Ryzhov)	V.V. Davydov (Ryzhov)
	L.F. Dobrov	
		I.G. Dvoretsky
		V. Fainberg
		F.Y. Finkel
		Yu. T. Galanskov
	V.L. Gershuni	V.L. Gershuni
Y.V. Glukhov		
	N.E. Gorbanevskaya	N.E. Gorbanevskaya
	P.G. Grigorenko	P.G. Grigorenko
		Gusakova
		V.V. Igrunov
		A.M. Ilchenko
		A.I. Ilyin
		Yu. Ivanov
		S. Karapetyan
		A. Kekilova
		V.P. Khailo
		V. Klebanov
	A.E. Komarov	A.E. Komarov
		N. Korablev
		A.P. Kozlov
	O.V. Kozlov	O.V. Kozlov
		L. Kravtsov
		A.F. Kutyavin
		Z.P. Kutyavina
		A.A. Kuzkin
		S. Kuznetsov
	V. Kuznetsov	
	P.Y. Lazda	
	P.A. Lysak	
		M.Y. Makarenko
		A. Malkhazyan
		Yu. Maltsev
		N. Margorin
		Zh. Medvedev
	G. Melngailis	
		A. Monakhov
		M.A. Naritsa
		B. Naudziunas

Table 1.1 (cont.)

West: Ill	*West: Sane*	*Soviet: Sane*
	V.N. Nikitenkov	V.N. Nikitenkov
	A.V. Nikitin	
	E.N. Nikolayev	E.N. Nikolayev
		V. Novodvorskaya
		A. Papiashvili
	S. Pisarev	
	S. Potylitsyn	S.A. Potylitsyn
		V.P. Rafalsky
		I. Rodionov
	A.F. Runov	
		A. Saakyan
		V. Salaty
	N. Samsonov	N. Samsonov
		A. Sarkisyan
		P. Shakin
		V.I. Shakina
	A.I. Shatravka	A.I. Shatravka
	Yu. A. Shikhanovich	
		L. Shtein
		A.V. Skobov
		Yu. I. Sobolev
		V.V. Spinenko
		G.N. Stetsenko
		G. Suprunyuk
		V.S. Timokhin
	V.G. Titov	V.G. Titov
		L.G. Ubozhko
	M. Varfolomeyev	M. Varfolomeyev
	Yu. Vineshnevskaya	Yu. Vineshnevskaya
		M. Voikhanskaya
		O.I. Vorobyov
		A.P. Zhipre
		B. Zoubok

Key: The 'Soviet: Ill' column is omitted since all hospitalized dissenters were found mentally ill by some Soviet examiner at some time. This table understates numbers of detainees sane at the time of hospitalization since it includes only individuals for whom the literature shows at least one psychiatrist's opinion on their mental state, and since the opportunity for Western psychiatrists to have seen most of these individuals was small. Individuals are reported sane if at least one psychiatrist found them healthy or, in a few cases, legally responsible or not in need of compulsory hospitalization. Individuals are listed as sane to Western observers if they were found healthy by Western psychiatrists or were described by Koppers as 'independently' found healthy after hospitalization. Those listed as sane to Soviet assessment have either been found healthy by at least one Soviet psychiatrist or responsible by a Soviet court. Some deteriorated in hospital.

Sources: Cf. Chapter 2 for complete information on the database; Bloch and Reddaway, 1977, 1984; Amnesty International, 1983; Koppers, 1990; Mercer, 1991, IAPUP, 1989, 1990. Cases reported by number only rather than name are excluded.

restraints, isolation, poor diet and arbitrary use of drugs might have undermined the mental condition of Yuri Oleynikov, Rail Nigmatovich Ozhegov, Lyubov Shtein and Vasiliy Nikolaevich Spinenko (Mercer and APA, 1991 *Releases* and *Internments*; see also Koppers, Bloch and Reddaway, Podrabinek).

Since new commitments created by hospital induction of disease were few – because most protesters were hospitalized only once in these data – it would be difficult for this consideration to have biased our statistical inquiry. In any event such examples should not be discarded from the evidence on political abuse of psychiatry since they represent one of its most extreme outcomes barring death: punitive or reckless generation of mental disease, or retaliatory exacerbation of existing mental conditions in an already vulnerable population. However we have no indication that this phenomenon was widespread enough to account for more than a few hospitalizations, though it might have lengthened some.

We have not found a Soviet counter-argument maintaining that the dissident population is *generally* mentally ill which derives from more than a few cases. Further, the fact that the 1989 US Delegation included four former Soviet psychiatrists makes it clear that divergent diagnoses are not merely the result of variations in assessment between East and West, but mirror political aspects of the time and place.

Systematic investigations by a British psychiatrist and a Soviet Politics specialist (Bloch and Reddaway, 1977, 1984 *et seq.*) substantiated the pervasive impression of mental stability if not well-being among Soviet dissidents, as did the reports of the Soviet psychiatrists A. Papiashvili, M. Voikhanskaya, and B. Zoubok *inter alia*. Since we have taken care not to count as psychiatrically repressed any dissenters whom we had reason to regard as genuinely unbalanced before forced commitment,[36] we doubt that the ineradicable lack of certainty in this matter has systematically affected our results. While errors in judgment of degree of mental health are catastrophic for individuals, they need not bias statistical findings. If the misjudgments are essentially random, their effects will tend to disappear in analyses of aggregate data such as those presented in later chapters.

Little evidence has been adduced to show that most dissidents who had been subject to involuntary psychiatric treatment in the USSR were ever mentally ill, or were sufficiently mentally ill in any intersubjectively diagnosed sense to require hospitalization. When interviewed in the USSR by Western mental health professionals and in several cases by Soviets or by former Soviets, and when seen in the West, most such individuals were found sane. In principle, émigré dissidents could have been suddenly 'cured' in the USSR as their visas were granted, or on arrival in the West or at other destinations, making it difficult to determine the degree of their illness while in the USSR. But material scarcities, poor living conditions and sketchy training of psychiatrists made the prospect of cures in Soviet mental hospitals remote. Certainly spontaneous cure on emigration was improbable, since the process of emigration out of the USSR was markedly more strenuous than daily life in the USSR, and real mental illness usually does not subside in a matter of a few jet-lagged days. Similarly it is unlikely that hospitalized dissidents who met with Westerners were instantly cured by exposure to Western medical experts, however talented. So it must be concluded that as a rule these individuals were hospitalized while mentally healthy.

Hypothetically it could be asserted that dissidents appear sane to Westerners because they were 'cured' in Soviet hospitals. Without any evidence that they were ill prior to hospitalization, this is difficult to assess. It is not even clear that many detainees met the minimal criteria in Soviet regulations for forced commitments, that they posed a social danger to themselves or others. Amnesty International and Dr Anatoly Koryagin interpret the 'social danger' hospitalization criterion as meaning that under Soviet law only those who posed immediate *physical* risks to their own lives or health or the lives and health of others could legally be committed involuntarily as socially dangerous (van Voren, 1987:45). This interpretation, that social danger represents a risk of violence, contradicts Reshetov's (1982) nebulous construction 'harmful to social relations' but is also implied in the 1973 letter from the All-Union Society of Neurologists and Psychiatrists. Further, in his defence of Soviet practices Alexander Sergeyevich Karpov, chief psychiatrist in the Ministry of Health in 1989, also claimed that individuals could not be committed unless they were aggressive and not only violent but potentially lethally so: 'able to put their own or others' lives at risk'.[37] Since no basis exists for alleging that those nonconformists detained after political or religious acts generally posed such a physical danger, even in the accounts of admitting psychiatrists, Amnesty International concluded (Amnesty International, 1983:4) that commitments must have been based on the temporally 'proximate exercise of political, civil or religious rights' interpreted as constituting socially dangerous behaviour. Our observations are consistent with Amnesty's conclusions.

2. Distinctive Aspects of Soviet Psychiatry: Structure

Structure of Psychiatric Clinics and Hospitals

Over the Soviet period many psychiatric institutions were created throughout the country, increasing accessibility of counselling[38] but also heightening the potential for societal control at a variety of levels. Local dispensaries existed in all republics/states throughout society including at the level of the factory, with their own treatment facilities and psychiatric panels with the authority to hospitalize (Babayan, 1985:304).

Although accounts of the structure of Soviet psychiatric practice are unclear, in the immediate post-revolutionary period a five-level structure was conceived, beginning with dispensaries, small hospitals, and extending to protracted care hospitals, agricultural labour colonies for chronic cases, and invalid centres. The agricultural colony apparently no longer exists, though some individuals under treatment for alcohol or drug use report serving terms in labour colonies. Psychiatric confinement in work camps of other kinds is recorded, and those held as alcoholics or drug-dependents were still pressed into forced labour as late as the early 1990s (Reddaway, 1991:48). The therapy-and-labour 'workshops' administered by the Ministry of Internal Affairs, in which those convicted of alcohol- or drug-related offences were held, in the early 1990s were struggling to be 'privatized' and/or transferred to the Ministry of Public Health; by 1994 they were being targeted for conversion to prisons and pre-trial detention facilities (Russian Federal Law on Institutions, No. 3, in Zheludkov, 1994). According to Zheludkov's report in *Izvestia*, the only practical effect of the new law on institutions appears to be that the names of the facilities might change and the minimum period of forced labour would increase from six months to a year, while so-called voluntary facilities would be administered by the Ministry of Health.

Babayan (1985:7) described the local dispensaries, evidently envisioned in the Civil War period as a method of providing outpatient psychiatric care, as '. . . capable of detecting in timely fashion the first signs of disease, *of keeping the patient under constant observation* . . .' (emphasis added). Babayan commented eerily, 'epidemiological screenings have been extended to one third of Estonia's population' by Estonian psychiatrists (1985:158), as though a pressing risk of mass insanity had faced Estonia just when the religious dissident movement was becoming particularly strong and active in the Baltics. Precisely the procedures and structures which allowed pre-emption and prevention of mental illness were most amenable to dispositional instrumental use, especially locally and in the short term.

Contemporaneous reports could be found of psychiatric clinics and hospitals in or administered by at least six ministries and Soviet agencies, among them the Ministries of Health,[39] Education, Social Security, and Internal Affairs (Gorman, 1969:843; Lukacher, 1991). Complaints of poor quality care, inadequate supplies, and poorly educated physicians were endemic in Soviet medicine. But the clinics of the Ministry of Internal

Affairs used treatment methods which a former detainee, the jurist Nikolai Sedov, distinguished from merely poor quality as 'barbaric' (Taranov, 1992:6).

Approximately 700 residential mental hospitals existed in late 1988 (Churkin in Yelin interview, 1988:43). Among these institutions Shifrin (1982:22–31) listed 81 psychiatric hospitals, clinics and prisons known by the early 1980s to house political dissidents, including 16 in Moscow, ten in Leningrad, and 55 over other regions, including the infamous one at Kazan apparently created to corral politicals. The number of special regime/strict supervision psychiatric hospitals was variously reported as perhaps 22 in the 1980s, while at least 11 purportedly still existed in 1991 (Baranovsky, 1991).

Most ordinary regime psychiatry[40] was practised under the Ministry of Health, though some was also reported under the Ministry of Social Affairs (Salvendry, 1975:229). Alcoholism and drug 'treatment' in 1991 remained with the Ministry of the Interior (WPA, 1991). The Ministry of Health psychiatric section authorized all general forms of treatment and also specified the procedures for psychiatric examinations, but might do so in collaboration with the Procurator, officers of the USSR Supreme Court, and/or the Ministry of Internal Affairs ((art. 51 Fundamentals of Legislation of the USSR and the Union Republics); Babayan, 1985:303). In effect Serbsky shared these prerogatives. Since both the Procuracy and the Ministry of Internal Affairs have been directly responsible for control of dissent, their link to psychiatric evaluation procedures and treatments via the Health Ministry opened up a powerful source of influence and abuse.

As the link to the Procuracy and the Ministry of the Interior shows, the structure of the Soviet mental hospital system reveals features evidently explicitly designed for control, deterrence and coercion, which are directly adapted to punitive purposes, and powerfully subject to regime pressures.

Structure of the Mental Hospital System: the Register

After release from a mental institution, dissidents might be required to register with and report to local or republic-level clinics or dispensaries periodically. Various reports in the eighties put the size of the register at around five or six million people. Because those registered could be required to present themselves at a clinic, the out-patient register thus compiled served as one mechanism of immediate recall to hospitals of those previously detained. This system included voluntary patients and those under compulsory 'dynamic observation' who could be trailed, 'visited' at home, telephoned at work, and forced to appear at the clinic (Reddaway, 1991:48fn; Bonanni interview with Aleksandr Aleksandrovich Churkin, then head of the Soviet Psychiatric Service, 1988; and the All-Union Society of Psychiatrists memo in AIPUP, 1990, No. 23:15). All nonconformists held to be socially dangerous fell into the dynamic observation group.

Those on the register were limited in choice of employment, and among other restrictions might find it difficult or impossible to obtain a driver's licence, go hunting, or travel outside the country.

Although the register was defended as being comprised only or mainly of voluntary cases, the WPA observed that those on the mandatory list usually outnumbered those on the voluntary list (WPA, 1991:32). Further it is unclear that many were voluntary in the sense accepted in the West. Even worse, one might be unaware of having been listed with the register. Possibly because of the historic primacy of the Plan in Soviet life, employers could place workers on the register, evidently without even the embarrassment of a psychological assessment (eds Shore and Keith, 1989:50), simply by complaining about real or conjectured behaviour at work.

The register served multiple pernicious functions. It facilitated rounding up the usual political suspects at times of domestic or international need, as before major Soviet holidays such as Labour Day and Revolution Day, before visits of foreign dignitaries, or in anticipation of increased international media attention. Further, it breached patient confidentiality. Security of information in the register at local and republic levels was unreliable, and the 1992 Russian law preserves access for some officials. Police and KGB access to register data was straightforward in Kiev (WPA, 1991:23), even if the requested information did not concern a purportedly dangerous person. Register information might also become available depending on the vagaries of local clinic physicians and directors, even though dispersion of information on one's psychiatric record could obstruct job placement, career advancement, driving certification and other livelihood and credential issues.

As part of the campaign to gain readmission for the Soviets to the WPA, the register was pared down. Rapid removal of superfluous cases began in 1987, so that perhaps 1–1.2 million had been erased from the registry over 1987–89. Allegedly 738 000 had been removed from the register in 1988 alone, while some 5.5–5.6 million were said to remain on record. Health Ministry authorities expressed a goal of reducing these numbers by at least two million in the short term. Ryan (1993:147) noted a distinct decline since 1987 in numbers of people under register surveillance, partly due to a reduction in the use of the mercurial diagnosis 'psychic disturbance'. Excluding the mentally retarded, the numbers of those first enrolled on the register declined from 619400 in 1985 to 352800 in 1990 as reported in *Narodnoye Xhozyaistvo RSFSR 1990*:270. Still, P. Morozov indicated that 5.5 million were left listed on the register in mid-1990 (IAPUP, 1990, No. 24:4). The psychiatrist and People's Deputy Yu. Popov estimated the size of the register at 4.5 million as late as mid-1991. If new cases enrolled were falling, and if hundreds of thousands or even millions had been removed, yet somehow the size of the register remained substantially the same as it was reported to be in the 1980s, about 5 or 6 million, either the 1988 report of the size of the register at about 5.6 million was incorrect or the numbers of those erased from the records are incorrect, or both. Reddaway observed (IAPUP, 1989, No. 22:5) that a State Statistics Committee tally of the size of the register cited in *Ogonyok* was 10.4 million in 1988. IAPUP reprinted an excerpt from *Ogonyok* 15–22 April 1989 in 'Not Afraid' giving a similar estimate of 10.2 million (1989, No. 22:41).

Structure of Academic Psychiatry

Among central academic institutions shaping psychiatry in the USSR was the USSR Academy of Medical Sciences' Institute of Psychiatry, formerly directed by the late Andrei V. Snezhnevsky. According to Babayan, the Institute of Psychiatry was the main research institution in the Union; and after 1962 its scholars concentrated on schizophrenia research in its clinical and biological aspects. A branch of the Institute opened in Tomsk in Siberia in 1981.

The Serbsky Central Scientific Research Institute of General and Forensic Psychiatry (Serbsky), also in Moscow, with a branch in Kiev, has been the single most powerful practice and research institute, functionally related to the Health Ministry. The 'prevention of socially dangerous activities' was its main task. Serbsky is known for its almost automatic findings of schizophrenia followed by recommendations of compulsory treatment. Ironically the Institute was named for a follower of S.S. Korsakov, Vladimir P. Serbsky, an opponent of restraints.

Serbsky was given supervisory power over all forensic psychiatric examinations in the 1954 Instruction on the Conduct of Forensic Psychiatric Expert Examinations in the USSR, ch. 1 section 2. Especially complicated – that is, political – cases were to be referred to Serbsky (op.cit., ch. 1, section 10). This nationwide legally authorized power of Serbsky was reinforced by Serbsky's practice of sending psychiatrists every six months to the strict supervision psychiatric hospitals to evaluate cases, present new cases, and apparently to treat.[41] Though local doctors could be named to this group as well, sometimes reducing the presence and potentially the known bias of Serbsky personnel (eds Shore and Keith, 1989:41), the power to oversee forensic psychiatric commissions throughout the USSR remained with Serbsky.

In 1991 the Serbsky Institute was directed by Tatyana Dmitriyeva, purportedly a specialist in 'litigation mania' or insistent appeal to legal rights as a form of dementia; the former Director (since 1957, retired 1990) and systematic apologist for abuse, Georgi V. Morozov, remained honorary director.

The Scientific-Statistical Centre at Serbsky amassed data for 'mass screening of all patients on the registers of neuropsychiatric dispensaries throughout the country' (Babayan, 1985:88). This provided the information base and the 1954 Instruction provided commitment and treatment power necessary for instrumental political use of psychiatry.

The All-Union Research Centre for Mental Health, another major psychiatric establishment institution shaping Soviet psychiatry, in 1991 was still under the direction of Marat Yenokhovich Vartanyan, who has defended punitive psychiatric practices for two decades.[42]

The Vladimir M. Bekhterev Psychoneurological Institute in Leningrad/St Petersburg (Bekhterev Neuropsychiatric Scientific Research Institute) was the oldest such institution in the former USSR. Created before the Revolution, in 1908, it has been Serbsky's main though largely unsuccessful rival for political and academic influence, advancing a biological/chemical view of the origins of some mental conditions. Bekhterev is known for recommending more modern treatments including family and group therapy, work therapy and rehabilitation. Its goal appears to have been to reduce lengthy hospitalizations and return patients to productive life as promptly as possible. Modest Kabanov is among the best known liberal psychiatrists there.

In the republics other centres of research and study were created, such as the Asatiani Institute of Psychiatry in Georgia, also with a biological as opposed to genetic orientation; and the Ukraine Institute for Advanced Medical Training, in Kharkov. Physicians could enrol for brief courses at these institutes, as at the Moscow and St Petersburg Central Institutes for Advanced Medical Training (Babayan, 1985:106).

Historically, the major professional guild of Soviet psychiatrists, the All-Union Scientific Society of Neuropathologists and Psychiatrists, has been characterized by Snezhnevsky-school directors, including Nikolai Zharikov, an associate of G. Morozov and of M. Vartanyan, and more recently by Alexander Tiganov, tied to Vartanyan. Though the mushrooming of independent psychiatric and psychological associations has changed this picture somewhat since the early 1990s, the Moscow-dominated All-Union Society of Psychiatrists and Narcologists remained the central professional organization of mental health physicians, undergoing a number of name changes.[43] After the collapse of the Union this Moscow-centred society[44] converted nominally to a CIS body.

Despite the perceived need in the outside world for professional medical organizations and practitioners to be independent of the government, from state agencies, and from law enforcement and investigative bodies – that is, to be professional, non-governmental and capable of advocating patient interests – the AUSPN appeared to remain affiliated with the Ministry of Health into the nineties, at least if point of origin of stationery is any clue. Observers believed the AUSPN to be government-funded since it cannot have been self-sufficient with annual dues of five rubles in 1991, when the ruble was subject to monstrous inflationary forces (WPA, 1991:28). However the 1992 Russian law on psychiatric care asserts the independence of psychiatrists, and the mid-nineties efforts of the Russian Society of Psychiatrists to create a self-regulating code of ethics testify to the efforts of Russian professionals to establish professional autonomy.

Since the late 1980s new local and regional professional organizations have proliferated. Psychiatrists, psychologists and investigators in Russia have publicized plans for a unified professional organization which would accommodate their diverse occupations. A number of new psychiatric associations have been admitted to the World Psychiatric Association (WPA), including Yuri Savenko's Independent Psychiatric Association (Moscow) as a full member, and the Estonian association, with provisional admission status (Reddaway, 1991:45).

Though the WPA readmitted the Soviet professional society conditionally in 1989, the WPA seems not to have employed well-defined admissions criteria in other cases since it has also admitted the PRC and the former Czechoslovakia, unanimously, despite repeated reports of psychiatric abuses in those countries.

Because academic and clinical psychiatry are not independent of the Ministry of Health, the Ministry's record of status quo attitudes and potential conservative influence on the profession and on relevant laws should also be noted.

Soviet psychiatry has evolved a complex organizational structure barely sketched here. Even so this outline of Soviet psychiatry as a research-oriented field and as a forensic practice profiles the forms necessary for information gathering to anticipate and monitor mass movements and for enactment of centrally determined policies concerning direction and control of mass movements.

Structural Vulnerabilities of Psychiatry: Links to the Communist Party, the Procuracy, and the State

Red v. Expert Problem The structure of Soviet psychiatry as a profession increased the possibility of regime use of psychiatric detention. Psychiatry was directly susceptible to Party and state pressures, not only because of the immediate connections to the Ministry of Health (MoH) through binding regulations but also because of the nature of professional advancement.

Because the Communist Party granted approval for rises, and issued recommendations on promotions for psychiatrists (Miller, 1985:22), psychiatrists and neuropathologists working as therapists could be seen in some capacities more as state (that is, Party) employees than as confidential advisors. Threats of firing could be employed to produce a desired diagnosis, as when because of an implied threat to her job Dr Snegireva at the Novinsky Ordinary Psychiatric Hospital in Minsk found Ivan Fyodorovich Petrashov insane (APA *Releases* 6/10/91). This powerful employer–employee relationship made the practice of psychiatry more centralized than in the West with some exceptions, *ipso facto* subject to simpler mobilization along ideological lines.

Diagnoses of sluggish schizophrenia, 'litigation mania', delusions of reform, and other political findings proliferated where Party approval was required for promotion within the medical establishment, where mental health policy was set by practitioners who tended disproportionally to be Party members, where academic instruction in some medical schools originated with professors chosen for their Redness rather than their academic soundness, and where Party approval could be obtained predominantly by following Snezhnevsky. The structure of Soviet psychiatry thus enhanced academic paradigm bias, which appears to be responsible for a number of reclassifications to find individuals insane. Structure also enhanced psychiatry's links to the Party, proliferating the mechanisms through which Party policy could be carried out.

Some analysts see the 1971 change in the Physicians' Oath made by the Supreme Soviet as symptomatic of directly available state options to pressure physicians, since the 1971 revision removed the phrases on 'healing of the individual' and explicitly added references to Communist morality, to physicians' responsibilities towards the Soviet people and to the Soviet state (Alexeyeff, 1976:103). The 1971 change also incorporated a pledge to keep undefined medical 'secrets' that do not seem to be those of individual confidentiality.[45]

Vulnerability of Psychiatry to MVD and KGB Connections Determining Initial Arrest, Regulating Diagnosis and Controlling the Special Regime/Strict Observation Hospitals

Institutional lines of Soviet authority and practice argue that the KGB and MVD might, at their discretion, have exercised a direct and prompt control on dissent via psychiatry, acting on their own or as an instrument of local Party officials. (Gelman indicates that some KGB officers may have followed instructions from local Communist Party authorities rather than the central KGB to control the behaviour of local political activists (1990:101–6).) Personal accounts of individuals bolster the conclusion of KGB effective power. G.M. Shimanov indicated that in his hospital admissions interview he was informed that the interviewer would phone the KGB directly to discover what accusations had been levelled against Shimanov (Senate Judiciary Committee, 1973:199). Koppers (1990) listed at least six individuals who were informed directly or through members of their families that they had been confined on instructions of the KGB at some level (F.Y. Finkel, A. Ilchenko, A.D. Ponomaryov, A. Statkevicius, G.N. Trifonov, and V.A. Tsurikov; P. Lukosevicius also alleged that the KGB dictated terms and length of treatment in his hospital). Mercer lists others including A.M. Ilchenko. Koppers found the KGB directly responsible for the charges and subsequent hospitalizations of V.V. Kuznetsov, P. Lukosevicius, Y. Kalinin, and A.D. Ponomaryov. N.N. Kryuchkov alleged that a KGB representative was present at what evidently functioned as Kryuchkov's commitment examination, which would suggest KGB responsibility for his detention also since the law allowed an agent of the 'appropriate' investigative body to appear at the psychiatric evaluation (Koppers, 1990:113). Further, a KGB officer evidently intervened directly to prevent N.A. Sorokin's transfer from an SPH to an OPH, which Sorokin's psychiatrists had recommended to save his life (op.cit.:155).

Another link to official channels, the special psychiatric hospital director was a KGB officer, and after the death of the Union, in Russia, a Russian Security Services officer, a major or a colonel, according to Alexeyeff (1976) and Grigorenko (in Reddaway, 1972:228). Grigorenko maintained that one department at the Serbsky Institute, 'the one which diagnoses political cases', was under KGB control and that the whole Institute was affected by the KGB. Since law prescribed Serbsky dominance over the review process throughout the country, KGB initiatives could be carried throughout the USSR via the mechanism of six-month reviews. Although Serbsky was put under the administration of the Ministry of Health, Pisarev (Reddaway, 1972:233) held that no subsequent change in the personnel administering the Institute took place. Reddaway also reported that KGB-detained Soviets were sent to Serbsky, where the 'professors' consulted with the KGB on a convenient diagnosis (1972:234). The IAPUP (1983:37) asserted that the KGB could set the duration and circumstances of hospitalization just as though it were setting penalties in criminal law. That the Kiev branch of the Serbsky Institute has published in *Kommunist* ((13) 1989), the Party's theoretical journal, suggested a close tie between the Institute and the Party.

Until the directive consolidating mental hospitals under the Ministry of Health in 1988, according to Sapiets *et al.* (1976:87–8, emphasis added), 'All *special* psychiatric hospitals in the USSR are, according to law, officially under the direction of the Ministry of the Interior . . . and the heads of psychiatric prisons are all MVD officers with military titles . . .' (See also Podrabinek, 1980:9, fn. 1.) The Ministry of Internal Affairs (MVD or Ministerstvo Vnutrennikh Dyel) connection provided a direct structural link to government or Party directives on treatment of dissidents.

Evidently the patient need not be present for a commitment order to be signed on instructions of the KGB or MVD. According to Yuri Sobolev, who escaped from Zagarinsky Psychiatric Hospital, the committing psychiatrist, implying he had been ordered to do so, admitted Sobolev without seeing him at all.[46] Other instances on record of findings of insanity on the basis of no evidence include telephone diagnoses without speaking to the alleged patient, and collective diagnoses of entire groups (*Izvestia* 28 June 1989).

Seeing a similar KGB connection to mental health practice, Boris M. Segal, former Director of the Department of Clinical Psychology and Psychotherapy at the Moscow Institute of Psychiatry, observed that Serbsky was tied to the police and the KGB (Segal, 1976:270). Further, chief physicians and administrators of psychiatric institutions tended to be 'members of local soviets' (Segal, 1976:268), providing a critical link to local Party officials and government agencies, until the results of more democratic elections by 1990 broke this connection in many locales including the pre-eminent Moscow and Leningrad.

The literature amply describes KGB pressures on psychiatrists dealing with Soviet dissidents. However, the argument implicitly assumes that a psychiatrist would know whether the KGB wanted an insanity finding on any particular individual, and that if psychiatrists preferred to err on the safe side for themselves, it was necessarily safer to assume that the KGB wanted insanity found. Bloch and Reddaway, Fireside, Amnesty International, and others support these assumptions in the Soviet case, as does much of the extensive crossnational literature on treatment of dissidents.

Bloch and Reddaway (1977b:29) reported 'psychiatrists prefer to opt for compulsory hospitalization when doubt exists about the level of dangerousness of a patient' in Wales and England, which tends to support the idea of a general predisposition to hospitalize in circumstances of doubt or risk, though one suspects that physical danger is referred to in the Welsh and English cases. If, as has been alleged, a general predisposition across societies to over-hospitalize those who are conspicuous irritants to the authorities can be identified, this tendency would have been especially powerful in the USSR, where the procuracy could bring charges of insanity and where the legal requirement of 'dangerousness' appears to have been interpreted as 'embarrassing' to the dominant ideology. Soviet psychiatrists themselves, including the chief psychiatrist of the USSR Ministry of Public Health, have identified a 'hyperdiagnosis' problem and a tendency to hospitalize too often and for too long (Yuri Reshetov in Keith and Shore, 1989:86).

Time pressure exacerbated this tendency, since admitting psychiatrists had to certify within 24 hours after hospitalization that a patient was ill and needed confinement,[47] even though time may not have allowed a rigorous preliminary assessment, or any assessment, or the evaluation may have found the internee healthy. Since they had to testify to the patient's imbalance initially to order hospitalization, doctors may have tended to protect their professional standing by confirming subsequently that individuals were legally admitted (Novikov and Razin, 1987:4), irrespective of the facts.

Structural pressures of these and other varieties would facilitate mobilization of courts and psychiatrists for political purposes, even relatively narrow interests such as factional disputes.

3. Inconsistent and Inappropriate Application of Non-Imputability (Incompetence) Criteria

Meaning of Imputability

The definition of 'imputability', or competence to be tried, is consequential for many reasons. First, those found incompetent or non-imputable by reason of mental condition are likely to spend more time incarcerated. In general in societies with both criminal imprisonment and psychiatric confinement, probability of eventual release grows over time for individuals confined to penal institutions, while it declines over time for those committed for long periods to psychiatric hospitals.[48] Though courts may define maximum prison sentences, they cannot specify the length of psychiatric therapy.

Second, those declared legally incompetent do not have the same rights as defendants in criminal cases. They are not formally 'sentenced', thus not setting in motion rights of appeal; they cannot be party to legal documents, and do not receive all the legal guarantees of normal trials, if in fact they go to trial. As Gershman (1984:55) notes, psychiatric detention in the USSR allowed trial to be bypassed indefinitely. Sentenced dissidents might be refused not only a copy of the charges against them but also a copy of their sentences. Interned critics of the regime might not even have been present at their own commitment hearings. Further, there had been no mechanism for judicial review of civil commitments (Salvendry, 1975:235) and few guarantees of due process until passage of a new law in 1988.

Third, definitions of legal competence may be consequential because the regime could use an insanity label to discredit an individual, or to prevent dissident issues from gaining adherents at home or abroad. Since a ruling of non-imputability could be made by either a commission of psychiatrists or by court order, two instruments of potential regime use existed. And they were blunt, since Soviet law recognized no degrees of imputability, or diminished legal responsibility, though it may have countenanced temporary accountability.[49] Further, as in the US, a defendant could be held fully imputable and yet mentally ill simultaneously.

Inconsistent Application of Criteria of Non-Imputability

Soviet press reports starting in 1986 noted the inconsistency in application of diagnostic criteria in resolving questions of imputability.[50] Some of this inconsistency derived from the broad construction of non-imputability to encompass not only an inadequate understanding of the purported crime, and diminished willpower or self-control, but also *any* mental syndrome in the defendant, and *any* behaviour construed as anti-Soviet. Ten of the 12 (83 per cent) released dissidents interviewed by the US Delegation in 1989 could not have provided a basis for their being held non-imputable in their forcible hospitalization cases, while only perhaps five of the 11 (about 45 per cent) still confined were either still non-imputable or may have been so at the time they were detained (1989:35–6). At a minimum these numbers show an over-use of the non-imputability designation. They imply that the Soviet rate of identifying non-imputables correctly among the dissidents may have been about 30 per cent, or even less, in view of the several releases which preceded the US Delegation's visit.[51]

As in the West, early Soviet law provided that individuals found not responsible would not be subject to the sanctions exacted in normal criminal cases, if the official view was that such people are genuinely insane and therefore not culpable. But a finding of incompetence due to mental state did not necessarily protect Soviet dissidents from penalties inflicted when the criminally responsible were convicted, and Soviet law provided for penalties to be exacted after a defendant was restored to mental health. This too parallels the practice in the US. However, the prosecution directed Soviet forced hospitalization, and under those circumstances the illogic of this procedure points to rational, punitive use of hospitalizations, since neither sanctions nor deterrence could be expected to succeed if their target populations were in fact irrational. Rubenstein pointed out that General Grigorenko, hospitalized in 1964, forfeited his right to a military pension and was ejected from the Party (1980, 1985:120–1), punitive measures which imply deliberate instrumental state use of these penalties as a means of social control, to punish the individual and to dissuade others from following his example. Three years later the 1967 Instruction[52] explicitly preserved pension rights for those undergoing compulsory treatment, as did the 1992 law. At least after 1967 pension confiscation was an illegal and especially severe sanction, reinforcing the provisions of the 1919, 1926 and 1960 Criminal Codes which held that unimputable people could not be punished. Whatever function Party membership may have served in this case, clearly an individual who was genuinely ill should still expect to receive his pension under law (Bloch and Reddaway, 1977:107).

In principle a potential correction for arbitrary application of competence criteria could be found in commitment procedures. For Soviet commitments to special psychiatric prisons/strict observation hospitals for two to ten years, a commission of experts and the criminal court had the option of recommending release; if the court denied release, the commission would reconsider. The reported speed of this reconsideration (15–20 cases per hour or three to four minutes per case, Alexeyeff, 1976:122; ten minutes or less in other sources) implies that it was barely pro forma and could not have constituted a real review of diagnoses or a meaningful avenue for release of accidentally hospitalized healthy people.

Other inconsistencies in the treatment of dissidents found insane add support to arguments that the state used insanity diagnoses and psychiatric hospitalization to try to direct the course of the dissident movement. Particularly salient is the inconsistency arising from political exchange of purportedly mentally ill dissidents as though they were espionage agents. If dissidents were genuinely mentally ill, non-productive, dysfunctional, required lengthy, costly treatment, and were not of interest as political detainees, it is unclear why they would have had any value enabling governments to trade them for assets in other societies, as when the Soviets exchanged Vladimir Bukovsky in December 1976 for the Chilean Marxist Luis Corvalán Lepe, and in February 1986 allowed Anatoly (Natan)

Shcharansky to emigrate to Israel in what is usually inaccurately described as a 'spy exchange'.

Another inconsistency arises when allegedly dangerously ill nonconformists were released for childcare. Evidently the prosecutor closed Natalya Gorbanevskaya's case, disregarding a recommendation from Serbsky and allowing her to be freed in 1970, 'because of her "insanity" ' and 'because of her two young children' (Rubenstein, 1985:105–6) who needed her, an irresponsible and baffling move unless the 'illness' was politically predetermined or was not dangerous in the first instance.

Further indications of non-therapeutic instrumental use of mental hospitals are the release of selected protesters as soon as they disavowed dangerous or disturbing views (ex. I.A. Yakhimovich in 1971), or increases in hospital confinement time after they refused to repudiate previous positions. Such cases strengthen the impression that the purpose of psychiatric incarceration is to produce declared changes in views and renunciation of causes (Reddaway, 1991).

These inconsistencies in application of imputability criteria are coherent with the hypothesis of instrumental use of mental hospitals as a means of social control.[53] At a minimum these cases imply a definition of mental illness whose extremes barely overlap with definitions used in the West, even in countries like the US whose practices are also vulnerable to criticism.

While competence criteria of mental state and age have been inconsistently applied in societies other than the USSR, the direction of the bias was different in the Soviet case. With some exceptions amenable to political interpretation, the bias in the US lies in the direction of finding questionable individuals competent so that they are dealt with in the prison system, and restricting their appeal options.[54] In the US (Bedau, 1964; Turk, 1969:20) the retarded and juveniles have been defined as legally competent, and have been and remain at risk of imprisonment and even of execution. It is not inconsistencies in treatment and classification themselves, but rather their peculiar direction and point of origin of cases, that made the Soviet experience remarkable. Although not all Soviet dissidents accused of political crimes were found unbalanced,[55] the Soviet tendency had been to find particular normal but socially salient individuals insane so that they could be hospitalized and their cases would not come to trial. Soviet allegations of insanity and possible social danger tended to originate with the prosecutor rather than with family members, co-workers, union representatives, guardians or local communities (see Reddaway in Sapiets, 1975:iv). (In an extensive literature, consult Thomas Szasz,[56] who writes that 'insanity' is merely a state-determined label; see also Franco Basaglia[57] and the 1960s Democratic Psychiatry Movement in Italy, which criticized mental institutions for inducing debilitation and disease.)

Not only did exercise of religious and political rights result in findings of mental illness, but overtly criminal behaviour might also result in a diagnosis of insanity. The literature sets out several examples of individuals whose apparently criminal behaviour critical of the Soviet state resulted in a diagnosis of schizophrenia rather than criminal prosecution.[58] Dr Avtandil Papiashvili, a Soviet psychiatrist who emigrated to the West, is one source of these accounts, as are visiting American psychiatrists.

4. Structure of Legal Practice and the Legal System

In the Soviet prosecutorial legal system the accused had no right to an attorney until after the psychiatric examination, even though the mere presence of a mental evaluation in the record might permanently prejudice future consideration of the person in question.[59] Further, a court order was not necessary for a psychiatric examination, which could be requested by the chief psychiatrist, any medical personnel, prison administrators, procurators and other investigators.

In the US, by contrast, mental health determinations usually are requested by lawyers for the accused,[60] and if the prosecutor is interested in obtaining a psychiatric evaluation, a court order must be obtained first. Since the prosecution does not guide the psychiatric evaluation procedure in the US, this structural feature of US law deters psychiatric reports from being used predominantly to bring about pre-trial forcible hospitalization or other penalties (see Bonnie), although the financial and opportunity costs of resort to the US legal system can be punitive in themselves.

In the Soviet case pre-trial hospitalization *could* be used as a punishment since psychiatric examinations tended to be conducted on an in-patient basis and thus already implied hospitalization. Further, for the evaluation the accused could be confined immediately even in strict supervision psychiatric hospitals.[61] Examinations could not legally exceed a 30-day limit,[62] contrasting favourably with the 180-day limits of some US states. However, pre-trial detention could last up to nine months, and no limit had been or perhaps could be set on duration of compulsory hospitalization (1967 Instruction, Part E, section 23).

The Soviet legal system exhibited all of the necessary structural attributes to allow political use of involuntary hospitalization. The procuracy could order forcible hospitalization during investigations, in the absence of a court order or other judicial oversight or meaningful subsequent review, and in any case the independence of the judiciary, which would have been necessary for real accountability, was not established. The procuracy itself was 'subject to Party discipline', its members being appointed by and serving at the pleasure of the USSR Procurator General even down to the city level, while the Procurator General himself was appointed by the President of the Supreme Soviet.

On the other hand, in this asymmetric relationship, the detainee did not even necessarily benefit from advice or representation from an attorney. The WPA found in 1991 that lawyers were generally not available to hospitalized dissenters, not only because of restriction of information about patient rights but also simply because of cost. Detainees might never see a copy of criminal charges or diagnoses brought against them, though Article 193 of the Code of Criminal Procedure of the USSR unambiguously required expert opinions be given to the accused. If a civil commitment were requested instead, no right to see any charges existed.

An ambiguity in Soviet law also facilitated political use of trials in general and findings of incapacity in particular. Though Soviet law guaranteed the presence of the accused at a trial (Article 246 of the Code of Criminal Procedure), Article 407 of the same Code provided only that the defendant be summoned to the trial 'if the character of his illness does not prevent this' (Berman, 1966:421; paragraph two of Article 407, Code of Criminal Procedure of the USSR as amended 1965), a cavil preserved in the 1992 Russian law (ex. article 34(2)). The Article 407 provision evidently granted to the judge in question the discretion to determine whether or not any individual should appear, thus legalizing trials *in absentia* of protestors whose presence would be newsworthy, awkward or embarrassing.

Political crimes' hazy definitions and the breadth of discretion in the Soviet legal system contributed further to the potential for political abuse. A number of articles in the RSFSR Criminal Code were written to allow flexibility in interpreting what behaviour or failure to act constituted a crime. Thus many articles could be given a political interpretation. While Articles 65–73 of the RSFSR Criminal Code were all nebulously written, Article 70, Anti-Soviet Agitation and Propaganda, was notoriously vague in prohibiting unspecified 'particular, especially dangerous crimes against the state' (Berman, 1966:180). Articles 190–1 were also criticized for their vagueness and surrealism, since they included penalties for failure to report crimes which have not happened yet ('known crimes which are being prepared', Berman, 1966:217; Art. 190 RSFSR Criminal Code). Conspiracy was already defined as a crime in a number of articles, so the need for a catch-all conspiracy charge is not obvious. And exactly how these future crimes would become known a priori is unclear.

Among the most crucial matters left to the judge's discretion was the choice of type of hospital to which allegedly mentally ill dissidents might be admitted. Involuntary criminal commitments could be made to ordinary observation hospitals, intensified observation in specific wards of ordinary hospitals, or to strict observation hospitals.[63] This choice of hospital, determining the living conditions of individuals forcibly detained – even, perhaps, the length of their lives – was based on a judgment of the degree of 'special danger' the particular dissident act represented for the larger society. Yet criteria for the degree of social danger were undefined, unoperationalized, and thus intrinsically subject to caprice.[64]

The US concern with due process[65] as a measure of fairness of treatment is raised in the Soviet case by the fact that both civil and criminal cases could be closed administratively, so that any procedural guarantees or rights of appeal which did exist might never be brought into play. The WPA raised questions in 1991 whether *de jure* guarantees were in effect at all in the USSR. Among the ten detainees they interviewed *none* had had any of the mandated reviews, yet 'a number' of them had been compulsorily interned, which should have set the six-month review process in motion. The WPA (1991:20) also noted that although in principle the law could serve as a check on arbitrary hospitalization, they knew of only 24 court cases brought in the Moscow area from 1988 through the summer of 1991 concerning compulsory hospitalization or placement on the psychiatric register. Of those, only two plaintiffs had won release or removal from the register (2/24 = eight per cent). To put these numbers in perspective, perhaps 80000 annually were hospitalized in the capital and environs, plus those assigned to the register requiring supervision by local or republic clinics.[66]

This discussion presumes that the law has the capacity to curtail political abuse of psychiatry. But this assumption may be overly optimistic. An excessive reliance on the law as a potential remedy for human rights violations ignores the aspects of arrest, trial and commitment which show state design for punitive purposes. (Cf. Reddaway, 1972.) Oleszczuk (1988a:114) noted that 'chastisement' was the first of several purposes of sentencing mentioned in Article 57 of the Criminal Code of the RSFSR, and mitigating factors which might have ameliorated this punitive aspect have been ignored frequently in the case of Soviet dissidents, despite the duty of counsel for the accused to try to exonerate the defendant or at least obtain mitigation (Article 51).

5. Punitive Transfer

The structure of psychiatric hospitalization allowed transfer among mental institutions along a spectrum of ordinary to strict observation regimes as well as transfer between levels of restrictions within hospitals and among hospitals and prisons. The possibility of transfer to more hazardous circumstances gave rise to allegations of punitive use of transfer. A court order was required for transfer or release of those committed following criminal trials, but this requirement would not necessarily prevent abuse of transfers. Since transfer to an ordinary psychiatric hospital might often signal release, transfers back from OPHs to strict supervision hospitals are particularly meaningful. For example, Koppers infers that Mikhail Nikolayevich Zhikharev's transfer from Sochi OPH to Chernyakhovsk SPH was due to 'failure to condone corruption' (1990:175). Zhikharev had written critical books after observing and futilely protesting against diversion of state building materials to private use. Zhikharev, charged with slandering the Soviet system, was hospitalized for over eight years, even though the maximum *prison* term under this charge was three years. Zhikharev was transferred to a special psychiatric hospital at about the time corruption cases in Sochi against local officials, which might have been furthered by his testimony, were under way. Anecdotal evidence beyond this case also attests to transfer to more stringent wards within hospitals for idiosyncratic reasons of relations with guards and physicians or simply for telling political jokes.

Irrespective of the purpose, individuals are also transferred between mental and penal institutions in the US, so transfer was not a unique attribute of the Soviet response to dissent. In interpreting transfers, Turk repeated that it should not be assumed penal institutions only punish and mental institutions only treat, since '. . . differences between the two categories of [US] institutions have never been as great as they are commonly assumed to be . . .' (Turk, 1969:21). Both have served some security and some rehabilitation functions in the US. In the Soviet case while the difference between prisons and strict supervision hospitals has been virtually nil, conditions improved vitally as one left a strict observation hospital for an open ward in an ordinary regime hospital or a local institution.

6. Punitive Use of Drugs and Treatments

Clearly at least some drugs, restraints, and 'therapies' not recognized in the West were inflicted on interned dissidents who did not 'need' them, for non-medical purposes. High doses of neuroleptic drugs were forced on those hospitalized under overtly political articles of the Criminal Code, such as Article 70 (anti-Soviet agitprop) or Article 190.1 (defamation of the Soviet system). At least three individuals observed by the US Delegation in 1989 displayed no psychotic symptoms, yet reported receiving antipsychotic drugs.[67] The allegations that drugs were used for explicitly punitive purposes against dissidents in mental hospitals included deliberate overdosing to create painful side-effects (Nekipelov, 1980), withholding drugs necessary to control secondary effects, and use of drugs to end hunger strikes, quash complaints, punish rule-breakers, force statements of guilt or abandonment of principles, or blackmail relatives who, without the threat of drugging their detained family members, might seek outside assistance or publicity.

Remarkable in the Soviet case was the use of accepted pharmaceuticals in large doses, evidently deliberately to induce side-effects in some cases, and use of industrial and other chemicals which do not have known medical applications to humans. Soviet defences of the first practice included assertions without substantiation that large doses of some drugs potentiate the effects of other medically necessary drugs or of other therapy. It has also been alleged that apparently punitive measures were simply well-meant behaviour modification techniques. No basis in the literature supports these defences and no clinical trials have been conducted along these lines to the best of our knowledge. Even drugs regarded as safe, which hold an acknowledged place in the psychiatric pharmacopoeia, such as antianxiety drugs (ex. phenobarbital), antipsychotic drugs (ex. promazine, chlorpromazine, haloperidol), antidepressants (ex. the tricyclicals), depressants, and stimulants have side-effects which can be deliberately induced as penalties, for rule infractions, and so on. The WPA reported that one interviewee from the US Delegation's visit in 1989 was subsequently subjected to punitive use of drugs, with the predictable exonerating notation in the file 'change in patient's condition'; that is, patient complained to Westerners. Excessive or unnecessary use of pharmaceuticals on healthy people supports the argument for deliberate Soviet punitive use of mental hospitals, *especially* since these allegations emerged from a country with unrelieved shortages of the most basic medicines including aspirin.

Retaliatory administration of drugs is difficult to document without internal hospital records since even first-person accounts necessarily lack precision. Even if dosage information were available, Soviet-prescribed doses of drugs were higher than those ordinarily prescribed in the West, complicating any empirical calculation of deliberate overdoses. Still it remains notable that drug treatment regimes do not vary much with the 'clinical presentation' of any individual (eds Shore and Keith, 1989:27). This uniformity is consistent with a small selection of available chemicals, poor education of physicians, and with a pre-designed political protocol based on punitive use of chemicals.

The example of Algirdas Statkevicius, a psychiatrist arrested for human rights work and critical writing, illustrates the arbitrary, vindictive role of drugs in political cases. Dr Statkevicius was given haloperidol, triftazine, and aminazine while detained, evidently in excessive amounts which caused to him to lose consciousness. When the chief psychiatrist at Chernyakhovsk hospital discovered Statkevicius could read English, he stopped purportedly necessary forcible drug treatment in return for Statkevicius' translating *Moscow News* from English into Russian for him (Koppers, 1990:157).

Benign explanations obviously can be advanced for the use of drugs with an internationally recognized role in psychiatric treatment, and for withholding, simply because of cost or scarcity, drugs which alleviate side-effects. It is considerably harder to explain Soviet use of chemicals which have no known therapeutic role and cannot be found in a modern pharmacopoeia. These included arsenic; phenazine ($C_6H_4N_2C_6H_4$), a dye base; and sulfazine, a one per cent solution of sulphur, described by Alexeyeff (1976:123) as producing 'a whole range of debilitating and severe side-effects' including pain, spasms and muscle necrosis at the injection site.

Though officials of the Health Ministry have said that sulfazine is no longer in use except with consent of those thus 'treated', its frequent mention in anecdotal accounts implies that sulfazine was used freely as a punishment in many hospitals, possibly in part because it was cheap and available. Sulfazine was used on ten of the 27 released or hospitalized individuals interviewed in 1989 by the US Delegation. The WPA found in 1991 that sulfazine was still used in the Kiev hospital, though purportedly only 'by [written] consent', an assertion which the relevant regulation published in 1990 has made more generally.[68] But free or informed consent cannot be obtained from those forcibly hospitalized, especially in a society which has not relied on collaboration and cooperation or even non-judgmental communication between patient and therapist.

Accounts of drug-related deaths and injuries are many. A.V. Nikitin died in detention in 1984 apparently as a result of repeated exposure to neuroleptics, as did N. Petrov (Koppers, 1990:131). A Hare Krishna devotee, Martik Zhamkochyan, died while hospitalized in 1986, apparently from tizercine. The IAPUP/Geneva Initiative lists multiple casualties of forced hospitalization by name, among nationalists, private enterprise advocates, asylum seekers and free press advocates including Emants Kcresh, Ivan Khomiak, Boris V. Lesnov, Alexander Lyapin, Maltsev, Vladimir Sergeyevich Maximov, Valerian Fyodorovich Morozov, Fyodor Parasenkov, and Shatalov, as well as a reference to some 30 deaths at Sychyevka SPH alone from 1987 to 1989 (IAPUP, 1988, No. 18:13–14 and 19:10–11; 1990, No. 24:17). N. Sorokin reportedly died in prison in the USSR as an indirect consequence of drug treatment (Gershman,

1984:57), and L. Plyushch was reported injured by injection of depressants (Sakharov in Sobel, 1978:38).

SUMMARY

While the USSR and the post-Soviet states are not alone in defining and prosecuting political crimes, the Soviet state had the most systematic record of political use of psychiatry for these purposes yet encountered (van Voren, 1989:13). The Soviet state tended to hospitalize rather than try turbulent individuals in lengthy criminal proceedings,[69] and, when a brief absence would be politically convenient, to hold nonconformists in ordinary psychiatric hospitals through civil/administrative procedures rather than arrest them. Complaints of irrationality in the Soviet instance tended to emerge from the prosecutor's office rather than from family members, co-workers, or others in immediate contact with nonconformists. Family involvement most often was directed towards *preventing* the hospitalization of family members.

That the Soviet Union made punitive use of psychiatry against Soviet dissidents is evident in:

- records on hospitalizing healthy regime critics;
- inappropriate and inconsistent findings of competence;
- The Party-, KGB-, and procuracy-influenced compliant structure of the Soviet mental hospital system.

In the Gorbachev administration, the government appeared to concede these points, since New Thinking implied dramatic reductions in arrests/hospitalizations for unabashedly political or religious charges. Aware of its public relations vulnerability, the Ministry of Health had announced plans by the late 1980s to reduce the population of USSR mental hospitals by 30 per cent (eds Shore and Keith, 1989:9). By 1989 seven of the special psychiatric hospitals or strict observation hospitals had been reported closed, 16 of perhaps 22 had been assigned to the Ministry of Health, and repeated claims had been advanced that all political or religious prisoners had been released from camps and jails, while perhaps 50 detainee dissidents had been discharged from hospitals.

Notwithstanding, the IAPUP/Geneva Initiative reported 'many' new cases as late as 1989 (ed. van Voren, 1989:10); Podrabinek reported 60 (op.cit.:99). IAPUP in 1990 recorded six current political detentions in Talgar SPH (Alma-Ata) specifically, denied by authorities. The Talgar detainees were transferred promptly after their cases were publicized

(1990(23):32). The Moscow Helsinki Watch Group as of 1 January 1990 was aware of 43 political hospitalizations still under way, the largest group of which was occasioned by the same sorts of 'anti-Soviet' writing, demonstrations, unauthorized meetings and distribution of critical printed materials which had been responsible for previous detentions before the era of glasnost, perestroika and demokratizatsia, and before Articles 70 and 190.1 were respectively revised and removed from the Criminal Code. The second most frequent catalyst of detention in this group, unauthorized border crossings or attempts, also reflects a pattern persisting from the pre-Gorbachev period.

Sporadic cases of compulsory psychiatric examinations and detentions for political or religious reasons have continued to come to light in the early 1990s, including a few not known in the West previously. If a predisposition to hospitalize critics persists across the post-Soviet territories, new incidents of forced hospitalization can be expected to develop, since many of the underlying causes of dissatisfaction among Soviet nationals were exacerbated by the breakup of the Union. If the Independent Psychiatric Association's records of reasons for consultations with the IPA from January 1989 to February 1990 are any guide (IAPUP, 1990, No. 24:12), clashes with psychiatrists continue to take place because of well-founded concerns over housing shortages, medical care, and whistle-blowing or other work disputes, as well as political criticism, all of which can be expected to continue or increase in frequency and intensity over the 1990s and into the next century.

2 Characteristics of the Evidence: The Database of Psychiatric Hospital Detainees

If you appeal to the anti-Soviet coalition for help, you will die in a strict regime psychiatric institution. Restructuring is not for 'khakhly' [ladies' men, fancy men].[1] Glasnost is for export.

Psychiatrist to Anatoly Mikhailovich Ilchenko, Ukrainian Central Information Service, in APA *Releases*, 1991:8

'Glasnost' extends only to those authors who do not say anything superfluous from the authorities' point of view. This means, first of all, authors who are dead . . .

Podrabinek in van Voren, 1989:93

DEFINITIONS OF TERMS

Who is a dissident? For our purposes, any individual known to have participated in any of the activities or organizations listed below was identified as a political dissident or a nonconformist active religious believer. Note that dissident activities spanned many aspects of political activism, religious work and observance, political and religious communication, protest, and creation and dissemination of self-published (samizdat) dissident journals and other materials, as well as possession and circulation of materials published abroad (tamizdat). Unofficial or illegal organizations included human rights groups, trade unions, political fronts, cultural associations, and religious societies.

Proscribed, even if in principle legal, activities defined as *dissident behaviour* are multifaceted. We include petitioning the government or other authorities, complaining to authorities, appealing for clemency or for adherence to rules to official organs, and signing collective petitions to government and other agencies. Public nonconforming behaviour is counted in such varied forms as demonstrating, including photographing demonstrations; conspicuous public speaking; writing slogans in public; meeting with officials in public to protest; participating in public nonconformist art exhibitions or poetry and literature readings; openly exhibiting dissident books, including mailing dissident books to authorities; and holding unauthorized political or religious meetings without authorities present as well as *en masse* gathering outside courthouses during well-publicized trials. We also include as dissenting acts deviant voting behaviour, such as refusal to vote, or refusal to vote for an approved candidate; and unauthorized electoral activity, such as running against an approved candidate or interfering with the ballot box. Hunger strikes in political causes such as national representation or human rights observances are included. Behaviour construed as direct refusals to acknowledge the power of the Soviet state, such as refusal to bear arms, to join the military, to be drafted or to go to a specific war would be counted, as are flag raising, lowering or burning; creating or joining an 'anti-Soviet' dissident group; renouncing Soviet citizenship; requesting non-Soviet citizenship or asylum abroad; and moving without authorization to a traditional homeland, or, in microcosm, moving as a prisoner into forbidden zones in camps and prisons. Behaviour overtly rejecting atheism, such as participating in religious processions (including 'Buddhist activities') is encompassed. Rioting and other violent behaviour with political objectives is counted, as are work stoppages or slowdowns when a political cause is clear; and plane hijacking or other unapproved border crossings or attempts.

Composition, production, circulation, and possession of self-published (samizdat) materials have been perceived as especially powerful dissident activities because of their potential to create uncensorable lines of communication and thus mobilize previously isolated sectors of society. We found this a frequent trigger act which functioned as a proximal cause of detention (Smith and Oleszczuk, 1989). Samizdat publications and literature date to the 1920s if not earlier as a post-revolutionary vehicle for explication of internal Party differences, though they did not flourish until after Stalin's death. They have been a fount of prohibited genre writing such as science fiction in the 1940s, and they remained a powerful versatile vehicle of social criticism. Thus samizdat possession, possession of unlicensed typewriter(s) or other duplicating equipment or printing presses, actual duplication of samizdat, distribution of samizdat including smuggling it out of the country, writing for, editing or signing samizdat, and creating new samizdat all comprise dissident behaviour.

Creation of unofficial groups, and membership or office-holding in such groups also is recorded as dissident activity. Examples of major unofficial or illegal groups and organizations include but are not limited to the Helsinki Watch (Monitoring) Group, the Committee for the Defence of the Rights of Believers, independent trade unions, the Working Commission on Psychiatric Abuse/Working Group for the Investigation of Psychiatric Abuse, the Working Commission on the Rights of Invalids (still apparently a taboo topic), other human rights organizations such as but not limited to Amnesty International, Group 73, the Action (Initiative) Group for the Defence of Civil Rights in the USSR, Committees for the Defence of the Rights of Believers, Baltic States Nuclear Free Zone organizers, political discussion groups, embryonic political fronts and parties, anti-Soviet Partisans, nationalist groups, nationalist youth leagues, prison camp underground groups, Mensheviks, 'Bolsheviks', EuroCommunists, unofficial peace activists, anti-nuclear protesters, cultural or literary circles, and religious societies such as parish councils or the Society of the Eucharist.

Other means of dissent, though real, are so varied as to defy accurate record-making. They have included *inter alia* testifying for the defence at trials of other dissidents, and assisting protesters to find lawyers. Some dissident behaviour is so frequent as to exceed the space boundaries in our dataset, although the format allows for up to 16 known dissident acts, eight arrests, seven trials, with charges and sentences including up to seven psychiatric commitments by court order, up to three non-trial psychiatric detentions, 14 interrogations, and a great deal of demographic and geographic information amounting to 117 or more variables per person. Some information which could not be captured in the format has been preserved in an overflow file (as of individuals arrested more than eight times, or especially active dissidents associated with more than 16 dissident acts). Other information was not coded because it appeared idiosyncratic, was judged unlikely to be repeated, or exceeded space available by some order of magnitude which made recording it impractical (such as the numbers of individuals sending congratulatory letters to Solzhenitsyn on his Nobel prize).

We have not countenanced defining armed insurrection as a dissident act, since dissenters preserve loyalty to certain idealistic features of the dominant society whereas guerillas or independence fighters do not. Therefore despite their intrinsic interest we did not record as dissent some cases of nationalist agitation in the Western USSR in the early 1960s which reflect sentences imposed for acts of war against the Soviet Union (see de Boer *et al.*), or the disparate acts of ethnic violence in Tadzhikistan, Georgia/Abkhazia, and elsewhere.

What is meant by 'state repression'? Several types of behaviour of individuals acting in the name of the state constitute state repression, and when directed against a particular protester allowed inclusion of the nonconformist in the dataset as a repressed dissident. All those included had been subject to at least one episode of forcible commitment to a psychiatric institution, but frequently had been the victims of other acts of state suppression of criticism as well. State repression includes any of the following, after at least one known dissident act.

Arrest; detention; forcible trial-ordered or administrative psychiatric hospitalization; interrogation by the police, Procuracy or KGB; criminal or civil trial; military tribunal or NKVD Special Commission hearing;[2] sentencing; or a record of prison, camp or exile term or other sentence or trial outcome including acquittal, pardon or amnesty.

Other measures of state persecution are more problematic to trace and document, and more difficult to attribute to particular authorities. Consequently such measures have been omitted from systematic data-gathering. These extend to arbitrary drafting into the military; expulsion from the University or denial of admission; expulsion from the Writers' Union or other professional associations; suspension from the priesthood; denial of Party or Komsomol membership and related privileges for those who wish to keep them; revocation of citizenship for those who wish to keep it (we do code renunciation of citizenship by individuals who wish to give up citizenship); failure to allow foreign asylum for those who wish to lose citizenship (we do code emigration and application for asylum/visa); search of living quarters and/or confiscation of property, rescission of residence permit, loss of housing or job even purportedly 'at own request', including cancellation of home purchase, reassignment to work in a distant or inaccessible place; destruction of art or other works; 'educational' KGB warnings; inexplicable auto accidents; apparently random street violence; restriction or deprivation of parental rights and forcible placement of children in boarding schools; annulment of marriages, and cancellation of maternity benefits.

In particular, *what constitutes psychiatric measures against dissidents?* Short-term administrative detentions of a few days up to two weeks; longer civil commitments to ordinary regime psychiatric hospitals or special regime (strict observation) hospitals; criminal commitments to locked wards in ordinary psychiatric hospitals or to special regime hospitals (prison hospitals); and required appearances at local clinics. While other measures can be interpreted as psychiatric restraint on dissent, such as requiring an indication of impaired mental status on identity papers, or including similar notations in work records, we have not coded such measures since they are less draconian than involuntary commitment, and, while they remain of interest, they are not systematically reported.

DATA COLLECTED

The cases of individual dissidents interned in psychiatric hospitals which are analyzed here are drawn in the first instance from a larger All-Union dataset on several forms of repression of political dissidents and practising religious believers in the USSR 1940–80, initially compiled by the author and her collaborator, Dr Thomas A. Oleszczuk. Dr Oleszczuk has extended this dataset through 1981, and with the kind permission of the respective researchers, Dr Smith has used Dr Andre Koppers' and Ellen Mercer's records to extend the dataset through 1991, to the end of the Soviet period. Dr Koppers is a historian with the Geneva Initiative on Psychiatry, which has compiled evidence on political use of psychiatry for over 20 years. Ellen Mercer, Director of the Office of International Affairs of the American Psychiatric Association and a participant in the 1989 US Delegation visiting Soviet psychiatric institutions, maintained data on dubious forcible hospitalizations and releases through 1991.

Selecting from the Smith–Oleszczuk Dissident Dataset all records for individuals against whom definite measures of administrative or court-ordered psychiatric detention or hospitalization can be documented yields a sample of 410 individuals from 1960 to 1981, when records are most complete, and 674 from the late 1920s to 1991 when our earliest observations are included and the Koppers and Mercer data are integrated. Less elaborate records on psychiatric detentions from the 1920s through the 1950s appear in the dataset but are not included in all the quantitative analyses because of the relatively less rich and detailed nature of the evidence for those decades.[3]

Data gathered for individuals include 117 possible observations, *inter alia* the name, birth date (and date of death where applicable), republic of residence, and religious[4] and ethnic affiliation[5] of political and religious dissidents; occupation;[6] the nature of their political or religious dissident behaviour; dates of arrest(s), detention(s), interrogation(s), and trial(s); charge(s) under the Russian Soviet Federal Socialist Republic Criminal Code or republic equivalent; length of prison term(s), camp sentence(s), and criminal/civil trial-ordered or administrative psychiatric detention(s); and emigration dates if any. Administrative commitments are recorded separately from trial-based criminal commitments presuming that they may reflect different aspects of the phenomenon, and merit separate study. Note is also made of pardons, amnesties, and commuted sentences, as well as cases reversed or thrown out on appeal.

We have not defined political and religious dissidents on the basis of charges levelled against them, but on the basis of their recorded behaviour.

Thus individuals in our dataset have been charged with far more and varied transgressions than the standard so-called 'political' offences, RSFSR Criminal Code Article 64 (treason), Article 70 (anti-Soviet agitation and propaganda, narrowed in 1989 to include only advocating the overthrow of the government), Article 190.1 (defaming the Soviet system, later repealed), Article 142 (separation of church, state and school), and Article 227 (infringement of others' rights via exercise of religion). The state has shown itself imaginative and flexible in the use of the civil and criminal codes to prosecute nonconformists. In our records, in the aftermath of dissident behaviour dissenters have been charged with allegations as creative as stealing library books, mooning rock musicians, inciting to suicide (better life in heaven), kidnapping, forging documents, assault, ritual murder, homosexuality, rape, illegal sale of icons, traffic safety violations, and vagrancy as well as the more usual parasitism and hooliganism. RSFSR codes and republic equivalents for criminal charges recorded in our dataset are set out in Appendices A.1 and A.2.

SOURCES OF DATA

For this inquiry, data were derived from multiple substantial sources in various languages, beginning with the *Chronicle of Current Events* and other dissident publications, and providing access to pre-existing collections such as *Arkhiv Samizdata, Sobranie Dokumentov Samizdata*, the archives of the Geneva Initiative on Psychiatry, and others. Sources include special interest and general coverage samizdat; emigré group publications; books, reports and data files from advocacy organizations such as Amnesty International; specialized human rights studies from academic research institutes such as the Centre for the Study of Religion and Communism at Keston College; a US national newspaper of record; and surveys of Soviet and former Soviet Union (FSU) popular and elite print and electronic media. They encompass:

1. *Chronicle of Current Events* (*Khronika Tekushchikh Sobytii*), Moscow. Issues 1–58 were examined, beginning in 1972 and covering the earliest reports from the USSR itself.

   The *Chronicle* reports arrests and psychiatric detentions mainly from April 1968 to November 1980. Sporadic coverage of incidents dating from the 1940s and earlier appears. By the early 1970s this source covered cases from all parts of the USSR, reducing any possible earlier geographic bias (Rubenstein, 1985:141), and was widely regarded as an 'all-Union dissident "newspaper"' (Oleszczuk, 1988:196). The *Chronicle* provides a continuing record except for a crackdown extending from October 1972 to May 1974. (See *Chronicles of Human Rights*, below.) Because in some periods the *Chronicle* has appeared not to concentrate on religious dissidents with the same intensity as on political cases, we have also included religious advocacy sources and other compendia which derive from religious sources.

2. *Biographical Dictionary of Dissidents in the Soviet Union 1956–1975* S.P. de Boer, E.J. Driessen, and H.L. Verhaar (1982).[7] Martinus Nijhoff Publishers: the Hague, Boston and London.

   This reference work draws its information from:

   a. the records from issues 1–38 (to 1975) of *Chronicle of Current Events*, providing the opportunity to verify reports in the issues through 1975 previously consulted.
   b. relevant records from the 30-volume *Sobranie Dokumentov Samizdata* compiled in Munich by the staff of Radio Liberty.
   c. *Samizdat Verein.*

   The *Dictionary* lists approximately 3400 individuals from among about 10 000 Soviet dissidents for whom at least partial information is available in the 1956–75 period. This *Dictionary* includes individuals as dissidents if they had experienced any of the following:

   - court trial for political activity
   - compulsory mental hospitalization for dissident acts
   - authoring at least one samizdat (self-published) item
   - joining a dissident political group or party
   - signing political petitions or collective letters of grievance to officials.

   This source includes additional precise information on formal charges made at trial, some of which were not initially available in samizdat since in some cases they had not been made public when detentions were first reported.

3. *Prisoners of Conscience in the USSR: Their Conditions and Treatment.* Amnesty International Report (Amnesty International: London, 1975, 1980).

   Two editions of this book, supplemented by Amnesty's 1979/1980 open external files for the late 1970s and early 1980s, kindly made available to us in the New York office, added access to unpublished information. Amnesty's many networks pick up group and individual accounts directly reported to them or referred to Amnesty through religious or political organizational connections in the erstwhile USSR.

4. *Chronicles of the Catholic Church in Lithuania* (*Lietuvos Kataliku Bazhnychios Kronika*) (Lithuanian Catholic Religious Aid Auxiliary Publications: Chicago). Later volumes in the series are published by the Society for the Publication of the Chronicles of the Catholic Church in Lithuania, Chicago.

   This is the central journal of the Lithuanian dissident movement, which proved itself resilient to repeated efforts to destroy it as a fount of information to the West. It summarizes other samizdat publications and extends coverage of repression of non-Lithuanians and non-Catholics into Belarus and Moldova.

5. *Chronicles of Human Rights in the USSR*, ed. Valery N. Chalidze (emigré dissident) (New York: Khronika Press).

   The *CHR* covers 1972 to the early 1980s, overlapping with reports in *Khronika Tekushchikh Sobytii*, appearing while the *Chronicle* was suppressed, and continuing after the *Chronicle* returned to print, adding some information from Western periodicals and emigré writing.

6. *ELTA Information Bulletin*. Washington, DC.

   The *Bulletin* is published by the Lithuanian National Foundation (prior to 1979, the Supreme Committee for the Liberation of Lithuania, (VLIKo)), an advocacy source devoted to mobilizing Western public opinion on behalf of Lithuanian independence. This source dates to 1956. After 1973 it excerpted samizdat materials as well as reports from recent emigrés to the US. Numbers 1–124 were included.

7. Keston College[8] research publications.

   Keston College, established by Catholic and Protestant religious authorities in England, monitors the status of observant Christians in the USSR. Among its research reports consulted are:

   Christian Prisoners in the USSR 1977: A Keston College Staff Study (Keston College: Kent, UK, 1977). General editor Michael Bourdeaux.

   Soviet Christian Prisoner List 1979 and *1981* (Keston College: Kent, UK, 1979, 1981). Society for the Study of Religion Under Communism.

8. *List of Political Prisoners* (1978, 1980, 1981). (*Spisok Politzaklyuchennikh SSSR*). Editor Cronid Lubarsky. First volume published in Munich, subsequent volumes in Paris.

The lists of prisoners are products of Lubarsky's private news service focused on the USSR's dissident voices, including religious as well as political protesters.

9. *Vesti iz SSSR/USSR News Briefs*. Editor Cronid Lubarsky. Published biweekly from 1982 onwards in Brussels: Cahiers du Samizdat; later, Munich: Das Land und Die Welt Publishers, Schwanthalerstr. 73/V., 8000 Munchen 2, Germany.

   This summary source combines reports from 'literally dozens' (Oleszczuk, 1988:197) of human rights organizations, advocacy groups, individuals and emigrés.

10. *A Biographical Dictionary on the Political Abuse of Psychiatry in the USSR* (first edition 1990).[9] Dr Andre Koppers. Amsterdam: International Association on the Political Use of Psychiatry, now the Geneva Initiative on Psychiatry (International Association for the Abolishment and Prevention of Political Psychiatry).

    Singularly useful for reports of cases since 1980, the *Dictionary* in addition can corroborate existing data since it derives from many of the same original samizdat and archival sources we have previously consulted. In addition to biographical, demographic, and trial information on those hospitalized, this *Dictionary* lists psychiatrists implicated in political use of psychiatry, and a directory of psychiatric hospitals which have served as psychoprisons.

    Dr Koppers, a historian trained in Eastern European History at the University of Utrecht, indicates that he researched all relevant open sources for his data, including *Arkhiv Samizdata* in Munich,[10] the appropriate collections in the Lenin Library in Moscow and in the State Scientific Medical Library in Moscow, as well as European and Soviet periodicals including scientific journals. Further, he had access to the extensive archive maintained for two decades by the International Association on Political Use of Psychiatry itself (Geneva Initiative on Psychiatry).

    Numbering among Koppers' periodical information bases are:

Izvestia	*The Observer*
Jewish Chronicle	*Pravda*
Komsomolskaya Pravda	*Sotsialisticheskaya Industriya*
Kontinent	*The Daily Telegraph*
Leningradskaya Pravda	*Tribune de Genève*
Literaturnaya Gazeta	*USSR News Brief*
Meditsinskaya Gazeta	*Vzglyad*
Novoye Vremya	*Die Welt*
NYT Magazine	

Koppers compiled additional information concerning actual practice of punitive psychiatry by travelling frequently in the USSR to interview numerous detainees.

11. American Psychiatric Association Office of International Affairs Lists of historical and current *Releases* and *Internments* (1991, Washington, DC unpublished), kindly made available by their Director, Ellen Mercer.

 Mercer's lists contain more recent information from the late 1980s and early 1990s than does Koppers and for this reason hers is the best available recent and most timely information in a single source up to the disintegration of the USSR. Ellen Mercer reports that her office kept the releases and internments lists up-to-date until 1991; dates on the lists indicate that they were revised as late as June 1991, though they, like Koppers, also include some early information from the 1940s and 1950s.

 The Mercer data also comprise an attempt at a universal sample of well-confirmed cases from many sources. Ellen Mercer has relied on her own individual and professional contacts in the West and in the FSU to generate her data. In addition, the *Schizophrenia Bulletin* special issue concerning the 1989 visit by a US delegation indicates that both the American Psychiatric Association and the US Department of State benefit from sources among Soviet human rights activists, the IAPUP, the US Helsinki Commission, Amnesty International, and the US Institute of Medicine/National Academy of Sciences (1989:12).

 Illuminating supplementary sources also consulted but not relied on exclusively for data construction due to known focuses in reportage or limitations in time covered are:

a. Antebi, Elizabeth (1977). *Droit d'asiles en Union Soviétique: Document* (Paris: Julliard).
b. Foreign Broadcast Information Service *Daily Reports* on the USSR and, after the breakup, on Central Eurasia. This source translates into English and summarizes the output of radio, television and print media in dozens of languages across the Union and subsequent independent states. Coverage is admirably broad across republics/states, making this source optimal for non-Slavic reports. But because inclusion of any particular issue or news item appears to be a function of priorities of a rotating crew of translators whose interests vary, we do not presume that it necessarily provides representative over-time reportage on psychiatric detentions.

c. Joint Publications Research Service and Foreign Broadcast Information Service global coverage of psychiatric issues as indexed in CD-ROM format. These transcriptions and translations of publications and electronic media information were consulted for global reports of political abuse of psychiatry, as well as for reports originating outside the USSR on Soviet cases of forcible commitments.
d. *New York Times* 1 January 1970 to 1 January 1982, for reports reaching the West to use in the bias study.
e. *Statesman's Yearbook*, for reports on internal exile as a sanction for dissent in the pre-revolutionary period.
f. Medvedev, Roy, *On Soviet Dissent* (London: Saunders, 1980).
g. *Tashkentski Protsess* (Amsterdam: Alexander Herzen Fund Press, 1976 *et seq.*). These accounts of Uzbek and Crimean Tatar dissident trials provide a degree of insurance against some risk to our sample of bias by location and by degree of publicity organized abroad.

POPULATION SIZE

Western estimates of the size of the misdiagnosed dissident population in Soviet mental hospitals until recently centred on a minimum of 200. Lebedev (1992) repeats that estimate for the number of writers forcibly hospitalized annually from 1975 to 1988. Amnesty International in January 1983 counted 305 since 1969. Bonnie (1990:328) referred to 'many hundreds' caught up only in court-ordered procedures in the 1970–90 period. Partial records led to allegations of at least 700 (Reich, 1978:31), though some estimates attributed as many as 1000 to a single psychiatrist (ed. van Voren, 1989:16, attributable to Serbsky director Daniil Romanovich Lunts). Since the population of political prisoners from which psychiatric detainees are drawn had been estimated as high as eight to ten thousand (Hubner, 1980:84, and De Boer, Driessen and Verhaar, 1982), and the numbers of Soviet dissidents who received warnings from the procuracy over 1967 to 1974 swelled past 121 000 (Lebedev, 1992), the potential for tens of thousands of psychiatric prisoners was real. A researcher with the American Psychiatric Association has indicated that internee numbers were once thought in the West to amount easily to 'perhaps thousands'. The International Association on Political Use of Psychiatry (IAPUP, now the Geneva Initiative) once estimated the total number interned at approximately 6000 (IAPUP, 1983:6).

However, credible Soviet psychiatrists thought detainee estimates in the thousands overstated (Mercer correspondence, 4 March 1992). Pyotr Morozov claimed in 1990 that the correct total number fell between two and three hundred, though this relatively low estimate may simply reflect an altered predisposition at the Serbsky Institute in the 1990s to send those considered ill to prisons and work camps instead of hospitals.

Our original sample includes over 400 well-confirmed cases of individual dissenters hospitalized during the period 1960–81 for whom records adequate for our analysis exist, and about 200 more from Koppers and Mercer data used to extend coverage to 1991. Given that we have examined a longer period of time, it is only to be expected that the resulting size of our sample after reconciliation of the respective datasets, 674, is somewhat larger than that encountered in Bloch and Reddaway[11] (1984), who found about 200 individuals detained from 1962 to 1976, and 300 or more since 1977.

CONSTRUCTION OF THE SAMPLE

For these analyses we have attempted to provide an approximation of a universal sample of the well-confirmed cases of the dissident population held in Soviet psychiatric prisons over 1960–91.[12] That is, we have made a virtually exhaustive search of primary and secondary printed material and some transcripts of electronic reports originating both in the West and in the erstwhile USSR to identify most if not all well-documented cases of named dissident individuals against whom psychiatric measures were invoked in the Union in this interval. We integrated the Koppers and Mercer data into our original dataset 1960–81 primarily to extend the data through the 1980s and into 1991, by which time the Union self-destructs and Koppers, Reddaway and others indicate that political use of psychiatry had virtually disappeared, though sporadic allegations in the media persist. One unanticipated result of the new data was additional information dating back to the late 1920s.

We argue that inclusion of the Koppers and Mercer data does not present a sampling problem, since they are derived from essentially the same sources used in our original data-gathering (with the addition of personal professional contacts), but instead substantiates our assertion that the use of multiple redundant sources of information in construction of the original datset in fact caught most cases of well-confirmed psychiatric detention of nonconformists. Oleszczuk shows (1988) that representative data on state repression in Lithuania could be derived by using merely two sources.[13] *Ceteris paribus* this may also be the case across the Union, and therefore the multiple diverse sources consulted here for the entire USSR would have generated a systematic sample of all well-documented cases of forcibly interned dissenters in the period under study.

While we cannot prove that omissions of well-confirmed cases have not occurred, just as we cannot prove any counterfactual, the result of our data-gathering is a dataset which we argue includes a high percentage of all substantiated cases,[14] which does not suffer from systematic omissions, and is therefore representative.

Some corroboration of the nature of the sample can be obtained from a comparison of the Mercer and Koppers additions with the original Smith–Oleszczuk data. Of the 428 cases Mercer and Koppers document, 190 do not appear in our dissident data. And altogether we show 181 cases which are not found in either the Mercer or Koppers data. Thus Koppers' and Mercer's lists extend our dataset by some 190 cases, of which approximately 117 are well detailed. These additions are mostly cases which either took place after 1981 or were in progress – under investigation or in trial – in 1980 and 1981 when our original data collecting ended, and not misses in earlier data-gathering of those dissidents who had already been ordered confined. Sixty-four of the 190 preceded our original cutoff date. Of these, 58 fell in the 1960 or later interval, and presumably should have been found in our sources. Keeping in mind the fact that Koppers' and Mercer's sources include direct personal contacts which were not tapped in our original data-making, it is surprising that as few as 58 of Mercer/Koppers cases were not recorded in our original data of over 400 people, although they took place when they should have been picked up in our original search.[15] The large area of overlap in cases reported continues to argue for a substantial degree of inclusiveness in our sampling strategy.

The numbers of political and religious psychoprisoners cannot be determined conclusively until arrest records and hospital documents become available. However it can be argued that the correct number of well-confirmed cases dating between 1960 and 1981 inclusive may be approximated by the sum of the unique cases in the Smith–Oleszczuk data (410) plus the previously undetected unique cases from Mercer and Koppers in the same period (58), or 468. Then 1 – 58/468 or about 88 per cent gives a crude measure of the inclusiveness of the Smith–Oleszczuk sample of well-documented cases before the additions to 1991.

The impression of inclusiveness in our original sample before the Mercer/Koppers additions is also bolstered by comparison of our sample with those independently compiled by Podrabinek and by Bloch and Reddaway[16] for somewhat different historical periods, using their personal observations, research and contacts in situ. Our early sample of more detailed cases as summarized in Appendix A.3 appears to include some cases (319) not encountered by Podrabinek, and about 281 not listed by Bloch and Reddaway, given some imprecision due to our transliterations and due to their conscious elision of already publicized cases. The final dataset used here with the Mercer/Koppers additions is of course most inclusive and covers some 674 individuals.

CHARACTERISTICS OF THE SAMPLE

Representativeness

The crucial question for our analyses is to what extent our sample of forcibly hospitalized political and religious protesters represents the total and unknown universe of all such individuals in the Soviet period, since our chief goal in this book is to examine the repression of dissent via this peculiar mechanism.

It is also a matter of interest to what extent dissent in general, and psychiatrically repressed dissent in particular, was a phenomenon of the larger Soviet society. For speculation on these matters, the similarities of our sample to the entire dissident movement or to the aggregate Soviet social structure are also pertinent, though we are not, strictly speaking, attempting to generalize any findings to these larger groups.

Similarities to the Dissident Movement

Psychiatric detainees are a diverse lot held for varying behaviour, such as workplace safety complaints, attempts to meet with foreigners, nationalist agitation, and failure to see the Soviet Union as a utopian society. In this diversity, detainees resemble the larger dissident movement. It may be tempting for simplicity's sake to make a false assumption of homogeneity in the larger dissident movement; but it, like the subset of psychiatric detainees, in fact exhibits diversity in proximal cause of repression, education level, occupation, ethnicity, religion, and ideology – including Marxism – among other indicators. Similarly, neither dissidents in general nor those confined to the psychiatric hospitals in particular can be assumed to be uniformly or generally maladjusted, or usually at risk of mental illness. As a rule these individuals are successful at their occupations or studies, and are at mid- or later points in well-launched careers.

Most psychiatric prisoners have a history of renegade political behaviour or overtly religious acts. Even though, while active dissidents, psychiatric detainees may have accumulated arrest records for political or religious activities, incurring an increased risk of losing their jobs and suffering other penalties, political arrests have not necessarily been a cause of major alteration in their political ideology. The Harvard Project found no effect of arrests on 'generalized political and social attitudes' (Inkeles and Bauer, 1968:37), all the more remarkable when one considers that their finding dates from the immediate postwar and Stalin era (1950–51).

In our hospitalized dissident data, as well as in the Harvard study, those arrested are not necessarily advocates of any particular ideology and do not appear to change ideology as a function of arrest or arbitrary hospitalization, although they may be more anti-Soviet than the population at large and may take measures to avoid a second or subsequent hospitalization by reducing subsequent dissenting behaviour. This observation implies that in the Harvard data the attitude-changing compellance functions if not the deterrence functions of political arrest as an instrument of state terror were not served, and suggests the same conclusion in our data.

Similarities to the Entire Soviet Population

Unlike the whole Soviet population, our sample is focused on adults, though minimum age at first arrest or detention falls in a few exceptional cases as low as 13 in these data, and is composed mainly of men. Of course the Soviet population, though ageing, included infants and juveniles, and displayed a distinct age-specific deficit of men, due largely to Great Patriotic War losses and more recent demographic disasters. A profile of socioeconomic status of the hospitalized nonconformists is probably not comparable to a similar distribution for the whole Union. For example, our sample has included relatively few farmers or peasants, though it does represent workers substantially (see Chapter 4 for more demographic information).

Perhaps dissenters entertain common sympathies with at least some age cohorts of the entire Soviet population, since the Harvard Project argues political *arrest* to have been a widespread phenomenon among the whole population in the early 1950s (Inkeles and Bauer, 1968:35–6). But many of those caught up in the dissident movement of the 1970s and later were not born until after the early fifties and cannot have participated in this generational experience. Although psychiatric measures of repression share some features with political arrests in general (for example, in focusing mainly on men (op.cit.:49; Smith and Oleszczuk, 1989)), nevertheless psychiatric repression displays its own characteristics of interest.

While some speculation along these lines may be fruitful, it is not necessary to show either that forcibly hospitalized dissenters are representative of the whole country or that they are representative of the entire dissident movement. These are empirical questions. We suggest that psychiatric detainees are not particularly representative of the larger society. Most likely the psychiatric prisoner population is not essentially representative of the larger dissident movement, since the former was singled out for a particularly poignant state sanction. We are not attempting to generalize findings to these larger populations but instead to explain a phenomenon – the application of politicized psychiatry – which occurred only against a selected subgroup of dissenters.

Potential Bias

Sample Bias by Occupation and Education If the probability of inclusion of any individual in our dataset is a function of the level of education or occupation of the dissident, the sample would be biased. It can be argued that among dissidents the less well-educated or less well-placed professionally may have fewer contacts and fewer options for publicizing their plight should they be forcibly confined. Therefore, for example, to the extent that some religious dissenters may have less formal education, they risk being under-represented in the sample. However the networks of Church-based contacts serve to include them in the sources we have used to construct our dataset. These limitations would suggest sample bias if dissent is mainly a phenomenon of the less educated or relatively unskilled. But in the larger dataset of dissidents from which our original psychiatric detainees were drawn, as well as among psychiatric detainees, many protesters were highly educated. Certainly in their occupations they were not mainly disillusioned failures.

Our evidence is consistent with the view of dissent as a phenomenon of the reasonably well educated, and consistent with the findings of the Soviet Interview Project that better educated Soviets were more alienated from their society. Interestingly, Inkeles and Bauer show for the early fifties a tendency for those with more material rewards, partly overlapping with more prestigious occupations, to express less hostility towards the regime (1968, ch. XI). Later generations as shown by the Soviet Interview Project did not repeat this pattern, if only because they had higher expectations for their standard of living and less experience with state sanctions – thus the researchers for the Soviet Interview Project see Soviet dissent later as a phenomenon of the relatively privileged (ed. Millar, 1987), though we find it broad-based even into the seventies (1989), and the final dataset compiled and analyzed here shows a diverse occupational profile among psychiatric detainees into the early 1990s.

Sample Bias by Location Moscow and Leningrad may be over-represented in these data, relative to the proportion of the Soviet population living in these cities. But this seems unlikely at least insofar as city of residence is an indicator, since those residing in the two major metropolitan areas never form more than 28 per cent of forcible political hospitalization cases and comprise a generally diminishing proportion of detainees over administrations, amounting to only seven per cent of known cases by the Gorbachev administration, consistent with a pattern of spread of dissent to outlying cities and even to some villages. On the other hand, given the possibility – though not the ease – of travel, proportionally more psychiatric hospitalizations may have originated in the two major cities, at least at the beginning of the dissident movement, since exposure of dissident causes and nonconformist behaviour to the foreign press and foreign nationals would be maximized. Outside major cities with universities and reporters from the international press, networks for publicizing cases of forcible commitments may have been less well developed for some time. However, in Oleszczuk's study of Lithuanian dissent (1988:39), even rural repression of dissent becomes known eventually, location serving simply to delay but not prevent the publication of these incidents in our sources.

Sample Bias by Nationality Apparent under-representation by nationality of cases from the Islamic republics may be due to a tendency for our sources to report dissident events and incidents of state repression in the Islamic republics collectively. Reports of mass arrests in which names are not provided, and reports of group dissident acts for which identification of participants was unavailable, though noted in our data-making, did not result in additions of cases to the dataset, since a case is a record for a named individual.

However some under-representation of Islamic regions seems to exist in our data for substantive reasons. The dissident movements in these regions prior to recent ecological and nationalist political group formation were relatively small and poorly organized, evidently not resulting in large numbers of cases of hospitalizations of prominent nonconformists from the southern republics. So under-representation of Islamic nationalities in the data compared to their prevalence in the total Soviet population in this instance may not be a defect in the dataset but a reflection of the true character of the phenomenon (Glebov and Crowfoot, 1989; Olcott, 1990; Motyl, 1992; Khamriv, 1994).

Source Bias by Ideology and Worldview Bias in the sources themselves can be fostered by the ideology of the compilers and by the dominant worldview of institutions sponsoring research.

Considering the effect of the worldviews of Radio Free Europe/Radio Liberty researchers on the content of *Arkhiv Samizdata*, since RFE/RL is an agency funded by the US government as part of Cold War public opinion and diffusion of information campaigns, its employees can be presumed to be motivated to include every possible case of punitive political use of psychiatry as part of a general predisposition to show excesses and abuses of the Soviet system. That RL may be motivated to find these abuses does not alter the fact that the abuses are real, documented in multiple sources including those originating from individuals who respect many values of the socialist world, and ultimately acknowledged at the highest levels of the Soviet mental health bureaucracy.

The most probable error for researchers of this stripe would be to include cases of undeniable mental illness without political significance among the political hospitalizations. They are unlikely for ideological reasons to have omitted cases of psychiatric detention of healthy Soviets. This orientation may actually be helpful for the inquiry in that it implies few omissions of cases of abuse and thus reduces any latent missing information problem that could result early on from maturation in samizdat reporting networks (while they are expanding their contacts), while maximizing sample size. Since worldview and ideology could be seen as potentially damaging to the inquiry by causing the inclusion of spurious cases, we guarded the data against spurious cases in two ways: a) the multiple sources consulted militate against inclusion of substantively spurious cases; b) we have omitted from the analysis any case intersubjectively known to be mentally ill whose illness precedes reprisal for political or religious observance and therefore appears unrelated to suppression.[17] Some questionable cases may remain. But at least some cases of genuinely mentally ill dissidents confined involuntarily remain of interest to this study – for example, those of individuals who became ill as a result of persistent violation of their human rights or as a result of earlier detention, and those who, while perhaps genuinely ill, are harassed in hospital/prison for political or religious reasons.

Compilers' ideology as a cause of potential bias on the Soviet side has two central aspects: the dominant ideology influences major figures in Soviet psychiatry to ignore, deny or explain away abuses, while the competing professionals and unofficial sources may have an interest in exaggerating the severity or frequency of unjustified hospitalizations. Since we do not use a dominant representative of Soviet psychiatry as a *source* of data,[18] this potential bias can have had little effect on the sample. The second question of bias in unofficial sources and later among competing professionals affects the sample centrally through the choice of samizdat as a data source.

With respect to samizdat, Oleszczuk finds in his study of Lithuania (1988) no evidence that factual errors in reporting are higher for samizdat than for elite media and no indication of bias by maturation of reporting networks in the major samizdat source for the whole Union, *Chronicle of Current Events*. Oleszczuk shows that if any bias exists in reporting little-known trials or shorter, less dramatic sentences, it lies in the direction of other sources (rather than samizdat) omitting the less spectacular or less 'newsworthy' cases.

Oleszczuk's empirical observation from the late eighties is coherent with the judgment made a decade earlier by Hubner (1980:85), who concluded that, because of serious penalties attached to exaggerations in samizdat, dissident writers throughout the Union were careful to preserve '. . . basic general qualities of the great majority of samizdat documents . . . the striving for the greatest possible objectivity, concreteness, adherence to facts, restraint . . .'

Reliability of Data

Because they are based on emigré interviews in samples with certain inescapable limits, both the classic Harvard Refugee Interview Project (Harvard Project on the Soviet Social System) and the extraordinarily rigorously designed and executed Soviet Interview Project confronted the same general issue raised here in our smaller study in the use of samizdat sources. That issue is whether reliable information can be obtained from the accounts of people who are at least in some respects self-selected and critical of or overtly antagonistic towards the state or society from which they come. Clearly the findings from these much larger studies have already proved insightful contributions to cumulative knowledge.

Concerning the reliability and validity of data derived in the first instance from samizdat, a foundation for these analyses, see Thomas A. Oleszczuk, 'An Analysis of Bias in Samizdat Sources: A Lithuanian Case' (1985), the quantitative appendix in *Political Justice in the USSR* (Oleszczuk, 1988), and Bloch and Reddaway's (1984:80) assessment of the *Chronicle* data alone: '. . . a large quantity of detailed, reliable and well-edited information was collected in conditions where the authorities were hostile and also exercised considerable control or even "veto power" over the basic means of communications . . .'

To our chagrin the record does show dissident behaviour and subsequent penalties including psychiatric repression which are not attributable to individuals by name. Such reports may mention '300 demonstrators' detained, 'a member of the Council of Representatives of the Free Trade Unions' arrested, 'another person' also interrogated, a 'pharmacist in Vladimir' hospitalized, etc. Despite their intrinsic interest, unless the name can be deduced from other proximal evidence, these cases are excluded from our data to enhance reliability, since it cannot be determined whether they overlap with named individuals already in the dataset or whether they represent new incidents.

This operational definitional requirement that cases of psychiatric suppression be identified by name probably results in some loss of information and may underestimate the true size of the detainee population, but it is necessary to make possible confirmation of cases in independent sources and thereby protect the reliability of the data.

Generalizability (External Validity)

The Harvard Project and the Soviet Interview Project also contended with the issue of generalizability of findings. The sample of refugees and emigrés interviewed in each instance was of perhaps maximal intrinsic interest and took advantage of historic opportunities to gather information, in the first case by interviewing a range of adult displaced persons in European camps during 1950–51, and in the second by interviewing a probability sample of predominantly Jewish emigrés arriving in the US in the shock wave of immigration between 1979 and 1982. Simultaneously, an interest arises in the question as to what larger population, if any, findings can be generalized.

External validity questions are a function of the population and time parameters to which we might wish to generalize. Clearly our conclusions apply only to the Soviet period, although evidence suggests some common patterns across administrations. Conjecturally we have implied some common features extending back into the Tsarist period. On the basis of this evidence we would not generalize to other types of governments or even necessarily to behaviour of independent states formed from the former Soviet Union. However, future research in related political structures such as those obtaining in Central/Eastern Europe and Cuba may show comparable patterns; and, at higher levels of abstraction, common features in reliance on state repression across time and polity type may be discovered.

Support for Statistical Inference: Sample Size

Due to increased accessibility and lower cost of information, our sample size in this study is more than twice the interview sample size of the classic Harvard Refugee Interview Project on emigrés (their n=329), and apparently it constitutes a larger proportion of the total number of psychiatric prisoners. Because sources of information proliferated, and we therefore did not have to rely as closely on targets of opportunity as did the early project, our sample also may be more nearly representative of the entire dissident movement and at least in some respects of the entire country, reflecting the all-Union character of political disaffection.

Statistical methodologists do not advance any single definite rule for the optimal size of a sample, though sample size is related to the precision of population estimates made on the basis of sample data. Hopkins and Glass note (1978:182) that a 'representative sample of 100 is generally preferable to an unrepresentative sample of 1 000 000!' For mailed-in opinion surveys, US social scientists may accept a response rate as small as five per cent. Our data clearly constitute a far larger proportion of the total recorded number of detainees than this, and would amount even in quite pessimistic circumstances to over ten per cent if the IAPUP high estimate of true population size at about 6000 is correct. If Bloch and Reddaway's estimate of perhaps 300 at any one time is accepted, and the average number of new hospitalizations per year in our dataset (15.8 with known dates) is a rough indication of turnover rate (release data are incomplete), our sample of 674 is a much higher percentage of the total detainee population. Therefore our data presumably yield a more accurate assessment of psychiatric repression.

The 'Quality' of Qualitative Information

We have argued that we have a sound basis for accepting the *quantitative* information used in our data-making. However our study is also coloured by more subjective, *qualitative* information obtained from secondary sources, primary sources, lectures, conversations, correspondence and published accounts of emigré experiences. We have confidence in the qualitative information conveyed by our sources, for example, of reports of punitive treatment while detained, because of its inherent plausibility, repetition and coherence with other known sources and cases, internal logical consistency, credibility of those making the reports, corroborations from professionals and outside visitors, and eventual if grudging corroboration from the Ministry of Health itself.

3 Four Explanations of the Political Use of Psychiatry

> Electroconvulsive therapy (ECT) is only used for exceptional patients who are 'highly charged' . . .
>
> (US Delegation Report from Kazan SPH, 1989:71)

> Crossing the border is a sign of mental illness, as is distributing religious leaflets.
>
> (Special psychiatric hospital official to US delegation, 1989:43)

As noted in the first chapter, many states confront episodic phenomena of widespread political, nationalist, ethnic and religious dissidence, or, like India, face a permanent risk of communal violence and dismemberment because of these social fracture lines. The Soviet experience with a dissident movement, remarkable for its duration, intensity, broad base of recruiting, and significance in the erosion of the Union, is also extraordinary[1] because of the state's response. The authorities have forcibly confined hundreds, possibly thousands, of the more vocal or irritating activists to psychiatric hospitals for extended periods as one coercive reaction to dissenting behaviour. Even pariah states such as South Africa at the height of its defence of apartheid and efforts to control inter-ethnic violence evidently did not resort to systematic psychiatric hospitalization in efforts to inhibit political upheaval in the townships. Perhaps equally inventively and more cost-effectively, the South African authorities did arrest thousands of children under 15, as a disincentive to political activity on the part of their parents and other relatives.

Large-scale psychiatric detention as a Soviet regime strategy for coping with criticism is disproportionally expensive compared with available options such as job and school sanctions, threats to professional qualifications, family and societal pressures, and imprisonment. Why the regime would move selectively towards reliance on punitive psychiatry then requires an explanation.[2]

The Western social science and comparative politics literature advances four principal explanations of psychiatric coercion, at varied levels of analysis and abstraction. Formally they comprise contrasting theoretical partial explanations for the use of psychiatry as a means of social control:

cultural predisposition, generational conflict, professional socialization, and instrumental regime use.

1. CULTURAL AND HISTORICAL PREDISPOSITION

Punitive psychiatry is a reflection of the paternalistic structure of the Orthodox Church and a repressive, autocratic political culture inherited from Tsarism, in the cultural and historical predisposition explanation. In this view political use of psychiatry during both the Tsarist and Soviet periods is a predictable consequence of an authoritarian political culture shrouded from the Enlightenment and enshrined in a centralized decision-making apparatus. Soviet society, according to this argument, inherited from Tsarism not only the forms of hierarchical decision-making structure but also narrow standards of acceptable behaviour and penalties for failure to conform to these rigid norms. This low societal tolerance for deviance and a broad and flexible definition of what constitutes deviant behaviour result in a penchant for arrest and detention – or exile and banishing – of societal irritants. Given this heritage of Soviet political culture, proportionally more arrests for political and religious dissidence would naturally arise in the USSR than in a society with a comparable level of dissident activity but without these historical and cultural antecedents.

2. INTERGENERATIONAL CONFLICT

The intergenerational conflict explanation holds that punitive psychiatry is a symptom of conflict among age cohorts, targeting teenagers and the elderly who are seen as nonconformist or obstructive. In this perspective expedient use of psychiatric hospitalization results when family or community members confronting younger (or, alternatively, elderly) socially deviant individuals request hospitalization, or force it on unwilling vocal nonconformists whose behaviour at certain crucial junctures of life events is seen as rebellious and politically or religiously meaningful (Turk, 1969; 1982). Teenagers treated as unemancipated and the elderly already dealt with as incompetent are unlikely to have access to a lawyer or other authoritative defenders. In this view nonconforming behaviour precipitating commitment is a consequence of life cycle events in the growth and development of individuals. Such behaviour would follow a U-shaped curve over time, since it would be expected to diminish over time as individuals mature, and then increase with ageing, though new individuals coming into the most susceptible age groups would provide continuing instances. Illustrative cases of this phenomenon can be found in many countries. In the USSR, since 'voluntary' commitments to mental hospitals could be initiated relatively freely by co-workers or by supervisors, voluntary commitments could be especially likely in cases of simple generational conflict.

In this view ideology *in se* is not a crucial element in the explanation of hospitalization of apparently healthy people, which is instead interpreted as normal life transition intergenerational struggle.

However, dissent, and consequently repression, may be generational in another sense not straightforwardly related to ageing and biological life cycle events. Nonconforming behaviour may well follow politicized 'generational' patterns in that it tends to characterize age cohorts of varying sizes who have experienced common political [or religious] formative events (Bahry, 1987:76), rather than age cohorts defined by 20-year intervals in standard demographic terms, as they pass certain growth and maturation milestones. Nonconformity not related to life cycle events would not naturally diminish over time,[3] but would be expected to continue over the active life of the cohort. If this is so, psychiatric repression might reasonably target certain age-cohort generations – and classes within them – disproportionally, since a disproportionate amount of nonconformist behaviour would originate within particular politically moulded generations and would not be expected to diminish over time or necessarily to increase with great ageing, ruling out a *laissez-faire* regime response.

In Soviet Interview Project data, Bahry finds the immediate post-war group born 1925–40 and the (mainly) post-Stalin age cohort born 1941–60 to be most active politically in the USSR, both in nonconformist behaviour and in socially encouraged compliant behaviour. Their tendency to nonconformist activity is not touched by life cycle events. Marriage and family have no effect on regime-critical behaviour, though retirement may have some influence by eroding resources and mobility (1987:78–81).

In contrast to the earlier Harvard Project from the 1950s, the Soviet Interview Project in the 1980s found generational differences in almost all statistical analyses conducted in a large stratified sample of emigrés (Millar, 1987:27), including opinion and ranking of different administrations in the USSR. The younger respondents who were successful and better integrated into society were *more*, rather than *less*, likely than older ones in the SIP data to have engaged in unauthorized and socially or politically unappreciated acts such as samizdat reading. The pervasiveness of this finding of generational differences, and its apparent unresponsiveness to material reward, or at least an insensitivity to material progress because of relative deprivation, described by Millar as 'a challenge for the Soviet leadership', suggests that a generational explanation of forcible hospitalization based on 'generations' defined as shared-formative-events age cohorts of varying sizes might have considerable power. In the politically-defined age cohort formulation rather than the life-cycle formulation, this generational explanation complements rather than contradicts the rational regime actor explanation, discussed below.

3. PROFESSIONAL SOCIALIZATION IN MEDICINE

Punitive psychiatry is a result of the normal training of psychiatrists in the USSR, according to the professional socialization explanation. Psychiatric training and definitions of morbid deviant behaviour vary across cultures as well as political systems, ideologies,[4] national experience, and competing schools of psychiatric thought. Thus no nation-state can claim to have defined mental illness without subjectivity. Among other vaguely constructed conditions, the theory of schizophrenia appears particularly poorly articulated (Scheflen, 1981). Clearly the identification of mental illness on the basis of societally deviant behaviour remains idiosyncratic among individual practitioners as well. Bloch's 1977 example, the conceptualization of homosexuality as deviant and morbid, is relevant still.

Therefore, in this view it is neither surprising nor sinister that the criteria operationally defining mental illness in general and schizophrenia in particular are far broader in Soviet and in some cases post-Soviet practice than in the US and elsewhere. In fact, cross-national comparisons suggest that a spectrum of diminishing definitional amplitude for serious mental disorders exists globally. In this spectrum US practice in diagnosing schizophrenia, while less inclusive than the Soviets', remains more inclusive than in Asia and Europe, according to the American Psychiatric Association (1987:192) and a World Health Organization study (1973).

One factor explaining the relative lack of precision in Soviet diagnostic criteria is that Soviet psychiatrists'[5] training as specialists is narrow compared with that prevailing in the West. The World Psychiatric Association asserts (1991:29) that the specialization in psychiatry in the USSR amounted on average from four months to one year[6] of additional study with no qualifying examination, and the Geneva Initiative asserts it might have amounted to a month of lectures or even less.

According to Joan Buchanan of the American Psychological Association, the Soviet taboo on clinical psychology and their rejection of Freud had prevented the development of formally trained clinical psychologists, and many other specialties in psychology were simply not taught at all, although Ph.D.-level social psychologists, sociologists and Pavlovian experimental psychologists were produced. An awareness of psychological dimensions in human problems has been maintained at think-tanks such as the Institute for the Study of the USA and Canada's Department of Politico-Psychological Problems, and the Laboratory of Small Groups Psychology, which produced among its notable works a study of adaptability to long-term residence in radioactively contaminated territories. Chernobyl and Afghanistan led to the 1993 creation of the Laboratory of the Psychology of Post-Traumatic States, at the Institute of Psychology of the Russian Academy of Sciences.

In view of shortages of training programmes and a history of sparse or prohibited inquiry in some areas, it is not surprising that even by 1991 the USSR had perhaps as few as 2500 psychotherapists and 1000 clinical psychologists (Popov, 1991:3 in *CDSP* 43(25):17). However the field has thawed since the fall of the Union. New centres of research and study such as the Laboratory of Engineering Psychology, opened in 1994 at the Institute of Psychology, have sprung up in the last few years, and new professional organizations such as the Russian Psychological Association, being formed in 1994, as well as new training centres such as the Faculty of Practical Psychology at the Kirov Pedagogical Institute, may make possible the training of larger numbers of psychologists in future. Numbering among the several new centres are the Psychological Institute of the Russian Academy of Education, the International Education and Psychological College, and the Moscow Higher School of Psychotherapy. Despite painful financial shortages, new journals are also appearing, including the *Bulletin of Psychosocial and Corrective-Rehabilitative Work*, disseminating foreign practice.

Mental health professionals in all specialties were disadvantageously trained in general in the USSR. In fact medical training itself was impoverished, scanty and superficial compared with its counterpart in the US, and was complicated by shortages of equipment, materials and every requirement such as soap, antiseptics, anaesthetics, and hot water. Generally medical school curricula have also created shortages of instructional time, sacrificing meeting time and energy to political courses, which in different periods may have amounted to a third (Golyakhovsky, 1984:8) or a fourth (Bloch and Reddaway, 1977:43) of total academic course time. Golyakhovsky contrasts this time devoted to Marxism-Leninism with the four *days* reserved for orthopaedics in the six years of his medical school instruction.

Medical instruction has also been biased in some periods by the predominance of Party instructors in some institutions. Golyakhovsky estimated that 50–75 per cent of his professors at the Moscow Medical School in the late 1940s and early 1950s were Communist Party members, as opposed to perhaps ten per cent of the population at that time (1984:22). Further, he asserts a pattern of preferential job assignment and promotion disregarding medical qualifications and instead rewarding Party work.

This training with its aspects of the Red v. expert problem implies potentially serious quality control deficiencies. Some practitioners still claim to be psychiatrists though they have never even attended medical school. It also defines a broader and potentially Party-dictated range of behaviour as indicative of insanity, and in particular defines as mental illness rejection of socialist values, and by extension Party guidance, which we will show in later chapters were severely penalized. Notions of social reform which might otherwise be seen as idealistic, and desires to emigrate which might be seen as either rational or romantic, are converted to symptoms of disease.

Variations in academic background of psychiatrists within the USSR may well account for some part of the psychiatric hospitalization and psychiatric prison detention of dissidents. Psychiatrists trained in the prestigious Snezhnevsky school (Moscow) have shown a distinct predisposition to overdiagnose political nonconformity as disease, in particular as asymptomatic – but genetic – schizophrenia. Without national-level certification for psychiatry (Salvendry, 1975:232), aspiring Soviet psychiatrists who are certified have instead been certified by the hospital where their residencies were completed, which is to say by their own instructors and supervisors. In-house certification creates a powerful basis for paradigmatic bias and for geographic idiosyncrasies. In the absence of a national credential, regional paradigmatic and other biases in diagnosis cannot be prevented, and presumably are propagated by professional socialization.

AN ASIDE: THE OBSERVER BIAS PROBLEM

The observer bias problem is related to all three previous partial explanations. While the literature on comparative psychiatric practice is not extensive, it does argue that in all societies dissidents and the less powerful may tend to be overdiagnosed as mentally ill. Because of this overdiagnosis the poor and less powerful tend to be over-represented among both voluntary and involuntary hospitalizations, because of behaviour challenging societal norms in the first case and because of greater vulnerability in the second. These two partially overlapping groups of people are also disproportionally subject to arrest. Further, prior political activity and arrest record may be taken into account when Soviet dissenters are detained for psychiatric examination, and may be evaluated as mental maladjustment or evidence of societal danger, leading to a greater propensity to find nonconformists mentally ill.

Therefore, any over-representation of dissenters and the relatively powerless among those forced into Soviet-era mental hospitals may be partially due to degree of observer bias in those calling for arrest, in arresting officers, and in psychiatrists. If observer bias accounts for a substantial amount of misclassification of Soviet dissidents as unsound, it would diminish the support for other hypotheses such as rational state manipulation, unless observer bias is only or mainly created by the regime. But as the previous three explanations suggest, multiple sources of observer bias may exist independent of regime pressure, as well as those several biases occasioned by the regime at varying times, such as a physician's desire to classify dissidents as mentally ill to prevent their being sent to Siberia or Afghanistan.[7]

Observer bias may be created by culture and ideology, enhanced by academic training, and may be particularly salient where new therapies or pharmaceuticals emerge,[8] or where prior police records, previous diagnoses, and information from the psychiatric register are easily accessible, especially if these have reached a conclusion of genetic basis for a mental abnormality or if they carry authoritative signatures. But dominant ideological line and to some extent the dominant academic paradigm can be affected by the regime, because of state and Party power over professional advancement in medicine. Thus some evidence tending to support the observer bias explanation for psychiatric repression of Soviet dissent could also be partially supportive of the instrumental use argument, or at any rate its consequences would be difficult to disentangle. We suggest that except when observer bias is regime-induced, it probably does not change rapidly. Thus if observer bias were the main determinant of detention of political nonconformists, the patterns of change in detentions should be relatively long-term and perhaps essentially generational as suggested above.

Our data are not consistent with this expected pattern, as can be seen in Chapter 5. Instead they show dramatic short-term fluctuations, and are not concentrated either on vulnerable age groups or on those of relatively easily victimized low socioeconomic status occupations. Neither are the data consistent with the presumption that relatively less powerful groups in society are over-represented among detainees, since detainees are not for example disproportionally women or minority nationalities. Because the observer bias hypothesis is a general one more specifically dealt with in the other explanations, and because at the level of abstraction expressed here it yields demonstrably false conclusions in our data, we do not deal with it further, except to note that in principle arrests and mental illness labelling may be two functionally interrelated societal responses to deviance.[9]

4. INSTRUMENTAL USE BY REGIME

According to the instrumental use explanation, psychiatric repression of dissent is an implement of the state, whose policy goals vary over time. When desired, punitive psychiatry can be a weapon of the state and the Party against human rights advocates, nationalists, True Believers of all stripes, embarrassing True Marxists and others. When expedient, psychiatric sanctions can be relaxed at propitious moments to show 'liberality' or 'reform'. This thesis is based on several assumptions: one, that at least with respect to this issue a ruling elite exists which approximates a unitary rational actor in its behaviour; two, that the ruling elite has many possibly competing or incompatible goals which may change over time; and three, that the elite can and does use its resources instrumentally to accomplish selected goals.

Idiosyncrasies appear in Soviet psychiatric diagnostic procedures and in the diagnoses themselves. While idiosyncrasies and variability in diagnoses are found in many countries, interpretation of them as deliberate follows from the fact that state and Party pressures could be brought to bear on psychiatrists via the structure of Soviet psychiatry, designed to facilitate government and Party manipulation. KGB authority over some hospitals prevailed until recently. Until the Communist Party fractionated, the Party influenced job assignments, approved rises and granted promotions for psychiatrists (Miller, 1985:22). Thus, even psychiatrists who were not Party members were employees of the Party to a significant degree and *ipso facto* subject to mobilization along ideological lines. The disintegration of the All-Union Party has had an impact on the practice of politicized psychiatry and is partially responsible for the decline in numbers of reported detainees as well as for continuing sporadic reports at the local level.

The process of detention and confinement in the USSR followed certain steps which allowed or even encouraged the participation of potentially politicized state agents at several points, including mayors, local Party officials, and others who could serve as instruments of state policy as well as of their own local objectives (see Bloch and Reddaway, 1977:ch. 5 for a description).

Until recently the legal recourse of individuals to combat political charges of mental illness was very limited, which is to say that they were the same rights as those enjoyed by all Soviet nationals to bring complaints against individual public officials. The outcome of Alexander Kolomna Kuznetzov's case charging unnecessary hospitalization, a lawsuit against the officer who signed his pre-internment arrest warrant, will be instructive (Koppers, 1990:117).

Additionally, as previously noted, because psychiatrists were not certified at the All-Union level, but if at all only locally, by the hospitals in which they have been trained, paradigmatic predisposition or discipline bias probably has a geographical basis and could in principle be mapped across the Union. As a result of the variations in diagnosis which these idiosyncrasies create, the same individual might be judged 'schizophrenic in Moscow, a psychopath in Leningrad, and healthy in Kharkov' (Novikov *et al.*, *Komsomolskaya Pravda*, 11 Nov. 1987). Since these diagnostic predispositions were known, they could be used politically simply by selection, for example, by ordering that a suspect individual be examined in Moscow or Kazan, where s/he is more likely, given the outlook of the staff psychiatrists, to be found seriously and possibly permanently ill. As previously mentioned, the Moscow Snezhnevsky school, dominant in Soviet psychiatry, trained specialists to identify a variety of schizophrenia which is 'sluggish' or asymptomatic, thus providing an irrefutable diagnosis applied to evidently sane dissidents, would-be emigrés, True Believers, and others.

The interpretation of punitive psychiatry as deliberate manipulation of medicine for regime purposes would be supported by evidence of state sanctions against psychiatrists who protest the hospitalization of healthy people, when such sanctions are not explicable as state penalties against incompetent practitioners who also happen to be vociferous. The cases of the Soviet psychiatrists Anatoly Koryagin and Semyon Gluzman, who opposed political use of psychiatry and were subsequently arrested and detained or imprisoned themselves, are among the most prominent which augur for the instrumental use hypothesis.[10]

SUMMARY

While elements of all four explanations may apply in particular cases, evidence from the data chapters, while varied, corroborates the rational use explanation. The most complete explanation of patterns in psychiatric detention of dissidents derives from deliberate rational use of psychiatry to deter, defuse and discredit dissent in the erstwhile USSR. In the next three chapters we describe the detainees themselves and set forth our evidence for a systematic state policy to direct dissent.

4 Who Are the Dissident Detainees? Some Observations and Descriptive Statistics

> Being a Jew, Kostya had been told by the K.G.B. – with whom he was almost on first name terms – that he had better leave for Israel soon. 'Otherwise', he quoted an officer as saying, 'we'll put you in another clinic, and return you to society as a totally healthy person . . .'
>
> Bonavia (1973:36)

Unlike political dissent at the close of the eighteenth century, which was a phenomenon of the relatively wealthy, well-educated, and well-travelled, Soviet dissent sprang from a broad base of political activism across and within social strata, and republics. Antebi (1977:120) observed '. . . ce n'est pas seulement une révolte d'intellectuels. C'est aussi une révolte diffuse, qui atteint toutes les couches de la population.' Workers and missionaries were swept up in it along with university students, white collar professionals, trade unionists, Hare Krishna devotees, environmentalists, and even police and erstwhile KGB employees. The cases of the taxi driver G.A. Bychkov, the shoe factory worker F.P. Dvoretsky, the hospital orderly F.N. Komarova, construction labourer Marchenko, and the manual worker V.A. Tsurikov provide examples of blue collar entanglement in the modern dissident movement. Soviet systematic persecution of the Evangelicals, often poor, also illustrates the class-inclusive nature of contemporary global political and religious repression of dissent,[1] as events in May 1989 in China corroborate.

SOCIOECONOMIC ORIGINS AND ATTRIBUTES

Shatz (1980) argued that most Soviet dissidents were university-educated, professional or artistic elites. Relatively few in his account were workers; scientists and writers predominated. Thus Shatz naturally drew a parallel between the dissenters he identified and the Tsarist intelligentsia. While our data show a more inclusive dissident movement than Shatz's,

Table 4.1 Occupations of Detainees v. All-Union Occupations in Percentage Terms

Occupation	*Smith–Oleszczuk Data*	*Narod. Khozyaistvo*
1. Artists, musicians, dancers Culture and the arts	3.8%	1.9%
2. Blue collar workers Industry, transport, construction	23.0%	54.0%
3. White collar employees Apparat. of organs of govt., administration, management; Communications	16.2%	3.0%
4. Intellectuals Health, teaching, sciences, services	35.9%	17.9%
5. Peasants/farmers Farming	1.0%	10.0%

Source: *Narodnoye Khozyaistvo: Statisticheskii Ezhegodnik* (Moscow: Goskomstat, 1982), pp. 357–8.
N.Kh. classifications appear on second and subsequent lines of each entry.

in which nearly a fourth (23 per cent) of our 674 cases are blue collar workers, we do find that the psychiatric detainees among dissenters in the All-Union data are disproportionally intellectuals and white collar employees. Among psychiatric detainees in the Smith–Oleszczuk data, more than a third (35 per cent) are from the intelligentsia, the single largest occupational category; and approximately 7.3 per cent are university students.

Sixteen per cent were white collar workers and professionals such as physician's assistants, engineers, practising journalists or technicians. Six per cent were religious such as ministers, priests, nuns, monks, or wandering holy people in rural areas. Four per cent were soldiers, militia or military officers, including an air force pilot. Another four per cent were artists, musicians, or dancers. Police and current or former KGB/NKVD officials together made up one per cent of all detainees. Peasants/farmers comprised only one per cent.

While it is difficult to conjure up an unambiguous method of comparing Western occupational structures to those summarized in Soviet sources, and we certainly have not done so here, some indication of the All-Union representativeness of psychiatric detainees' socioeconomic strata can be obtained by comparing the reported occupations of the individuals in our dataset with the closest corresponding or partially overlapping rough proportions obtaining in *Narodnoye Khozyaistvo* reports of employment in various branches of the Soviet economy for 1970, approximately a midpoint in our data.[2] As this preliminary examination attests, psychiatric detainees are not distributed across occupational categories in proportions which reflect the reported All-Union structure, but instead are employed in fewer blue collar and agricultural jobs, and more intellectual, white collar, arts and culture positions.

In contrast to Shatz and to the distribution in our All-Union data, in his case study of the Lithuanian dissident movement, Oleszczuk did not find a predominance of intellectuals among those forcibly interned in Lithuanian psychiatric hospitals. Oleszczuk found (1988b:116–18) that dissidents subject to psychiatric detention in Lithuania were generally similar on dimensions of occupation, gender, type of dissent, and kind of trigger act which was followed by arrest to other accused brought to regular trials. Given the enormous disparities among republics/states, presumably other republic-level studies would also show significant variations from the All-Union findings.

CENTRAL CONCERNS AND ORGANIZING ISSUES

Insofar as their concerns are revealed in the content of demonstrations, samizdat, protest letters, and other messages, a substantial majority (82 per cent) of the psychiatric detainees in the Smith–Oleszczuk data for the whole USSR were dedicated to one of seven major substantive issues. These are, in decreasing order of prominence, emigration and visa concerns (21.7 valid per cent); religious freedom (17.2 per cent); nationalist and anti-Communist goals (13.3 per cent); human rights advocacy (10.6 per cent); general anti-system dissent (5.6 per cent); samizdat (5.2 per cent); a cluster of workplace complaints, anti-corruption efforts and environmental campaigns (4.7 per cent), and True Communism (4.1 per cent). Our prior analysis has suggested that emigration and visa concerns mounted in the eighties, which may well reflect an accurate assessment among detainees not only of their own future life chances in the USSR but also of the future of the Soviet economy. Religious freedom is the cause accounting for the second largest group of psychiatric prisoners. That some 13 per cent of detainees are essentially pure nationalists and critics of the Union – and in fact were so before 1985 – presages the powerful nationalist upsurges of the M.S. Gorbachev period which facilitated the separation of the republics into states and fuelled the wars in Moldova, Nagorno-Karabakh, Tadzhikistan, and Georgia.

These substantive concerns are partially exposed in first known dissident acts used to advance selected causes, which can be summarized as samizdat and provocative writing in about 21.3 per cent of cases; creation of new political groups (joining, registering, holding meetings), about 19.2 per cent; publicity/agitprop (demonstrations, news conferences, petitioning), about 17 per cent; attempts to leave the USSR (illicit border-crossing attempts, hijackings, asylum requests), about 15.5 per cent; religious activity such as public processions, roughly six per cent; and anti-Party or anti-Soviet symbolic gestures (returning Party card, refusing to vote, running unauthorized candidates, offences against the USSR flag, and so on), about four per cent.

Bloch and Reddaway (1984:73) show that in the 1977–83 period about 50 per cent of psychiatrically detained dissidents were human rights or democracy advocates. Bloch and Reddaway also discovered that about ten per cent were nationalists; would-be emigrants comprised approximately 20 per cent, church activists amounted to about 15 per cent, and about five per cent were comprised of sociopolitical irritants, individuals 'inconvenient' to the Party or to the State because of multiple complaints against bureaucratic malfeasance. When forcibly hospitalized dissenters in our data are classified over an overlapping period 1960–81 by the meaning of the trigger act evidently precipitating their detentions – that is, by the dissident act closest in time to their arrests – a majority, a notable 55 per cent, are human rights advocates, when literary and samizdat 'offenders' are included. However, again indicating the growing wave of national sentiment, 21 per cent are nationalists. Only about 0.4 per cent appear emigration-related in these terms, about nine per cent are religious dissidents, and about eight per cent chronic 'complainers' and domestic political critics. Our findings for this overlapping period 1960–81 are coherent with those of Bloch and Reddaway, though emigration-related trigger acts may be under-reported in the Smith–Oleszczuk data.

OCCUPATION AND HOSPITALIZATION

Higher prestige work may have provided visibility which exposed nonconformists to additional risks of forced psychiatric hospitalization, as indicated by a weak but highly significant association between numbers of all detentions and our occupation categories when ranked by Soviet-perceived prestige (($\alpha = 0.000$); see Yanowitch, 1977; Lane, 1982).[3] This relationship is due to a connection between prestige of occupation and frequency of the more serious *court-ordered* commitments, since, when detentions are broken down by type, no significant association between prestige of occupation and numbers of *administrative* detentions can be found. Further analysis with more precise job titles would be necessary to establish this connection.

Other observations denote some protection for individuals whose contacts and networks of support within and outside the country may have been extensive, and especially severe sanctions in some cases for individuals who had been seen as unreliable enforcers of societal norms, for example in national security, though not, apparently, police.[4]

For psychiatric detainees whose occupation is recorded, the average duration of all forcible confinement was 5.4 years. Nonconformist police were fortunate in averaging less than one year of hospitalization; the cases of an invalid and a farmer at two and four years' respectively also show some leniency. No special protection existed for blue collar workers, who typically were hospitalized somewhat longer than average (6.07 years). Especially lengthy terms of hospitalization were inflicted on a musician (11), those in the military (6.8), and KGB/NKVD personnel (6.6).

Similarly in duration of *administrative* hospitalizations alone, police averaged detentions of less than two weeks (11 days). Blue collar workers were again held somewhat longer than average. The military, at 2.8 years, and religious professionals, 3.8 years, were penalized the most heavily in these terms. In this measure some indulgence towards artists, who average about 1.4 years of administrative detention, is suggested, though it does not exist in the total detentions data or in the sums of court-ordered detentions.

Musicians were especially favoured in that their average frequency of administrative detention was less than half that of the whole group of psychiatric detainees. Current or former KGB, invalids, and peasants/farmers were held administratively more often than average; KGB personnel were also detained under criminal law at higher than average frequencies.

Average *court-ordered* time in hospital for those dissenters whose occupation is known was 6.6 years. Police again are lightly sanctioned in these terms (1.9 years on average), while the military are not (8.6 years). Students and blue collar workers are harshly treated, averaging 7.7 and 7.5 years respectively in court-ordered confinement.

In the workers' state no special protection was extended to blue collar workers, in that workers were subject to at least as many administrative detentions as average in the group of all hospitalized dissenters, and perhaps more court-determined ones. A partial umbrella for peasants and farmers can be argued, since their average rates of court-inflicted hospitalizations are only about one-third the number characterizing the whole group of detainees. Perhaps unexpectedly in a declaratory atheist state, religious professionals' average numbers of court detentions were only about half the group mean, possibly out of respect for the extensiveness of their support networks and their ability to mobilize opinion on their behalf. But religious professionals' administrative hospitalizations were especially lengthy. This divergence between the two types of commitments may be due to the potential for large-scale publicity and embarrassment from religious communities which sustained court trials would arouse, an outcome that would be unlikely from a brief administrative commitment procedure. (See the more extensive discussion in Chapter 6.)

RELIGION

Among the cases for whom religious adherence is known,[5] approximately 21 per cent of psychiatric detainee dissidents in our data are Jewish, 20.3 per cent are Russian Orthodox, 13.4 per cent are Evangelical Christian and seven per cent are Roman Catholic. About two per cent are identified simply as Christians without further denomination.

Plainly Jews are over-represented among those interned, whether counted as an ethnicity or as a purely religious group. They also begin to appear in court at an earlier age than other dissidents, as early as 25 at the time of first court-ordered detention. A few cases (4) of Zionist Jewish Pentecostalists are recorded. The remainder of hospitalized dissenters whose religion is known include among Christians the Adventists (3.5 per cent), Mennonites (1.2 per cent), Pentecostalists (5.2 per cent), True Orthodox (3.5 per cent), Uniates (1.7 per cent), and others. Hare Krishna followers (4.1 per cent) and Buddhists (roughly two per cent) also appear. While some detainees are culturally Islamic as indicated by nationality (Bashkir, Uzbek, Tatar), we have no direct evidence of their adherence to Sunni or Shiia Islam and therefore no basis to consider Islamic influences on dissent and forcible commitment.

An analysis of penalties attached to dissident behaviour indicates that psychiatric prisoners are *not* treated equitably irrespective of religious affiliation. In the population for which religion and length of both court-mandated and administrative detentions are known (n = 106), average length of all detention is 4.2 years.[6] In these data True Orthodox believers average a stunning 7.5 years' compulsory hospitalization. Roman Catholics also receive substantially longer detentions than the group average for all cases where both religion and the length of enforced hospitalization are known, 6.9 years. Russian Orthodox adherents on average are hospitalized for 5.8 years. This sanction may reflect concerns that departure from the stabilizing role fulfilled by Russian Orthodoxy posed a particular societal risk, and that the Roman Catholic Church is a powerful source of authority which could challenge that of the state in some parts of the former USSR where the Catholic population is substantial, as in the Baltic Republics. Hare Krishna followers and Uniates also suffered lengthier detentions than average. Although these results may be an artifact of small sample size in the two categories, it is worth noting in corroboration that Uniates also were detained about twice as often administratively as the average for the whole group.

Distinctly shorter detentions were visited upon Mennonites (0.25 years), Adventists (0.38), Jehovah's Witnesses (1.0 year), Pentecostalists and Buddhists (both 1.3 years). Jewish dissidents' detentions are slightly shorter than the group average in these data (3.6 years), but this measure does not reflect severity of hospitalization, for example, the regime in force at the hospitals concerned.

Subdividing by detention type, non-judicial internments show some similarities to patterns obtaining in the total hospitalization data. Administrative hospitalizations among Russian Orthodox (3.3 years long on average) and True Orthodox (7.3 years) again were substantially more extensive than the 2.1 years typical for non-judicial internments, and Roman Catholics (2.2 years) and Evangelical Christians (2.3 years) were held marginally longer. Adventists (0.38 years) fell well below the group mean, as did Jewish detainees (0.27 years), Mennonites (0.25) and in this case Uniates (0.47) and Pentecostalists (0.78), though these last two findings may be the result of small sample size. A Buddhist detainee also shows a shorter than average hospitalization (one year).

In court-ordered proceedings, with a mean of five years, some of the same targeted severity is preserved. Under court directives, Roman Catholics (8.5 years on average), Russian Orthodox (8.2 years) and Uniates (7.7) suffered markedly longer than average hospitalization terms, suggesting that when they are tried, as opposed to detained administratively, their activities posed a serious enough risk to attract a stringent penalty. Pentecostalists (1.4 years) join non-denominated Christians (3.1), Jehovah's Witnesses (one year) and Buddhist (one year) dissidents in receiving shorter than average court-sanctioned sentences.

Some variations across religion in average age at first detention appear in the Smith–Oleszczuk data. For *court-ordered* commitments, average age at first detention for those whose religion is known is 34. Jews and Buddhists were somewhat younger than average (30), perhaps due to the early emphasis in both religions on responsibility for right action and curing the ills of the world. The one Pentecostalist was decidedly younger than average at 28. Both Russian Orthodox (38) and Evangelical Christians

(43.4) were notably older than average, usually not becoming activists until they had achieved some professional status as priests or ministers.

Average age at first *administrative* hospitalization for those whose religion is known is 36. Buddhists (29.5 years old on average), Jews (33.3), a Hare Krishna devotee (27), and Mennonites (25.5) hospitalized were substantially younger than average for all cases showing both religion and age at first detention, while True Orthodox (49) and Uniates (45) were substantially older than average, in part a result of their tendency to be religious professionals before they became involved in the dissident movement.

NATIONALITY

Victims of psychiatric repression mirror the nationality characteristics of the overall Soviet population, with some notable exceptions. Russians predominate (55 per cent) among the victims of forced psychiatric confinement, as they did in the population of Soviet activists and dissenters generally, and in the entire Soviet population (53.4 per cent in 1970).[7] Ukrainians made up 16 per cent of nationality-determined cases, while accounting for about 17 per cent of the Soviet population in 1970, approximately at the midpoint in the 1950–91 data.[8] The Balts, 2.1 per cent of the All-Union population, account for a disproportionate 12.4 per cent of internees, of whom 7.4 per cent are Lithuanian, 2.6 per cent Latvian, and 2.4 per cent Estonian. Other concentrations in our data which are not necessarily proportional to their presence in the whole Soviet population include Armenians (three per cent of detainees and 1.5 per cent of the Soviet population), Belarussians (two per cent of detainees and 3.7 per cent of Soviets), Georgians (1.5 per cent of detainees and about 1.3 per cent of Soviets) and Germans (approximately 1.5 per cent).

Considering major nationality groups, detainees of Slavic ethnicity make up nearly three-quarters of the total psychiatric prisoner population (73 per cent), at parity with their proportion of the whole Soviet population in 1970 (74 per cent). Balts, at 12.4 per cent of all detainees, are notably over-represented since they made up merely 2.1 per cent of the population of the USSR in 1970. Transcaucasian nationalities,[9] comprising 4.5 per cent of all psychiatric prisoners but only 2.8 per cent of the Soviet population, were also distinctly over-represented, even though we have no confirmed Azeri cases.

Most striking in the nationality data is that the Islamic nationalities together account for less than one per cent of all cases of psychiatric repression, yet this group amounted to 14.5 per cent of the USSR's population in 1970 and certainly was growing at a rapid rate. Central Asian nationalities may therefore seem significantly under-represented in these figures, especially in view of the strength and history of regional national sentiment which might have been assumed to have given rise to many nationalities dissidents in the area. Much may still remain unknown in these regions. However, Kreindler concluded even in the late 1980s (1986:401) 'Up to the present, the native Central Asian nationalities have not produced a visible dissident movement of their own', or perhaps simply not one visible to Western media, although the Meskhetians and Tatars, with their own organized groups, could be catalysts of such a transethnic movement.

Considering Jewish people as a nationality, as is done in Soviet demographic theory, we can make several observations. One, in most years in the Smith–Oleszczuk data, Jewish nationals *are* detained discriminatorily, in that they are forcibly hospitalized considerably more frequently than their proportion in the whole Soviet population would indicate (1.1 per cent in 1959; 0.9 per cent in 1970 and about 0.7 of one per cent by 1979), but perhaps not out of proportion to their presence among dissidents in general in this period, roughly 25 per cent in our incomplete demographic data. Among psychiatric detainees Jewish nationals comprise five per cent of the total. Second, a precipitate decline occurs after 1973 in the percentage of dissident detainees who are Jewish, especially notable in the mid-seventies, reflecting the tide of emigration which had already relocated approximately 280 000 people by the late 1970s. (See Reuschmeyer, Golomshtok and Kennedy, 1985.)

Relatively little variation across nationality in average numbers of administrative or court-set hospitalizations can be found in these data. Some small tendency for Armenians, Estonians, Georgians, Germans and Latvians to suffer fewer administrative detentions can be argued. Similarly the averages show a slight tendency for Armenians, Belarussians, Georgians and Lithuanians to be the victims of fewer court-mandated hospitalizations than are other nationalities. In any case the most typical experience for all detainees is one detention. This might have been either one administrative or one court-ordered confinement, but tended to be administrative.

Psychiatric detention was not focused on only one or a few nationalities. Instead the scatter of cases of internment across nationalities is noteworthy. Thus among others represented in the data but comprising a smaller proportion of our total than those mentioned above, in this case less than one per cent of those hospitalized, are a number of Czechs, Dagestanis, Finns, Kazakhs, Moldovans, Poles, Romanians, Tatars, Turkmens and Uzbeks.

That no particularly powerful differences in average numbers of detentions by nationality can be documented, and that no consistent favouritism towards Slavic linguistic groups exists, suggest a uniformity in rate of application of this social sanction across ethnic groups. That 13 of the 15 major domestic nationalities and some less populous ones as well as some border ethnicities are represented here is an indication of the wide sweep of repression, and the broad demographic base for political dissent in the USSR. It attests to the potential that nationalities dissent has shown for rapid escalation to violence, as well as for political organization, coalition-formation, political party creation, and ultimately for independence of the states which used to comprise the Union.

Nationality exerts a powerful effect not on frequency but on *length* of detention in these data where both variables are known (n = 270). For the whole group of cases showing both nationality and length of court-ordered as well as administrative internment, average length is 5.4 years. Estonians and Finns experience the shortest average hospitalizations (1.3 years or under). The other Baltic nationalities (Latvian, 3.8; Lithuanian, 2.9) also average somewhat less than the group mean. A group of nationalities clusters within a year of the mean (Armenians, Belarussians, Germans, and Jewish). Russians' average detention is almost identical to the group average. The longest average forced confinements by specific nationality are imposed on a Dagestani (15 years), a Tatar (13), Georgians (11) and Ukrainians (7.1).

These results are altered by considering the court-mandated hospitalizations separately from those arising from civil/administrative procedures. Court commitments among those whose nationality is known average 6.8 years. Among dissidents for whom both nationality and court-ordered detentions are known, again Georgians (11) and Tatars (13) suffer the longest court-ordered detentions on average, and Germans (1.4) the shortest. Both Lithuanians and Ukrainians undergo longer than average terms (7.5 years each). Among persistent dissenters repeatedly ordered hospitalized, five nationalities survive to endure a third court-directed commitment. They are Jews; two Baltic nationalities, the Latvian and Lithuanian; and two Slavic ethnicities, Russian and Ukrainian.

Non-judicial detentions, which tend to be shorter, average 2.4 years for the whole group whose nationality and length of administrative detention are known. Two nationalities stand out for the severity of their administrative sanctions, Belarussians (8.1 years) and a Dagestani (15). German, Romanian, Russian and Ukrainian administrative detention terms are also longer than average, but sample size in some groups handicaps any generalizations. Armenians were almost exactly at the average. Estonians (0.27),

Finns (0.01) and Jews (0.33) experienced the shortest average administrative hospitalizations for any nationality group in these data. Latvian and Lithuanian terms fall under one year, 0.91 and 0.66 respectively. Among persevering nonconformists subject to repeated administrative detentions, Jews, Armenians, Russians and Ukrainians experienced three or more episodes of administrative confinement.

Some results of this disaggregation may be artifacts of the small sample size in some nationality groups. Finns, for example, are not the focus of most Soviet-era efforts at socialization or political control, if only because the ethnic Finnish population of the erstwhile USSR was small.

The tendency to give Belarussians relatively short court-imposed hospitalizations but pronounced long administratively-ordered ones may be meaningful. Some differences in nationality targets for court-directed as opposed to administrative compulsory hospitalization such as the Belarussian one also suggest that the two procedures fulfil different functions. The tendency to apply short detentions of both types to Balts and Finns, yet to repeat them three or more times, suggests that in some instances both types of detention may be inflicted in a controlled way but reapplied if the desired results are not obtained. It is notable that Russians tend to be detained roughly as long as average in both procedures, yet they are not detained normally in the sense of frequency: while one or two detentions is most typical, Russians (and Ukrainians) are represented among detainees held three or more times.

DEMOGRAPHICS: GENDER

Most (92.7 per cent) psychiatric detainees are men, disproportionally many not only compared to their presence in the larger population of political activists but also obviously to the whole Soviet population, especially considering the demographic deficits in the USSR population among older male age cohorts. Men are somewhat more likely than women to be detained under court order (the average relative frequency is significantly higher), and men are more than twice as likely as women to receive a second court-mandated hospitalization. Perhaps predictably, women are significantly more likely than men to be detained administratively. After initial detentions, both men and women face similar risks of a second administrative detention. The average number of psychiatric detentions undergone is 1.49 for men and 1.44 for women.

In general in these data at the aggregate level few statistically significant differences in psychiatric penalties extracted from men and women can be isolated. Duration of first court-ordered psychiatric hospitalization, for example, which averages 5.7 years for men and seven years for women, appears to show a sizeable difference in treatment by gender, yet this difference is not large enough to be interpreted as non-accidental.

However the illusion of uniformity of treatment by gender vanishes when data are disaggregated by detention type and by numbers and duration of hospitalizations. Then a meaningful pattern consistently but not exclusively favouring females can be documented. Total duration of incarceration, which is the sum of all time served in prison, camp, exile, psychiatric detention and pre-trial detention combined, is nearly twice as long on average for men psychiatric prisoners as for women. This measure, which averages 7.5 years for men and 4.2 years for women, can be interpreted as reflecting a significant bias in favour of women nonconformists across five types of penalties for political or religious deviance ($\alpha = 0.02$).[10] The same significant inequality exists in duration of total administrative hospitalizations, averaging 2.7 years for men and 1.4 for women. Duration of first court-ordered camp or prison sentence, to which psychiatric detainees may have been subject before, during or after hospitalization, averages 6.9 years for men and 3.3 years for women, also indicating a non-accidental difference in means (significant at 0.08) documenting more lenient treatment of women dissidents, *ceteris paribus*.

While average length of all detentions combined does *not* show a meaningful, statistically non-accidental difference by gender (4.0 years for women and 5.3 years for men), disaggregation by court-ordered v. administrative commitment again does reveal a statistically significant difference in total administrative hospitalization time, averaging 1.4 years for women and over 2.7 years for men. This difference is due not to first administrative detentions, which do not favour women, but instead to the length of second administrative detentions, which bear out a disparity favouring women, the average for men being 1.16 years and for women 0.26 years ($\alpha = 0.02$).

On the other hand, when frequency of compulsory hospitalization is calculated, women tend to experience marginally more administrative detentions than do men, averaging 1.04 as opposed to 0.88. But the frequency of court-ordered detentions reverts to the typical pattern of greater severity towards men, who average about a third more detentions than women in these data.

Some failures to show significant differences between men and women detainees in consequences of psychiatric confinement are remarkable in themselves. Since in general women's life expectancies exceed those of men, it is exceptional that the difference in recorded lifespan in this case, as indicated below, is too small to be presumed not to be artifactual. It may simply be too early to find this pattern in view of the age structure of the dissident and former dissident populations.

In general in these data, men are significantly over-represented among those dissidents subject to psychiatric measures, and typically are dealt with more harshly. They also tend to be somewhat younger at initial detention, 34 as opposed to 37.5.

DEMOGRAPHICS: AGE

Soviet dissidents' average age at first psychiatric detention of either type is approximately 35 (34.6) for the incidents of detention for which year and age of dissident are known. The age data show a wide standard deviation of 11.9 years, indicating a considerable range in age among typical first-time internees. Exceptionally young detainees are found among students (24) and the military (28.5) while the older detainees have been KGB (41), ministers, priests and other religious (44.8), and a musician (49).

Average age at first court-ordered psychiatric commitment is approximately 33.4, the most frequent observation being 32. The oldest detainee at first hospitalization in these data was 66; the youngest, 13, yielding a range of 53 years between the oldest and youngest dissenter or religious observer detained by court order. Nine were under 21. The wide standard deviation (10.8 years) indicates some dispersion, skewed in the direction of younger detainees. A majority of cases fall within seven years of the mean, or between 26 and 40 years. Predictable variations in age at first criminal detention follow from occupation: students are distinctly younger (24.5 years) than average in the whole detainee group showing both variables, and KGB officials (46 years), ministers or priests (40.3 years), and white collar workers in general are older than average.

The patterns in age at first *administrative* detention resemble those for first court-ordered hospitalizations. Average age at first administrative hospitalization is 35, and the most frequently observed age on admission is 27. Half are younger than 34 and half older. The youngest hospitalized is 13, the oldest 79. Most incidences of first administrative detention were visited on those between 27 and 43, or those whose ages ranged within eight years of the mean. A wide standard deviation of 12 years again shows dispersion, also skewed towards younger detainees, but this distribution is more nearly normal.

Age alone is not strongly linearly related to numbers or durations of forcible commitments. Age at first hospitalization and total number of all detentions are only weakly, though significantly, associated in a linear measure ($r=-0.16$; $\alpha=0.000$). The small value and negative sign on the r are consistent with a minor grant of leniency to older protesters, or interpretable as a consequence of fewer dissident acts, hence lower risk of detention, after retirement. As we will argue, some significant differences in hospitalizations do emerge when politically defined generations are separated in the data.

LIFESPAN

Unprecedented even for an unevenly industrialized country, age-specific death rates began to creep up in the USSR in the sixties and have accelerated since, marking dramatic drops in life expectancy for both men and women over this period and since the collapse of the Union. Despite this aspect of the Soviet and post-Soviet continuing demographic disaster, since many participants in the dissident movements of the sixties, seventies and eighties were young adults at the time of their political activism, they are not yet at maximal risk of normal mortality. Thus most known psychiatric prisoners from the dissident movements who appear in our records may be presumed to be still living. For those known to be dead whose birth and death dates are also known,[11] including four individuals born in the 1880s or 1890s, average lifespan was approximately 45.5, with a median of 43. Sample size is too small to support a definitive conclusion on the meaning of this small lifespan. However since those individuals, like the whole sample of detainees, on average spent almost five and a half years forcibly hospitalized, even as many as 16, it may be more than speculative to assert that psychiatric detention shortened their lives, to a span not much different from that prevailing during the Roman Empire.

GEOGRAPHICAL LOCATION

Altogether for 515 of 674 individuals (76 per cent) confined to psychiatric hospitals, location or republic of residence of the dissident is known. In view of the size and population of the Russian republic, it is not accidental that 59.6 per cent of incidents of psychiatric detention of dissidents known to us took place in Russia. Some 21 per cent transpired in the Ukraine, 4.7 per cent in Lithuania, 3.1 per cent in Latvia, and 3.1 per cent in Estonia, while about two per cent each took place in Kazakhstan, Belarus and Armenia. Other incidents were scattered over Azerbaijan, Georgia, Kirghizia, Moldova, Tadzhikistan, Turkmenistan, and Uzbekistan.

Republic-level data show that percentages of psychiatric hospitalizations of protesters are roughly proportional to the percentage of the total Soviet

Table 4.2 Distribution of Detainees by Republic

Republic	*% USSR Population*	*% of Detainees*
Russia	54.00	59.60
Ukraine	19.00	20.60
Lithuania	1.30	4.70
Estonia	0.56	3.10
Latvia	0.98	3.10
Belarus	3.70	1.90
Armenia	1.00	1.70
Kazakhstan	5.40	1.60
Georgia	1.90	1.00
Moldova	1.50	1.00
Azerbaijan	2.10	0.60
Kyrghizstan	1.20	0.40
Tadzhikistan	1.60	0.20
Turkmenistan	0.89	0.20
Uzbekistan	4.90	0.20
Total	100.03	99.90

population residing in the republics named, with some exceptions. That is, in these data psychiatric repression of dissent relative to the population is not focused on any particular republic of the USSR, but instead is widely dispersed across the Union. (Consult Feshbach, 1982:10 for population tables; see also Glebov and Crowfoot (eds), 1989:178–82.)

When Feshbach's tables of Soviet population by republic are consulted for 1970 (1982:10), an approximate mid-point in the Smith–Oleszczuk data at hand and the closest available Soviet census, and when the proportion of the total Soviet population residing in the republics is computed in the 1970 figures, the proportions of total population to percentage of total psychiatric internees are as displayed in Table 4.2.

Table 4.2 indicates that residents of the Baltic republics were over-represented among those forcibly hospitalized, since they comprise larger proportions of the detainee dataset than of the comparable Soviet population. Residents of Belarus, Kazakhstan, Azerbaijan, Kyrghizstan, Tadzhikistan and Uzbekistan are somewhat under-represented. These figures may suggest some lenience towards Belarus.

However roughly, these percentages evince a degree of proportionality in psychiatric detentions across republics. On average, in absolute values, the difference between percentages of detainees and percentages of the Soviet population living in each republic is less than two per cent (1.86). One reason for some disparity in the proportions reported above, besides variations in activity level of dissidents across republics, is that some republics may have been more effectively organized to publicize detentions within the USSR and in the West.

The rough correspondence between the proportions of internees per republic and the proportions of Soviet population comprised by each republic provides evidence for the society-wide extent of the use of psychiatric measures of control.

Distribution of detentions across major Soviet cities also shows some regularities. Within Russia most detentions in absolute numbers rather than in relative terms are concentrated in the two largest cities. Despite a greater diagnostic bias in Moscow towards finding political or religious nonconformists to be mentally ill, more in absolute numbers were actually confined for a time in Leningrad/St Petersburg, the site of a comparatively liberal school of psychiatry.

The predominance of Leningrad in absolute numbers of detentions remained throughout the 1960–81 period, which also shows powerful growth of detentions in other regions. However, during the 1980s the predominance shifts to Moscow, so that by the end of the Soviet period the largest known group of forced hospitalizations of nonconformists and religious practitioners has taken place in Moscow (22.8 valid or non-missing per cent), followed by Leningrad/St Petersburg (11.4 per cent) and Kiev (4.8 per cent). Though documented instances are spread over 114 cities, about 40 per cent of the well-confirmed psychiatric detentions took place in the three major metropolitan areas just mentioned, distantly followed by Vilnius (2.6 per cent), Yerevan (2.2 per cent), Sverdlovsk and Novosibirsk (1.8 per cent each), Riga and Sochi (1.5 per cent each), and Dnepropetrovsk, Kuibyshev, Minsk, Odessa, Tallinn and Vladimir (all 1.1 per cent).

On the basis of data on degree of urbanization of detainees' residence, psychiatric confinement of nonconformists can be described on the whole as a powerfully urban as opposed to rural phenomenon. Eighty-two per cent of detainees whose residence is known (63 per cent of the total) were from major or central cities such as Vladivostok in Primorski krai, Petropavlovsk in Kamchatka, Rostov na Donu in Rostov, Kazan in the Tatar ASSR, and so on. Seventeen per cent were from lesser cities, and only two per cent from villages.

SUMMARY

In contrast to the dominant ideology of the Soviet state, the lack of privilege or immunity from psychiatric imprisonment for blue collar workers stands out. Whether measured in lengths or frequencies of administrative or criminal commitments, no particular protection is obtained for non-conforming workers in the workers' state. Some shielding of peasants and farmers from egregious excesses of psychiatric commitment can be shown, but sample size is limited and in any case this tendency is not substantial enough to suggest either a real normative bias in their favour or a pragmatic concern with solving the agriculture problem.

The presence of juveniles as well as sexagenarians and septuagenarians among psychiatric prisoners is remarkable, as is the evident lack of lenience towards these age cohorts in most measures. A pattern of lenience towards women dissenters can be demonstrated, possibly a result of some lines of mitigation in Soviet law or beliefs about women's responsiveness to mental health treatment, but it is not a function of relative youth since women on average are older than men at first forcible hospitalizations.

Punitive psychiatry was not mainly an instrument of Russification or of oppression of minority nationalities. The consistency of its use across republics and nationalities, including substantially but still proportionally against Russians, is one of the most pervasive observations in these data. Politicized hospitalization was a systematic society-wide phenomenon which generated proportions of internees in each republic roughly corresponding to the proportion of the All-Union population within the republic.

Within this general pattern of consistency across republics and nationalities in psychiatric detentions, some anomalies can be found. Though psychiatric prisoners have encompassed 13 of the 15 major Soviet nationalities, some less populous nationalities, and several border ethnicities as well, few detainees figured among the Islamic nationalities. Disproportionately many Balts and Jews were forcibly committed over the 1928–91 interval covered by this study. Some traces of lenience towards Balts in *length* as opposed to frequency of administrative detentions might be interpreted as a reflection of the importance of this region to the economy of the USSR. But Balts, Georgians, Tatars and Jews are disproportionally severely sanctioned via long court-ordered detentions, as are Ukrainians perhaps to a lesser extent.

The observations on nationality illustrate the scope and risk of nationalist divisiveness over several decades in the USSR as the empire staggered and fragmented. They also hint that a believable or more timely programme of democratization might have had potential for pacification of the nationalist dissident movement, though democratization is not democracy and perhaps was not intended to approach it too closely. By the time incremental changes such as overt legislative representation of nationalities were instituted, they could no longer be effective.

While patterns in all politically suspect hospitalization are of interest, disaggregation by detention type is instructive since the terms of court-edict hospitalizations are based in criminal law and may be relatively stable over time, while administrative rulings for emergency confinement have not been directly regulated by law until recently (see Bonnie) and may be more versatile and discretionary. Some variations in methods of detention of nationalities, such as the flexibility towards the Balts, and the tendency to assign long administrative and short court detentions to Belarus nationals, suggest adaptability, selective leniency and a rational search for time-sensitive responses to dissidence. These variations combined with the selectivity in detentions with respect to occupational groups, in which heavy sanctions fall on those entrusted with upholding state norms, and some lighter sanctions on those capable of arousing mass opposition, suggest that the two forms of psychiatric incarceration, administrative and criminal court-ordered, were intelligently directed to serve different functions.

At the same time the consistency found here in both administrative and court-ordered detentions of targeted religious groups implies a uniform strategy towards religious behaviour in the USSR, especially towards those religious communities capable of mounting a political challenge or posing questions of legitimacy, the Russian Orthodox, Uniate and Roman Catholic in this interval. The religious diversity among psychiatric prisoners, as well as the variety in occupation and nationality, testifies to the breadth of the dissident movement and the inclusive nature of the use of medicine to cope with activities perceived as pernicious.

5 Trends, Changes with Administration and Spatial Dispersion

> So evidently the upper, visible part of the iceberg has melted considerably. But, as we all know, an iceberg also has a hidden part . . .
>
> (N. Safronova, *Izvestia*, 29 March 1990)

TRENDS: PATTERNS IN FREQUENCY OF PSYCHIATRIC REPRESSION

Psychiatric repression of Soviet political and religious agitators peaked in 1971[1] and 1972, measured in terms of new forced hospitalizations in this examination of the 1928–91[2] period (see Figure 5.1). After a drop to low levels in 1974 and 1976, court-ordered compulsory hospitalizations again built slowly to another relative maximum in 1982, when a December amnesty carefully excluded political detainees. Unlike court-mandated commitments, new *administrative* detentions did not subside in the mid-seventies. They show at least a local peak in 1974, for President Ford's trip to Vladivostok, with local hospitals at capacity. As an evident effort to avoid World Psychiatric Association censure, which nevertheless took place in August of 1977, administrative hospitalizations were reduced in that year, but rebounded exponentially over the next three years. (See Figures 5.1–5.3.)

The curve of all new hospitalizations fluctuates over time, showing distinct increases in 1962, 1964 and 1966 with a general pattern of growth. In 1967 a precipitate drop is recorded. A steep increase follows from 1967 though 1971. Then from the 1971–72 highs through 1978 new hospitalizations plummet. A short interval of exponential increase from 1978 to 1980 is followed by a drop in 1981 to a low not seen since 1964. The early and mid-eighties are characterized by an upsurge from 1981 through 1986 and a decline from 1986, the year of the Gorbachev–Reagan Summit, through 1991, the year of the WPA visit. The pattern of decline is consistent with timing of known releases, following the 1987 Decree of the Presidium of the Supreme Soviet, and anticipating the visit of the US Department of

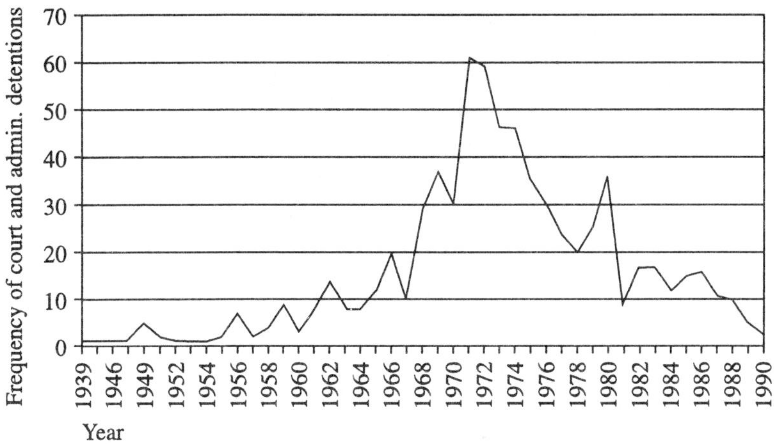

Includes only cases for which date is known.

Figure 5.1 All New Hospitalizations

State delegation in March 1989 by discharging detainees beginning in December 1988.

An increase in political hospitalizations also takes place in 1980 in Bloch and Reddaway's data, vanishing in 1981. This increase is probably correctly attributed to a temporary street-clearing regime move anticipating the 1980 Moscow Olympics (Bloch and Reddaway, 1984:73), especially since the administrative detentions in this interval were brief.

When these observations are broken down by type of new forcible commitments, differences in timing emerge. A small peak in court commitments in 1963 is followed by relative minima in 1964–65, remarkable since the minima coincide with surges in dissident acts and with the widely publicized Sinyavsky–Daniel trial and conviction for anti-Soviet thought and actions. (See Figure 5.2. Administrative detentions, shown in Figure 5.3, begin to pick up in 1964.) A massive leap in court-ordered hospitalizations begins in 1967 and increases monotonically until 1972, followed by an abrupt drop during 1973–74. These features correspond roughly to the frequencies of year of first arrests. However after 1974 first arrests fluctuate around a general pattern of decrease, to vanish in 1991, with two relative maxima in 1967 and in 1971. In the court-mandated hospitalizations a new pattern of fluctuation around a general *increase* begins after 1974, which persists until 1986–87, notwithstanding the signing of the Helsinki Accords in 1975. Bilateral discussions in 1988 between the US and the USSR, and the January 1988 new Soviet regulations on provision of mental health

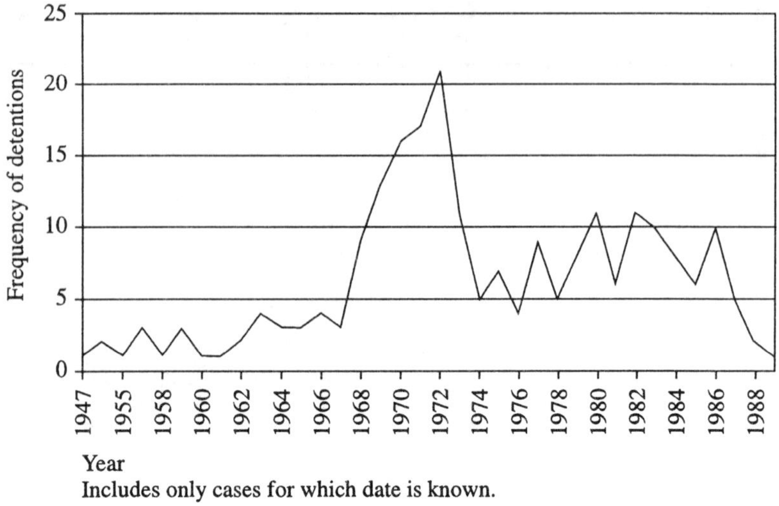

Figure 5.2 New Court-Ordered Forcible Hospitalizations

care, led to numerous other releases from prisons and psychiatric hospitals. These developments not only ushered in a decrease in new court-ordered commitments but also a predictable new reliance on administrative admissions, which increased in 1988. The later pattern of general increase in criminal commitments derives from an upsurge in second arrests, which can be shown in these data from 1974 until at least 1981, with 1984 and 1985 relative maxima in the second arrests data. Third arrests show relative maxima in 1970, 1974, 1977, with the values of these three maxima decreasing over time so as to suggest increasing fatigue among experienced human rights protesters in this period. Both first and third arrests show a relative maximum at 1980, coinciding with a peak in the data on all new hospitalizations.

Increases in *criminal* commitments up to 1972 may be due to coincidences of both internal and external factors. The Nixon visit in 1972 probably increased the risk of short-term criminal as well as administrative detentions. The elevation of KGB head Yu. V. Andropov to the Politburo may also have signalled a tendency to resort to criminal commitments as a means of dissuading others from joining the dissident movement.

The first notable upsurge in administrative detentions takes place in 1962. The sudden drop in 1963 is followed by an exponential increase to 1966 and another precipitate drop in 1967, probably in preparation for the visit of the American delegation and clearing the diplomatic stage for

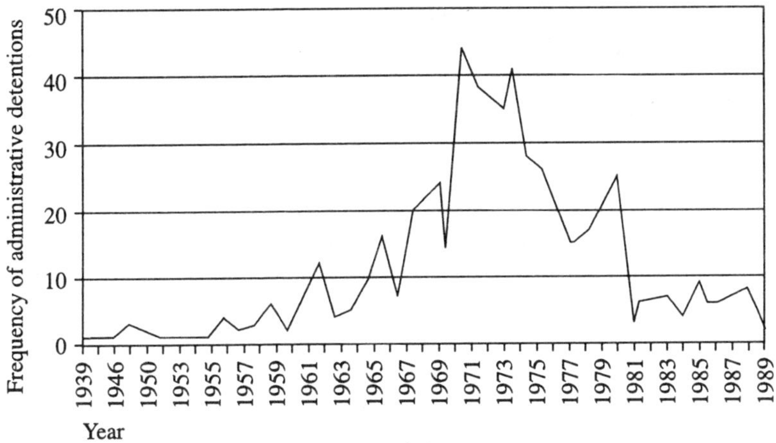

Includes only cases for which year is known.

Figure 5.3 New Administrative Hospitalizations

the historic meetings at Glassboro State College. A relative maximum in numbers of new administrative hospitalizations appears in 1969, followed by the absolute maximum in 1971.

One reason for the increase in 1971, indicated in our administrative hospitalizations data and also reflected in total numbers of new commitments, is the use of the *Instructions on Urgent Hospitalization of the Socially Dangerous Mentally Ill* released in 1961 and again in 1971 (Podrabinek, 1980:70–1). These instructions expedited detention without trial or even the involvement of higher-level authorities, and suggest central governmental interest in use of short-term administrative detentions as a means of social control.

Another peak in administrative detentions appears in 1974, after which the numbers slide to a relative minimum in 1977, following the Brezhnev visit to the US in 1976, which at least in terms of human rights policy appears to have been counterproductive. The 1977 through 1980 period shows exponential increase, reflecting among other forces the crackdown which began in 1977 and 1978 in which Natan Shcharansky, Yuri Orlov and other well-publicized human rights activists were detained. A drastic drop in 1981 to nearly the absolute minimum in the data is followed by a small increase from 1981 through 1988.

The patterns in all new hospitalizations naturally share some common features with new court-ordered detentions and new administrative detentions, as the figures indicate. Administrative detentions show a peak in 1962 sufficient to generate a relative maximum in the all new hospitalizations as well. The exponential growth from 1964–66 is also shared. In 1967, administrative commitments fell so far that even though court-ordered procedures leapt ahead, all new hospitalizations combined still show a distinct drop.

All three hospitalization curves share steep growth up to 1969, tracking the acceleration in numbers of recorded dissident acts. Similarly 1971 is an absolute maximum for administrative commitments and for all new hospitalizations, as well as an increase if not a maximum for court-ordered detentions.

In 1973 court-mandated commitments decrease so swiftly, and administrative detentions drop enough, to result in all new hospitalizations plummeting. Similarly 1976–77 either constitutes a period of decrease or includes a relative minimum for all three curves. By 1978 an exponential increase in administrative holdings and all new hospitalizations accompanies a general increase in court commitments as well.

While 1981 shows a drop to near absolute minima for administrative procedures and for all new hospitalizations, court procedures have already begun to increase. By 1983 so have administrative figures and the totals for all new commitments, which do not drop definitively in these data until after 1986. 1981 also appears to mark a departure point beyond which repression spread more rapidly outside major cities and tourist areas to outlying towns, allowing a measure of control to be exerted while still contributing to the rehabilitation of the international image of Soviet psychiatry (IAPUP, 1983:52). The visit of the US Delegation to selected Soviet mental hospitals in 1989 may have provided an additional incentive to reduce numbers of new commitments, as did the World Psychiatric Association visit in 1991.

Although psychiatric hospitalizations of nonconformists respond to both internal and external events, the responses are not necessarily intuitively obvious. An uncompromising Soviet foreign policy would not necessarily be matched by repressive practices at home, since control and prosecution of Soviet dissidents have been in different hands from the conduct of foreign policy on some issues, though not with respect to the campaign for readmission to the World Psychiatric Association. Thus the détente period at its height, 1970–72, would not necessarily correspond with a conciliatory Soviet domestic policy. Given the influx of foreigners into the country, with consequent perceived increases in security risks, it is not accidental that in fact peaks in arrests and psychiatric hospitalizations of protesters coincide with the apex of détente, 1970–72, as well as with superpower achievements in arms control and other substantive issues at other times. In 1969, a relative maximum in the administrative detentions data, the US and the USSR began the Strategic Arms Limitation Talks (SALT), and the US ratified the Non-Proliferation Treaty. 1972 marked the second *highest* point for all Soviet forcible hospitalizations, but also signalled an epochal year for arms control. The superpowers in 1972 signed and brought into force SALT I's Interim Agreement on Strategic Forces; signed, ratified and brought into force the Anti-Ballistic Missile Treaty, widely interpreted as the most meaningful arms control measure in the postwar era and an official acknowledgment of mutual risk in deterrence relations; and signed the Biological Weapons Convention. In 1975, coinciding with a high level of administrative detentions and a relative maximum in court-ordered commitments, the Helsinki Accords with its human rights protections were signed.

As Figure 5.1 of all new hospitalizations corroborates, international events could exert an influence on the levels of domestic psychiatric repression in the USSR. International visits, such as those of the US Delegations to Soviet mental hospitals in 1967 and 1989 and the World Psychiatric Association visit in 1991 (by which time detentions had dropped off the chart to effectively zero, representing only some administrative detentions of a few days), were met by the lowest levels of punitive political hospitalizations obtaining since 1960 or even earlier. Some decreases in frequency of forced commitments also precede or coincide with international conferences, in particular the WPA meetings of 1977 (but not 1971), at which appearances mattered. This illustrates the sensitivity of some internal Soviet events to external influence.

We have shown elsewhere (Oleszczuk and Smith, 1986) a negative relationship between Soviet exports to the US and arrests for dissent under détente, when increased trade and technology diffusion were valued Soviet foreign policy objectives, and hard-line policies towards domestic political activists were seen as counterproductive to the larger societal needs of foreign economic policy. At least in the short term Soviet *imports* of US goods might have been associated positively with domestic political repression, since increased trade brought more business contacts, students, and intellectual exchanges from the West into the USSR, with perceived intrusion of dangerous ideas. Those trade findings as well as the patterns seen here in the psychiatric repression data imply that the Soviet Union made internal concessions for specified foreign policy goals, initially in the disappointed search for most favoured nation status and trade in high technology items, as well as later in the ascribed-status-laden quest to be readmitted to the world community of mental health professionals.

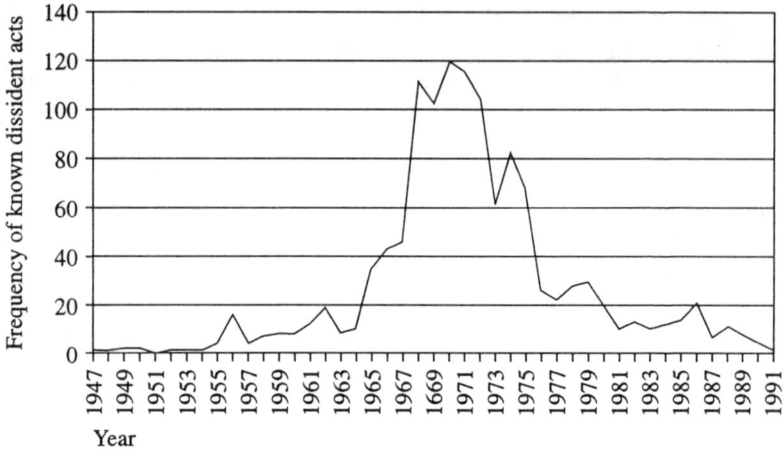

Includes only cases for which dates are known.

Figure 5.4 Total Numbers of Dissident Acts

TRENDS: THE RELATIONSHIP BETWEEN DISSIDENT BEHAVIOUR AND PSYCHIATRIC REPRESSION

The frequency of known dissident acts illustrated in Figure 5.4 describes a pattern quite similar to that of the hospitalizations data, but precedes hospitalizations slightly. This similarity in the curves means that new forcible hospitalizations of political and religious dissidents are strongly and significantly associated statistically with total numbers of known dissident acts in our data.[3]

Our records of known dissident acts soar after 1964 (see Figure 5.4), coherent with Medvedev's view of the origins of the contemporary Soviet dissident movement in the October 1964 ouster of N.S. Khrushchev and the Central Committee Plenum's consideration of rehabilitating Stalin. A pattern of increase in administrative hospitalizations had already begun by then, and a generally increasing trend in court-mandated commitments appeared a few years later, at the latest between 1967 and 1968. The court detentions are later characterized by a trend of roughly bell-shaped increase and decrease over 1977–87 which does *not* correspond directly to the numbers of known dissident acts. Increases in frequency of court-ordered hospitalizations signals some increased repression in the mid-eighties just as administrative detentions had been becoming relatively less frequent as well as shorter.[4] The court-ordered detentions in the late

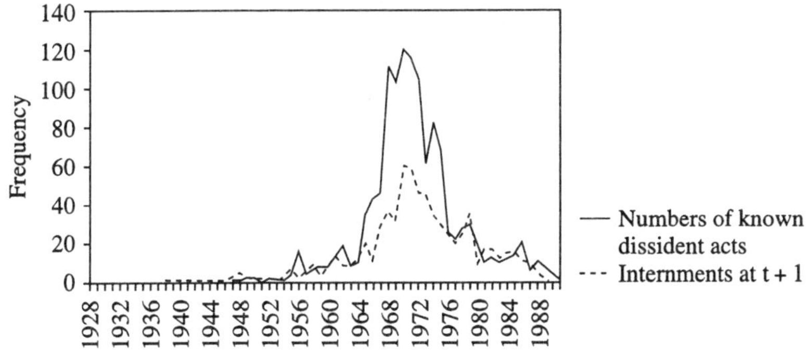

Includes only those dissident acts for which date is known.
Includes only those new hospitalizations for which date is known.

Figure 5.5 Dissident Acts and Subsequent Hospitalizations

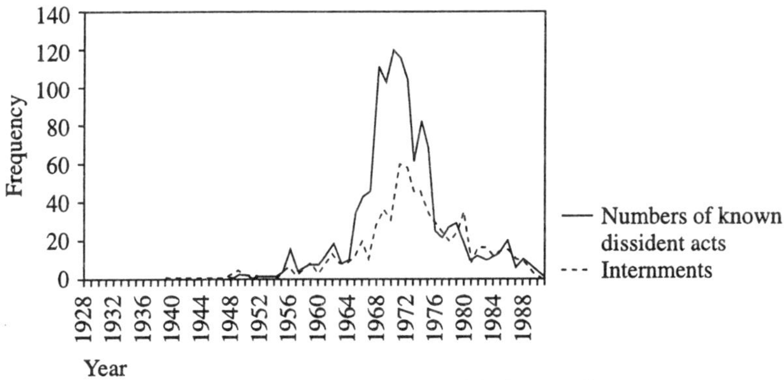

Includes only those dissident acts for which dates are known.
Includes only those new hospitalizations for which dates are known.

Figure 5.6 Dissident Acts and Current Hospitalizations

seventies and early eighties may be due in part to attempts to quell the anti-Afghanistan war movement.

Figures 5.5 and 5.6 plotting both phenomena highlight how closely trends in hospitalization frequency resemble the general patterns in numbers of dissident acts. This resemblance in shape of the two curves is powerful enough to be captured preliminarily in linear measures of association despite the curve in the data, Pearson's r between frequency of all hospitalizations and numbers of dissident acts recorded in any year amounting to

0.835 ($\alpha=0.000$). When a time lead is introduced into the analysis to represent the response time of the authorities to changing levels of dissent, the correlation between frequency of dissident acts in one year with number of hospitalizations in the subsequent year rises to 0.89 ($\alpha=0.000$), supporting via statistical association the theoretical contention that *forcible hospitalization was a direct response to levels of dissident activity*. Figure 5.5, in which frequency of dissident acts and numbers of subsequent hospitalizations track each other closely, reflects this high correlation.

A linear regression analysis predicting total number of political hospitalizations one year after dissident acts yields a highly significant multiple R of 0.89 and an R squared of 0.79 at $\alpha=0.000$.[5] About 80 per cent of the variation in numbers of political and religious detentions can thus be explained simply by examining changes in one variable, number of known dissident acts in the prior year, which provides evidence that hospitalizations respond directly and proportionally, with a short time lag, to levels of political and religious agitation. On average, hospitalizations were sensitive to numbers of known dissident acts such that one additional recorded dissident act yielded about 0.4 new hospitalizations, or just under three documented dissident acts could be expected to result in a future hospitalization, as indicated by the b coefficient on numbers of dissident acts.

TRENDS: AGE OF DETAINEES

Average age of psychiatric prisoners at first detention changes across Soviet administrations. For cases in which date of birth and year of first detention are known, separating individuals by administration yields an average age at first hospitalization of 41.9 under Stalin, 35.4 under Khrushchev, 33.7 under Brezhnev, 39.4 under Andropov, 35 under Chernenko, and 29.4 under Gorbachev. We suspect sample size under Andropov and Chernenko is small enough to question the precision of the estimates for these two administrations. Thus, the other numbers probably represent a general decline in average age at first hospitalization across Soviet administrations.

Some exceptions to this trend may be found if a more specific analysis is conducted. In the Smith–Oleszczuk data before the Koppers and Mercer data were added, we found (1989) that as the dissident movement was consolidated in the sixties, a natural secular trend for average age at first detention to increase could be seen in annual data. The increase initially exceeded that which passage of time alone could account for, and then levelled off. The increase in average age of internee Soviet dissidents between 1960 and 1970 exceeded ten years; the increase between 1970 and 1980 did not, and instead began to flatten out. So in the sixties the rate of increase in average age was not just a function of the ageing of the nonconformist population likely to be drawn into dissident acts and subsequent arrest, but also was probably a reflection of recruiting somewhat older individuals. The increase between 1970 and 1980 was somewhat less than ten years, consistent with the loss of many individuals from the dissident movement and with recruitment of some younger dissidents as is seen in statistics cited later in this chapter.

TRENDS: PATTERNS IN LENGTH OF FORCIBLE HOSPITALIZATIONS

The average length of psychiatric detention tends to decline over 1950–91. This pattern is particularly strong and persistent since it is sufficient in average terms to overcome the influence of a few Stalinesque terms of two decades or more which end in this interval. (Earlier records from the mid- and late fifties include a number of hospitalizations of 15 and 25 years or more.) Mercer and Koppers show some releases in the late 1980s of individuals who had served 20-year terms dating from the sixties, including an individual who fired a gun at Brezhnev,[6] and others.

The pattern of overall decline in length of detention is persistent and evidently responsive to external as well as internal events, but becomes more complex when administrative and court-ordered durations are plotted separately (see Figures 5.7 and 5.8). Drops in average length – but not frequency – of administrative hospitalizations coincide with or anticipate the December 1971 World Psychiatric Association meeting, formal détente announcements, and the public opinion consequences of freeing Leonid Plyushch in 1976. The 1977 meeting of the World Psychiatric Association, at which Soviet practices were condemned, coincided with relative lows in length (and frequency, as mentioned earlier) of court-mandated detentions in this period. Other low figures occur in the average length of administrative holdings during 1980 prior to the Moscow Olympics, again in 1985 around the time of the International Youth Festival in Moscow, and in 1988. 1986 is a relative minimum for duration of court-directed detentions.

Some increases can be seen at other understandable points. In 1972 the average administrative sentence and court term lengthened slightly, presumably in anticipation of the Nixon visit to Moscow, and coinciding with a decision (Bloch and Reddaway, 1977b:287) not to release more *well-known* dissidents to avoid appearing to make too many concessions. Bloch and Reddaway report that every well-known dissident then detained had

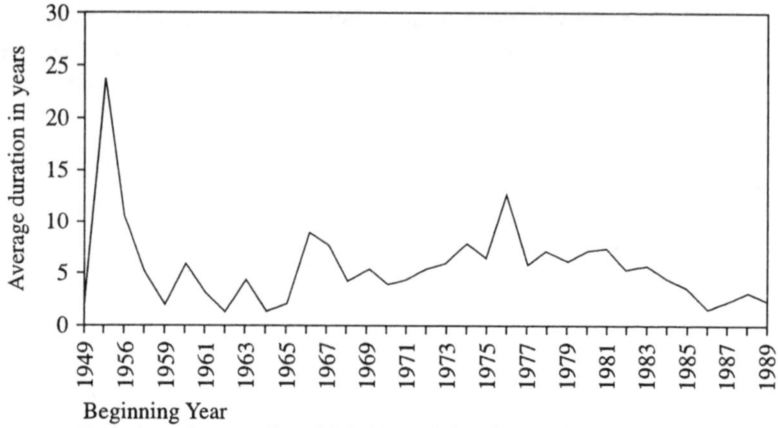

Includes only cases for which date and duration are known.

Figure 5.7 Average Length of Court-Ordered Hospitalizations by Beginning Year

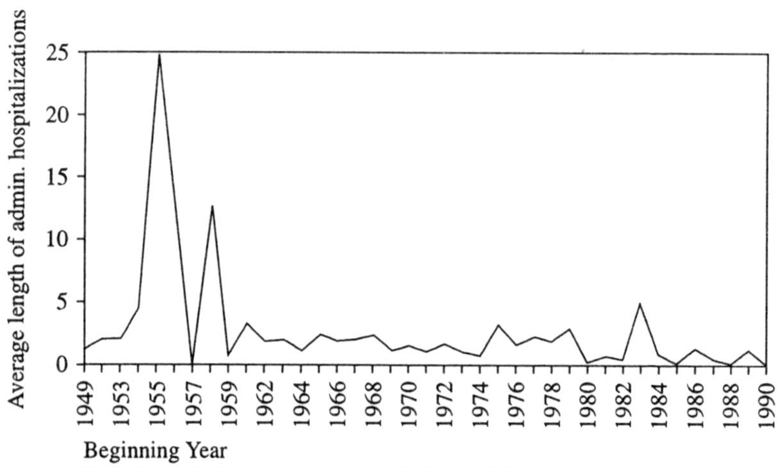

Includes only those cases for which date and duration are known.

Figure 5.8 Average Length of Administrative Hospitalizations by Beginning Year

been released by 1974 (1977b:288), a relative minimum in new court commitments and the second highest point in the new administrative detentions in our data.

Among those first detained or still held in psychiatric confinement into the eighties were Vladimir Gershuni, the editor of a samizdat journal who was picked up in 1982 and released in 1987; Natalia Atulienok, a pacifist

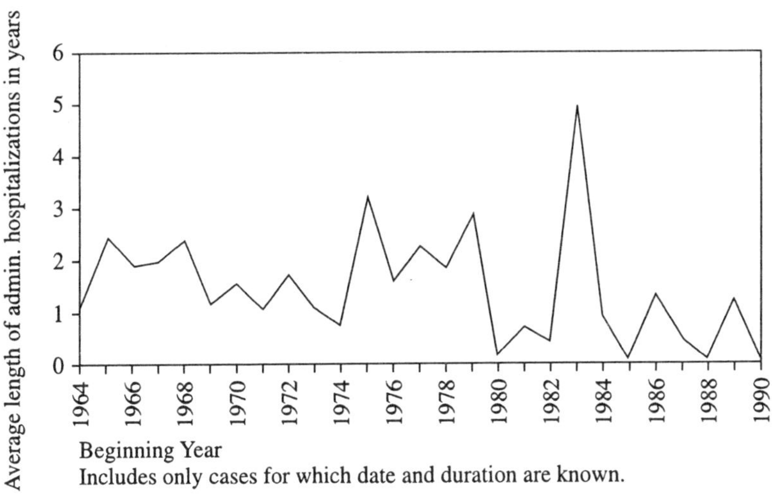

Figure 5.8a Average Length of Administrative Hospitalizations since Khrushchev

discharged in 1985; Dmitri Prigov, artist and poet detained in 1986 for attending an 'anti-Soviet' meeting; Serafim Evsukhov, hospitalized in 1987 after demonstrating for emigration rights; Yuri Sobolev of Slavkino, detained in 1990 on the instructions of the Nikolayevsky Party raikom because of his 'nasty plans' for the election (Razboynikov in *Izvestia*, 1990); and Oleg Kozlov, sent to Serbsky by the Latvian KGB after hijacking a Riga–Murmansk flight to Finland in 1990.

Podrabinek found a greater reliance on administrative detentions under Gorbachev, which we also show in some terms in this chapter. Podrabinek reported (Van Voren, 1989) a list of 60 political prisoners in hospitals in the late eighties, as well as 90 whose location was unknown, many of whom were presumed released.

Separating administrative from court-ordered hospitalizations reveals that while administrative detentions preserve a rough pattern of decrease in average length of internment seen in the entire dataset, with an anomaly in 1983, *no moderating trend exists in* court-ordered *detentions until as late as 1981*. (See Figures 5.8, 5.8a and 5.9; cf. Reddaway, 1987.) As expected, since the average duration of court-ordered commitments does not tend to decline uniformly over time, separating court-ordered detentions by Soviet administration reveals no statistically significant differences across varieties of leadership in the severity of this particular sanction until almost the end of the Union. On average, no significant differences emerge until Gorbachev, for whose administration average length of first

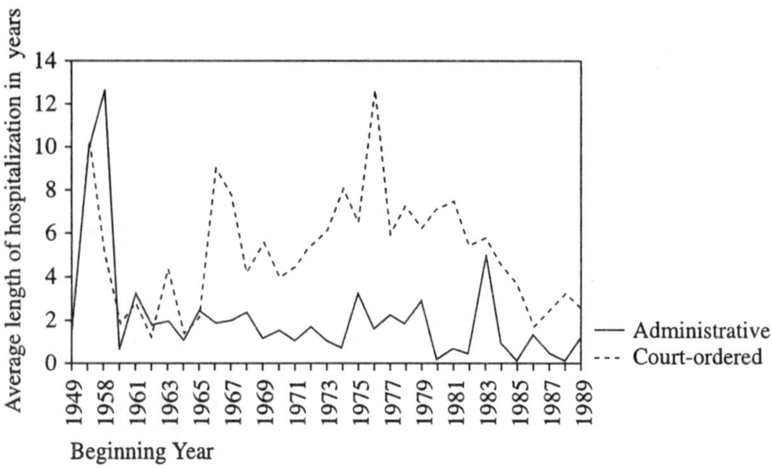

Figure 5.9 Average Length of Court-Ordered and Administrative Hospitalizations by Beginning Year

(and usually only) court-ordered commitment per dissident was 2.6 years as compared to 6.7 years under Chernenko ($\alpha = 0.000$).

Viewed over time, Soviet judicial detentions of dissidents reached maximal lengths in the late 1950s, as did their administrative counterparts. Administrative hospitalizations moderated in the 1960s to an average detention of about two years while court-ordered commitments climbed. After 1970 the length of average court-ordered psychiatric detention of nonconformists again grew, remaining distinctly longer than administrative hospitalizations. After 1971 the length of administrative detentions began to show some averages of one year or less, whereas court-ordered detentions fluctuated around six- and seven-year terms and rose as high as 13 years' average duration.

This divergence implies that at least since 1968 court-mandated commitments of political and religious dissidents served a different function than non-judicial hospitalizations and might have been reserved for dissidents who presented more serious risks to regime values or who failed to be deterred from further activity by a previous prison camp term or administrative detention. (See the deterrence discussion in Chapter 6.) However Figure 5.9 does show a seven-year interval in the Brezhnev administration over which the patterns in frequency of both types of detentions track each other so closely as to imply that they were responding to the *same* stimulus (one year apart) and probably served the *same* function in that interval – 1974–81 in administrative detentions and 1973–80 in criminal court-ordered hospitalizations.

In the whole dataset the contrasting and consequential difference between the durations of administrative and court-mandated hospitalizations is preserved. Court hospitalizations are generally much longer than administrative ones. Counting instances for which both length and commitment type are recorded, court-ordered hospitalizations extend for more than six and a half years on average (6.53), with half the cases falling above 4.7 years and half below. Administrative detention time for individuals, like court-ordered detentions, ranges from a few days to over 25 years, but unlike court-mandated cases averages approximately two and a half years (2.56), or only about 40 per cent of the duration of court hospitalizations. A few longer administrative commitments extend the average more than is truly typical, since many cases fall in the one- and two-week range. The median administrative hospitalization only slightly exceeds five months, and the most frequent observation is about 29 days. Thus administrative commitments were usually significantly shorter and tended to decline over time, again implying that in general the two types of commitments served different functions.

Other reasons besides anticipated duration of detention may predispose authorities to seek one kind of commitment over another. Speed militates for administrative hospitalizations on an emergency basis. Another reason to choose administrative methods, as indicated by Podrabinek (1980:117, 135), is that administrative detentions could be concentrated on dissidents against whom a legal case would be weak, embarrassing, or non-existent.

RELEASES

Our data on releases and escapes are incomplete. Considering only the Mercer and Koppers information on cases from 1980 onwards, the central observation, on which Mercer and Koppers agree, is that conspicuous numbers (34) of political and religious psychiatric prisoners still held in the late eighties were discharged in 1987 after the Decrees of 2 and 9 February of the Presidium of Supreme Soviet. At least 20 releases in 1988 are shown, and 16 in 1989, while in the Koppers and Mercer records no more than eight had been set free in any prior year in the eighties.

POLITICALLY ENGAGED GENERATIONS?

Our evidence is indicative of uniform and evidently centrally directed processes of political practice of psychiatry, rather than of life-event generational conflict patterns. However, in Bahry's analyses of Soviet political activism (in Millar, 1987), generational explanations do affect Soviet dissent when generations are defined according to shared experiences of life-shaping *political* events such as the purges, rather than demographic events such as teen rebellion, marriage and the birth of children, or ageing. Bahry found that Soviet age cohorts born between 1925 to 1940, and between 1941 to 1960, were the most active politically, both in societally approved groups such as Komsomol and as dissidents in societally sanctioned political protest groups. If her observations hold in these data, we should find that numbers of known dissident acts differ significantly between this group of active participants in Soviet life and those born into earlier or later generations as defined by watershed political events. If the state responds rationally and predictably to dissent, and proportionally to levels of nonconformist activity, we should also expect these age groups to have borne proportionally heavier penalties for their nonconformity, other things being equal. Bahry's elaboration of generational arguments is thus compatible with a rational actor explanation of state use of psychiatric repression.

In fact we do confirm that those born into Bahry's activist age groups were more active as dissidents than the whole group of psychiatric detainees, exhibiting an average of 2.7 as opposed to two known dissident acts per person in our data. This difference is due to the contrast between the 1925–61 cohort's activity level and the much reduced level of dissident acts attributed to those born after 1961, 2.7 as compared with 1.2 reported events ($\alpha = 0.003$), since in our data no statistically significant difference in average number of dissident acts per person can be found when comparing the activist groups born 1925–61 with those born *before* 1925 (2.7 compared with 2.3 reported dissident acts).

These groups born 1925–60 also paid a higher price than their younger confrères for their nonconformist activities. In our data those born after 1925 and before 1961 were hospitalized on average nearly five years, while those born later than 1961 were confined for barely more than one year on average ($\alpha = 0.000$), approximately a 500 per cent difference in the penalty although the frequency of their documented dissident acts amounts to only 135 per cent of the later group's (2.7/2). In measures of frequency of repression, such as number of court-ordered detentions, although the heavier penalties are preserved to some degree, only marginally significant differences between these age cohorts and those born later can be observed. Mean numbers of administrative detentions are almost identical. The differences between groups exist instead in the *durations* data.

Because earlier detentions tended to be extremely long, no statistically meaningful difference exists between the 1925–61 groups and those born *before* 1925 in total time hospitalized on average. Mean time forcibly hospitalized for those born pre-1925 equals nearly eight years (7.67). No significant differences between these groups in frequencies of total detentions are found in our data.

Dissenters and religious observers born into the most active age cohorts identified by Bahry are significantly older at first arrest in our data (30.8 years as opposed to 20.6) than are those born after 1961, as well as significantly older at both first court-ordered commitment (31.9 versus 20 years) and first administrative detention (32.7 versus 21.2 years). Comparing the Bahry activists with those born earlier, however, the pre-1925 protesters are distinctly older, averaging 50 at first arrest ($\alpha=0.012$). The pre-1925 dissenters are generally so much older than their later counterparts that this divergence in age is sufficient to generate significant differences between the two cohorts in age at first administrative confinement (51.3 years; $\alpha=0.002$) as well as first court-ordered detention (50.2 years; $\alpha=0.017$).

These findings support an explanation of dissent, political participation, and calculated state penalties based on generations as defined by major political watershed events rather than by lifecycle events. It is noteworthy that the divisions set out by Bahry repeatedly generate highly significant differences in dissident activity levels and in subsequent penalties in a variety of measures,[7] and therefore make a meaningful contribution to a complete explanation of dissidence and state response.[8]

DIFFERENCES ACROSS ADMINISTRATIONS: TREATMENT OF DISSIDENTS

While the modern Soviet dissident movement is usually understood to have begun in the sixties, as a large-scale societal response to the ousting of Khrushchev and the signs of re-Stalinization, principled political opposition and unauthorized religious practice did occur as early as Stalin, and arrests and psychiatric hospitalizations for political and religious reasons can be documented into the late twenties. In that sense it is possible to define contrasts and elements of continuity in policy towards dissent across the entire Soviet period. As for dissident policy during the Stalin administration, the continuing discovery of mass graves into the 1990s speaks for itself. Khrushchev, who allowed enhanced freedom of expression, was seen as decidedly more progressive with respect to human rights. In the Brezhnev era, dissident activity reached its highest documented levels. The Brezhnev administration, under pressure from the outside world, authorized a massive exodus of nearly half a million people, never previously permitted. But it also carried out maximal numbers of arrests and detentions in the early seventies, and enforced a crackdown in the late seventies and early eighties which imposed new restrictions on communication and travel. Chernenko, Colton notes (1986:215) 'showed the odd flash of compassion' but more typically was repressive. Andropov, seen by some Western observers as liberal, was in some terms an anti-dissident activist. His administration made ample use of administrative detentions, facilitated re-sentencing of political detainees, and criminalized new political acts or enlarged the range of old behaviour to be defined as criminal. Gorbachev, perhaps correctly preoccupied by the economic catastrophe, also relied on administrative detentions but appeared committed to real progress on human rights issues such as family reunification and emigration.

Brezhnev and Andropov averaged far more arrests of dissenters per year than other administrations, when only psychiatric detainees are considered and when the Stalin years are excluded for reasons of missing data.[9] This is proportional in the first case to a drastic increase in recorded dissident acts, and probably in the second case to a harder-line policy on dissent.

Khrushchev's administration averaged 10.2 well-confirmed dissident acts annually with a mode and median of eight, maximum of 19 and minimum of four. As expected, given the numerous arrests in the Brezhnev administration, recorded dissident acts rose to maximal levels in that period, averaging 57.7 each year with a median of 44.5, an annual maximum of 120, and a minimum of ten, certainly not a period of stagnation in these terms. Recorded dissident activity was so high under Brezhnev that its *lowest* points characterized a normal year in the Khrushchev period, and were more or less representative of an average year in the regimes which followed. Andropov's administration, like Khrushchev's, was characterized by ten known dissident acts per year on average, and Chernenko's by 12. Gorbachev's typically averaged 9.3 known dissident acts per year, with a mode of 11, median eight, maximum 21, and minimum one.

A comparison of the activity levels and penalties exacted from dissenters first coming to the attention of the authorities in different administrations can help illustrate the risks of beginning political activism at different times. While this method of comparing administrations may seem to confound the effects of several factors which changed with governments, because especially persistent dissidents remained active and could be repeatedly penalized across two or more administrations, most nonconformists in our data were not long-term activists. In fact in these data the most typical experience (72 per cent) is one arrest and a prompt administrative detention, or one arrest and a trial-based detention. And the most *representative* experience where evidence exists is one dissident act per person, which catalyzes arrest. Although the circumstances of arrest and forcible commitment make clear that all individuals in our data were engaged in a number of dissident acts, many of which by virtue of exigencies of the circumstances were not recorded, well-documented records of dissident acts exist for about 60 per cent (403) of the 674 nonconformists in our dataset. Thus the sum of known dissident acts per person reaches an average of only two in our data, and the single most probable number of dissident acts for those whose activities are well-confirmed and dated is only one per person on average,[10] although persistent dissenters may be on record for 16 or more dissident acts.

Comparing administrations sequentially, those whose first known arrest occurred under Stalin were subject over the course of their nonconformist activities to significantly more arrests than those first arrested under Khrushchev (3.1 compared with 2.2 arrests; $\alpha=0.02$), as well as significantly more administrative detentions (1.5 v. 0.9 administrative confinements, $\alpha=0.01$). On average they spent more than twice the amount of total time incarcerated or hospitalized than did those first detained under Khrushchev (21.6 as opposed to 9.6 years, $\alpha=0.001$).

Those first arrested under Khrushchev were committed by court order almost twice as often as those first arrested under Brezhnev ($\alpha=0.03$) and were also at a higher risk of incarceration in all forms ($\alpha=0.000$). On average they were likely to be arrested twice rather than once ($\alpha=0.000$), consistent with a higher level of political and religious activism shown in the differences between their average numbers of dissident acts (3.4 as opposed to 2.2, $\alpha=0.08$). Those first arrested under Khrushchev were held in prisons, camps and hospitals on average a third longer than those first picked up under Brezhnev (9.6 years as opposed to 6.1; $\alpha=0.011$).

The comparison between those first arrested under Brezhnev and those first arrested under Andropov is the first to show a meaningful difference in occupation ranked by prestige, the later detainees being drawn on average from significantly *lower* socioeconomic groups. Although the Andropov administration was short, some other non-accidental differences in treatment of psychiatric detainees can still be shown. Those first arrested under Andropov were on average to spend almost six and a half years hospitalized, as opposed to their counterparts first arrested under Brezhnev, who experienced somewhat less than five years' psychiatric detention on average ($\alpha=0.05$). Administrative commitments were somewhat shorter in the Brezhnev administration ($\alpha=0.03$). These differences are not due to declines in use of later arrests and detentions which persist into the Chernenko and Gorbachev administrations: the observed differences are in the opposite direction.

On the other hand, those first held under Brezhnev suffered somewhat more detentions on average (1.5 as opposed to 1.1; α=0.001), possibly a consequence of their undergoing about twice as many administrative detentions (0.9 per person as opposed to 0.4; α=0.01), since the court-mandated hospitalizations average virtually the same in the Brezhnev and Andropov administrations. Similarly those first arrested under Brezhnev averaged a slightly but still significantly higher number of arrests over the course of their activities (1.4 as opposed to 1; α=0.000), as would be expected since their level of dissident behaviour was also distinctly higher (2.2 as opposed to 0.6 known dissident acts on average; α=0.000).

Those nonconformists first arrested under Chernenko may have been at somewhat higher risk of both administrative detention and court-ordered hospitalization than those first held under Andropov. Small but significant differences in averages point to that finding, but sample size makes a definite conclusion unclear. Socioeconomic status definitely differed significantly; those first arrested under Chernenko were drawn from higher strata, and on average they spent more time in court-ordered hospitalization (6.4 years compared to 2.4; α=0.000).

Considering the records of those who were first arrested under Chernenko or Gorbachev, Chernenko detainees spent far more time hospitalized in any facilities (6.4 as opposed to 1.9 years; α=0.000), due to a comparable predominance in the court-ordered hospitalizations data (6.4 years as opposed to 2.4 years, α=0.000). This difference also appears in the measures of total time incarcerated or hospitalized, at about the same level, 6.3 years compared to 2.1, α=0.000). However Gorbachev's first arrestees were subject to significantly more administrative detentions than were Chernenko dissenters (roughly one versus none on average, α=0.000), just as Podrabinek has observed (Van Voren, 1989), and significantly *fewer* court-ordered confinements (α=0.000). Those first arrested in the Chernenko administration averaged slightly, but still statistically significantly, higher than their Gorbachev counterparts on occupational prestige rankings.

If the Andropov and Chernenko administrations are set aside as too brief to have generated much data in the first case, or to have implemented systematic policies on dissent in the second, comparisons of the groups first arrested under the longer-lasting Khrushchev and Brezhnev administrations with those of the Gorbachev era are also revealing.

Those first picked up under Gorbachev were significantly younger at first forcible hospitalization than those first arrested under Khrushchev, 29 as opposed to 36 (α=0.04), consistent with a general observation of falling average age among hospitalized dissenters over time. They were also victims of substantially shorter compulsory psychiatric confinements, 1.9 as opposed to 6.6 years ($\alpha = 0.000$), again due to drastic differences in court-ordered hospitalization duration (7.4 years as opposed to 2.4; $\alpha = 0.001$). The administrative detentions also differ significantly but not as dramatically as the court-mandated hospitalizations, averaging 3.6 years in the Khrushchev administration case and 1.2 years for those first held under Gorbachev ($\alpha = 0.09$).

Gorbachev detainees spent significantly less time in any incarceration or hospitalization (2.1 compared to 9.6 years on average, $\alpha = 0.000$). They endured significantly fewer detentions overall (1.2/1.8; $\alpha = 0.003$), due to their lower average numbers of court-mandated hospitalizations. Numbers of incarcerations for those first arrested under Gorbachev are significantly less than the one per capita usually experienced by those first arrested under Khrushchev ($\alpha = 0.000$). Similarly the counts of all arrests are decidedly smaller on average for those first stopped under Gorbachev, about 1.1 as opposed to 2.2 under Khrushchev ($\alpha = 0.000$).

These observations are associated with the predictably smaller average number of known dissident acts for political activists under Gorbachev (1.2 as opposed to 3.4 under Khrushchev, $\alpha = 0.002$) as the dissident movement waned, metamorphosed, and national separatism became a reality.

The comparison between those first arrested under Brezhnev with those first stopped under Gorbachev is proportional to that obtaining between the Khrushchev and Gorbachev detainees. Again those first arrested under the later Gorbachev administration were significantly younger than those detained in the Brezhnev period (29 v. 33.7; $\alpha = 0.06$). Brezhnev arrestees endured significantly longer hospital stays (4.9 as opposed to 1.9 years; $\alpha = 0.000$, due to both longer administrative detentions and longer court-ordered commitments, averaging 6.3 years), as well as nearly three times the average total incarceration time, 6.1 compared to 2.1 years stagnating, $\alpha = 0.000$. Predictably those arrested under Brezhnev also underwent a slightly but significantly higher average number of arrests, detentions and incarcerations of all types.

DIFFERENCES ACROSS ADMINISTRATIONS: IDENTITY OF DETAINEES

Dissident Type

Consistent with the diversity of the dissident movement, central issues characterizing nonconformist behaviour varied across administrations, as well as within administrations. No one particular cause accounted for more than ten or 20 per cent of known detainee dissidents as a rule. The largest group of dissenters for whom major issues can be known or inferred from content of writing, public speaking and other evidence under Stalin were human rights advocates or visa and border crossing contenders, 17 per cent each.[11] The largest single cluster of nonconformists in the Khrushchev period were religious believers, 17 per cent. Under Brezhnev the most numerous group was made up of those seeking visas or attempting unauthorized border crossings, 16 per cent. Under Andropov, the forces of nationalism had coalesced and nationalists with or without anti-Communist sentiments were the more numerous (19 per cent), as they continued to be under Chernenko (50 per cent of a small sample) and Gorbachev as well (22 per cent).

The issue areas represented by at least some protesters in all administrations or in at least five of six were 1) generalized human rights concerns, 2) religious causes, 3) visa/emigration concerns, and 4) nationalism including anti-Communism, whose advocates more than double in percentage terms after Brezhnev.

Gender

Women remained an approximately constant small proportion of psychiatric detainees across administrations, roughly five per cent of cases for whom a first arrest year is available, never amounting to more than 8.6 valid per cent, in the Brezhnev administration.

Nationality

Consistently present among internees across all or all but one administration were Jewish, Latvian, Russian, and Ukrainian nationals. Lithuanians were represented in four of six administrations. As expected given their predominance in the Soviet population and in the larger group of dissidents, Russians made up the single largest group of detainees by nationality in every administration, never amounting to fewer than 32 valid (non-missing) per cent of cases for which both administration and nationality are known. Russians comprised 69 valid per cent of forcibly committed dissidents in the Khrushchev years, and 60 valid per cent under Brezhnev, although their proportions declined over administrations after Khrushchev, presumably reflecting the rise of non-Russian nationalism. The Ukrainian presence among detainees, second largest in three of six administrations, also predictable in view of their proportion of the whole Soviet population, did *not* tend to decline across administrations, fluctuating between 14 and 25 valid per cent. Consistent with the exacerbation of the Nagorno-Karabakh conflict, Armenians were the second largest nationality group of detainees under Gorbachev.

Religion

Religion of detainees exhibited the same variety as dissident type, and which religious affiliation conferred an enhanced risk of hospitalization responded to changing conditions. As newer religious groups gained adherents in the USSR, their members began to appear among detainees. Thus, first with Brezhnev and still under Gorbachev the data show hospitalized Hare Krishna members. Zionist Jewish Pentecostalists are hospitalized in the Gorbachev years, as well as those more typically systematically arrested and detained under most administrations, the Evangelical Christians, Jews, Pentecostalists, and Russian Orthodox. Even though Gorbachev sought support from the Russian Orthodox hierarchy in return for no more state persecution, at least one known Russian Orthodox believer was hospitalized in his administration. However no Catholics appear in our data among Gorbachev era internees, perhaps because of the arrangement signed with the Vatican in 1989.

Occupation[12]

An occupational profile of Soviet psychiatric detainees shows some stability across administrations, given difficulties in interpretation posed by small sample size in the Andropov and Chernenko years. In each administration intellectuals (professors, writers, researchers, diplomats) accounted for a third to half of interned nonconformists whose occupation is known and for whom dates of arrest are available, though they did not make up half of the dissident movement. Blue collar workers made up about a fourth of the psychiatrically repressed population in each administration except Khrushchev's (17 per cent) and Gorbachev's.[13] Students comprised a growing proportion of those forced into hospitals from Khrushchev to Brezhnev to Gorbachev, while white collar workers represented about 19 per cent on average across administrations. Remaining cases showing no particular pattern across administrations include artists, musicians, police, military, KGB/NKVD, those following religious vocations, peasants and farmers, and invalids.

Rankings of occupation by prestige indicate that Andropov-era detainees were drawn from lower socioeconomic strata than those held under

Brezhnev or Chernenko, and those hospitalized under Gorbachev may also have come, on average, from lower-status occupations.

SPATIAL DISPERSION: URBANIZATION AND METROPOLITAN RESIDENCE OF DISSIDENTS

Urbanization

Concentration of dissent in urban areas generally declined across administrations when measured in terms of degree of urbanization of nonconformists' residence. Although relatively few cases were reported at the village level, the proportion concentrated in provincial central cities as opposed to other cities declined over time in terms of valid per cent from near 90 per cent in the Stalin and Khrushchev years to about 70 per cent under Gorbachev, and the percentage reported at other smaller city levels rose from about 11 per cent in the first two administrations to the low twenties by Chernenko and Gorbachev. Since the proportion of cases in which residence is unknown does not tend to diminish over time, the shift out from major cities is probably not mainly due to more information on residence becoming available, but to diffusion of dissident activity, and secondarily to a desire after 1981 to obscure the mechanism of psychiatric repression without retiring it.

Metropolitan Residence

Psychiatric repression was a widespread phenomenon not exclusively concentrated in the two major cities, Moscow and Leningrad. Even when detentions taking place in Kiev are added to those recorded in the capital and in Leningrad, only 40 per cent, not a majority, of well-confirmed psychiatric detentions can be accounted for. As mentioned in Chapter 4, although many arrests and detentions took place in the two major metropolitan areas of the USSR, well-established detentions spread across at least 114 cities. Insofar as city of residence is known, the percentage of detainees from the two central metropolitan areas tends to decline across administrations from about 28 per cent in the Stalin administration to seven per cent under Gorbachev. This decline is consistent with a general decrease in the degree of urbanization of the phenomenon, and with its spread to smaller cities, without evidence of widespread 'contagion' to the village level.

City of First Detention

Sixty-six cities across the Union were sites of first hospitalizations of dissidents.[14] Clusters of first forcible commitments are found in Moscow (25 per cent of valid or non-missing cases), Leningrad (11.6 valid per cent), Dnepropetrovsk (9.0), Kazan (8.7), Chernyakhovsk (5.5), Alma-Ata, Volgograd and Yerevan (all 2.3 valid per cent). At least the first six cities are sites of major well-known psychiatric hospitals. No other city shows more than two valid per cent of cases. Notably, five of the cluster cities fall in the Russian republic, and one each in Ukraine, Kazakhstan and Armenia.

City of Second Detention

Compared to first detentions, second detentions show a smaller scatter across cities, 48 in all, consistent with the smaller number of second hospitalizations of either type among this group of dissidents. Larger clusters of forcible commitments again appear in Moscow (28.3 valid per cent), Leningrad (10.5), Dnepropetrovsk (9.4), Kazan (5.2), and Chernyakhovsk (4.2), in the same order as for first detentions, probably again reflecting the location of major psychiatric prisons and geographic patterns of referral. But the smaller clusters of second detentions are more numerous and not in the same places as for first hospitalizations. They include Sychyovka (3.7), Mordovia (3.1), Tashkent (2.6), Vladimir (2.6), and Vilnius (2.1). Again only three clusters lie outside the Russian republic, in Ukraine, Uzbekistan, and Lithuania, these regions possibly coming to the fore as a function of elapsed time and changing focus of dissent.

In general Russia predominates in all data on republic of detention, through at least the fifth compulsory hospitalization per individual, when sample size shrinks to 45.

SPATIAL DISPERSION: DISTRIBUTION OF DISSIDENT ACTS ACROSS REPUBLICS AND TIME

In the whole dataset, over 1229 dissident acts whose date is known can be documented across 14 republics,[15] as well as hundreds of others whose location or date are not recorded. Some indication of nonconformist activity level can therefore be found in the average number of known dissident acts per year in each republic.[16]

Low average levels of activity characterize Azerbaijan (0.33 per nonconformist per year), Georgia (0.6) and Moldova (0.8), while moderate levels typify Estonia (1.3) and Kazakhstan (1.0). Higher levels of dissent are seen in Uzbekistan (averaging 2.0 dissident acts per year), Ukraine (2.1), Armenia (2.3), Latvia (2.4), Lithuania (2.5), Belarus (2.5), and Russia, with a meaningful maximum of 2.7. Turkmenistan in these data averages four dissident acts per dissenter per year.[17]

Examining the timing of first dissident acts[18] makes it clear that dissent began at different times across the Union. Our earliest reports of political and religious protest by republic date from 1947 in Russia, 1949 in Latvia, 1954 in Ukraine, 1955 in Lithuania, 1956 in Kazakhstan, 1959 in Georgia, 1960 in Belarus, 1962 in Moldova, 1966 in Azerbaijan, 1968 in Armenia, and 1969 in Estonia.

Across the whole Union 1971 was the most typical year for a nonconformist detainee to begin dissident activity. When average date for first dissident act is calculated by republic,[19] Georgian and Latvian residents lead the movement in these data, on average tending to begin recorded dissident activity in 1966 or mid-1967. Russian dissidents typically made themselves known first in early 1970, followed by Ukrainians in late 1970. Those living in Belarus and Lithuania on average undertook their first dissident acts in early or mid-1972, Kazakh residents in early 1973, Moldovan residents in mid-1974. Nonconforming inhabitants of Estonia tended to begin recorded challenging behaviour relatively late, in 1977, and those in Armenia, in 1979.

SPATIAL DISPERSION: DISTRIBUTION OF REPRESSION ACROSS REPUBLICS AND ADMINISTRATIONS

Forced mental hospitalizations are distributed widely across republics under all administrations for which an adequate sample of information on republic of residence and dates of detentions is available.[20] As in the case of nationality of the individuals committed, and in city detained, Russian residence predominates in these data. In each administration the largest group of detainees lived in Russia, although the residence data fluctuate rather than decline across administrations as do the statistics on Russian *nationality*. The second most frequent republic of residence is Ukraine in four of six cases, and Lithuania in one.

In each administration, psychiatric repression extended over at least six or seven republics in the whole sample for which dates and republics are known. These numbers may be artificially depressed by the relative paucity of information from the Andropov and Chernenko periods. When these two administrations are omitted along with the Stalin period for reasons of relatively small confirmed sample size, the average number of republics from which detainees come in the remaining administrations rose to nine, so that more typically 60 per cent of the republics were implicated during the lengthier better documented administrations.

Reflecting the widespread nature of the phenomenon of psychiatric repression, no republic fails to produce a number of hospitalized dissidents in at least one administration. Again, however, the appearance of underrepresentation of the Islamic republics arises, since the five republics which evince psychiatric repression in one administration only are all culturally Islamic. These are Azerbaijan in the Brezhnev period, Kirghizia also under Brezhnev, Tadzhikistan under Gorbachev, Turkmenistan under Brezhnev and Uzbekistan under Andropov. Republics in which psychiatric repression persisted over five or six administrations are Slavic (Russia and Ukraine), but cultural bias is probably not the explanation for their centrality in these data since they also accounted for the majority of the Soviet population and therefore had a higher prior probability of serving as residences for any Soviet citizen. Baltic republics, Latvia and Lithuania, were the homes of psychiatric detainees in four administrations.

Typical numbers of detentions per dissident vary across republic. In the All-Union data where republic of residence and numbers of hospitalizations are known, the All-Union average is 1.6 court or administrative hospitalizations per protester. Azerbaijan, Armenia, Estonia, Kazakhstan, Kirghizia and Moldova were more indulgent in these terms than other republics, averaging only 0.67, 1.2, 1.2, 1.1, 1.0 and 1.0 known detentions per dissident respectively.[21] Latvia (1.8), Lithuania (1.63), Russia (1.65) and Turkmenistan (2.0) were more exigent, although these numbers do not differ much from the all-Union average.

These variations flow directly from the republics' respective experiences with level of dissident activity. All of the republics which ordered substantially fewer hospitalizations also experienced smaller average numbers of known dissident acts, well below the All-Union norm of approximately two, with the exception of Armenia (2.33 dissident acts on average). Azerbaijan (0.33), Estonia (1.3), Kazakhstan (1.0) and Moldova (0.8) all exhibited low levels of known dissident acts.

The republics in which *more* detentions than average were observed experienced elevated levels of dissident activity. Latvia on average shows 2.38 dissident acts per individual nonconformist; Lithuania 2.54; Russia 2.68 and Turkmenistan 4.

The observed correspondence between levels of dissident acts and levels of hospitalization is exactly what would be expected if psychiatric repression was a rational state response to rising levels of behaviour challenging state values and expectations for behaviour.

The most characteristic psychiatric repressive measure against nonconformists in these data is an administrative detention; thus, the average number of *court*-ordered hospitalizations per person when republic of residence is known falls below one, at 0.64.[22] Considering all administrations together, the average numbers of criminal court-mandated detentions across republic show relatively little variation, tending to lie within plus or minus 0.10 of the all-Union mean of 0.64. Distinctly fewer court-ordered procedures were used in Azerbaijan (0.33), Georgia (0.40) and Moldova (0.20) in these data. Distinctly more than the all-Union average were used in Latvia (0.75). But these variations are small enough to suggest a similarity rather than a pattern of differences in application of this penalty across republic.

The mean numbers of *administrative* detentions by republic also show such a close pattern around the usual average of one detention as to suggest a uniform policy of use of this measure, one time per identified nonconformist across republics. Most of the cases for which data are not missing fall within plus or minus 0.07 of the average, and the range is small. The largest average number of administrative detentions in any republic is found in Lithuania at 1.08, and the smallest is 0.33 in Azerbaijan.

Average age of psychiatric detainees at their first arrest is another repression indicator. Average age at first arrest can be so interpreted because it measures arrest and because it also captures some elements of discretion in the process of repression. That is, in a population of known dissidents it can document whether juveniles or elderly protesters are selectively targeted or selectively ignored. Like the frequency of detentions data, average age at first arrest shows relatively little variation across republic around the mean for the whole Union, about 32.4 years. For most republics the average age of political and religious protesters at their first arrest falls within plus or minus three years of the all-Union average, 32.4. Georgia and Kirghizia show unusually young average dissident populations, 24.3 and 27 years old at first arrest respectively. Azerbaijan (37 on average), Turkmenistan (46), and Uzbekistan (55) had dissident populations which were appreciably older at first arrest. However, for both the notably younger and older detainees, sample size is small enough to raise questions of the stability of the results in future testing. The most powerful observation in the data on age at first arrest is again the similarity across republic rather than the dissimilarities, suggesting a uniform nationwide strategy on how and when to respond to dissent.

Incidence of psychiatric repression is thus spread across republic and across administration with some uniformity in average rates of application. Severity as a function of length of repression can also be traced across republic.

The sum of all time hospitalized, whether via administrative or criminal court procedures, is one indicator of severity of psychiatric repression. Where both republic of residence and durations of detentions are known (n=288), the average length of all hospitalizations per individual dissident is 5.2 years. Belarus, at 8.4 years, and Kazakhstan at 9, show distinctly longer than average hospitalizations. Latvia (3.6), Lithuania (3.7), Moldova (2.3) and Tadzhikistan (3.5) show averages per detainee which are perceptibly shorter than usual across the Union.

Breaking these figures down by detention type among those actually held via each procedure reveals an average in total administrative detention time of 2.2 years per dissident across the Union. Belarus at 5.6 and Kazakhstan at 11.0 years show extremely long average administrative durations; Estonia (0.34 years), Lithuania (0.82) and Armenia (0.93) relatively short ones.

Average length of total court-ordered hospitalizations reaches 6.6 years across the Union. Extremes are exhibited by Estonia (10.8 years), Kazakhstan (8.8), and Belarus (7.9) as well as Latvia (4.7), Moldova (3.6), Tadzhikistan (3.5) and Uzbekistan (4.6).[23]

Similarly measures of total time incarcerated, imprisoned in any type of camp or jail, or hospitalized show some differences across republic which appear meaningful. The average across the Union in total time incarcerated reached 7.3 years for those psychiatrically repressed dissidents whose republic of residence is known. Azerbaijan (12.7), Belarus (10.7), and Georgia (13) experienced the highest averages by republic, and Moldova the lowest (2.3 years on average).

SUMMARY

This chapter documents the broad-based and extensive practice of Soviet psychiatric repression across decades, republics, and political administrations. Some evidence for the diffusion of repression out from central cities over time is presented, probably following the spread of major branches of the dissident movement and changes in geographical foci of arrests. Publicized releases from larger urban areas 1983–89 which did not seem to extend to smaller cities may have contributed to the growth of cases in smaller cities over time, as Helsinki Watch researchers have surmised. More detailed study of this aspect of the geographic spread of repression may show regularities in the process which follow epidemiological models of contagion or geographical contiguity models of propagation.

Age of psychiatric detainees at first hospitalization tended to decline over administrations and across age cohorts as defined by Bahry, auguring for the recruitment of younger members into dissident groups over time. Students comprised a growing proportion of those compulsorily hospitalized, while the proportion of women among psychiatric prisoners remained low and roughly constant. In contrast to some studies, we show a sizeable component of psychiatric prisoners to have been blue collar workers, who received no special protection in the workers' state. Some leniency may, however, have been extended to Balts among the nationality groups, perhaps because of their role in the Soviet economy. Russian nationals' proportions among detainees, always substantial, declined after Khrushchev.

The rise of nationalism and anti-communism is clear in the nature of dissident acts recorded in our data. Under Andropov, Chernenko and Gorbachev these issues accounted for the single largest groups of psychiatric prisoners, displacing the human rights and emigration concerns which had predominated in earlier periods.

If R. Medvedev (1980:118–19) is correct that the size of the dissident movement declined in the last half of the sixties and through the seventies, the base of recruiting from which psychiatric detainees were drawn became arguably smaller. If the numbers of forced psychiatric hospitalizations do not conform to this pattern but instead show increases, this would imply a higher risk of detention of activists, and even greater enhancement of reliance on psychiatry to dissuade in the latter sixties and the seventies. In fact we do show dramatic increases in frequencies of compulsory mental hospitalization from 1967 to about 1972 depending on the measure used. Also coherent with Medvedev's interpretation (1980:68), our data reveal increases in duration but general decreases in incidence of detentions from 1971 through 1976, as well as a surge in exits from the USSR, evidently because forced expulsions grew over this interval as an alternative response to dissidence.

Incidence of psychiatric repression was sensitive to major external as well as internal events in these data, including human rights activism in the West, but did not necessarily respond immediately or in the direction preferred in the West, as the considerable increases in forcible commitments during the height of détente show.

In these data frequency of hospitalization at the All-Union level is well described as a simple linear function of level of previous dissident activity, as measured by the sum of dissident acts in the immediately prior year. This relationship reappears at the republic level, even though disaggregation to the republic level would not necessarily be expected to show the same general pattern as that obtaining across the whole country. The tendency for frequency of hospitalization to follow frequency of dissident acts nation-wide and within republics, and the necessity of using both administrative and criminal internment measures together to predict hospitalizations well from prior dissident acts, argue that both means of detention were part of a *unified* coherent policy to respond to dissent. This evidence supports our argument that the mechanism of psychiatric repression relying on frequency of hospitalization was rationally centrally directed.

At the same time the variations across republic in *duration* of detentions, both administrative and court-ordered, as well as in total time incarcerated, support interpretations of psychiatric repression in which considerable discretion was left to the republic or lower levels to respond to varying needs and contrasting regional or local policies. Bonnie (1990b:335–6) concluded that especially after the 1988 regulations providing for review were promulgated – but were still not in effect as late as 1990 – power over psychiatric commitments remained with local psychiatrists. Therefore local Party officials could still affect who was detained, and for how long.

6 The Risk of Psychiatric Detention, Demographic Variables and Deterrence of Dissent

After all the (KGB) investigator, too, is an ordinary Soviet citizen – more ordinary than most . . .

Reich (1978:36)

This chapter examines a set of demographic variables and other attributes to determine which characteristics and political causes presented the greatest risk of frequent and lengthy forcible hospitalization among a group of dissenters known to be detained at some point in their nonconformist activities. We also investigate the extent to which state response to dissidence may have served deterrence functions in Soviet society. The calculations reported have been derived from two datasets, the Smith–Oleszczuk data on psychiatric detainees used in the previous analyses (n=674), and our larger dataset on Soviet Repressed Dissidents (n=2749), also structured as described here in Chapter 2.

Occupation may have conferred some protection against frequent or lengthy hospitalizations for Soviet dissidents. Nationality may also have provided some protection, since a pattern of relative clemency towards Baltic groups is verified. Dissenters' causes and behaviour also were related to risk of forced hospitalization. Dissidents who rejected Party guidance, created or joined new political groups, or attempted unauthorized border crossings faced the greatest risk of long and repeated commitments.

Punitive transfer among hospitals cannot be documented in the aggregate in these data. But a pattern of heavy penalties exacted from those charged with particularly 'political' offences is found. Individuals committed via criminal trials who were charged with 'political' violations are transferred among special regime hospitals more frequently than others.

Punitive hospitalization tends to generate new waves of protest in these data, rather than to succeed in deterring new dissident acts. Little evidence can be found of either specific or general deterrence effects as defined by Western criminologists. Instead, reinforcing effects appear, revealing a core of persistent dissenters who *increase* their level of activity after a first sanction. It is even possible that psychiatric repression propagated dissent.

CHARACTERISTIC EXPERIENCES

Frequency of Hospitalization

The Smith–Oleszczuk data show 674 dissidents in psychiatric detention at some time during the period under study, and almost a thousand (997) detentions for which dates or durations can be confirmed. Of these 674 individuals, 467 were detained once, 126 twice, 49 three times, 20 four times, 8 five times, and 4 six times. The most characteristic experience, obtaining in 67 per cent of all cases, is one detention per dissenter, predominantly administrative. Some 88 per cent of dissidents experienced two or fewer detentions, 95 per cent three or fewer.

All Time Hospitalized

Total time detained in psychiatric hospitals[1] varied in these data from a few hours to 34 years per person. Average duration of forcible hospitalization reached 5.2 years, with one year the single most frequently observed term, and three years the median. Other common durations of detention in these data were one month, six months, two years, four years, six, seven, eight, nine, ten and 11 years. Including only those cases for which duration of hospitalization is documented, Soviet protesters experienced 1839.1 years' total forced hospitalization time.

RISK AND SEVERITY OF DETENTIONS AND DEMOGRAPHIC VARIABLES

Detention Risk as a Function of Social Stratum

The risk of psychiatric internment not only varies over time, as argued in the previous chapter, but also by socioeconomic stratum of the individual as indicated by occupation, as sketched in Chapter 4. Here we consider the relationship in more detail.

Especially harsh treatment fell to current or former KGB employees, followed by blue collar workers, students, the military, white collar workers and intellectuals. Those in these occupations (except for white collar

Table 6.1 Frequency and Range of Hospitalizations by Occupation

Occupation	*Average Frequency*	*Maximum*	*Minimum*
KGB/NKVD*	4.0	6	2
Blue collar	1.9	6	1
Students	1.8	5	1
Military	1.7	5	1
White collar	1.7	4	1
Intellectual	1.6	5	1
Artist, dancer	1.6	3	1
Police*	1.5	2	1
Peasant/farmer*	1.5	2	1
Religious professionals	1.4	3	1

* Small sample size; estimates may not be stable.

Table 6.2 Psychiatric Detainees' Occupation

Occupation	*Number Known Detained*	*Per cent of Total*
Intellectuals	142	36 %
Blue collar workers	91	23 %
White collar managers	64	16 %
Students	29	07 %
Religious vocations	25	06 %
Military	15	04 %
Artists and dancers	10	03 %
Musicians	5	01 %
Peasants/farmers	4	01 %
Police	2	0.5 %
KGB/NKVD	2	0.5 %
Invalid	1	0.3 %
Totals	390	98.3*

* Percentages do not sum to 100 because of rounding error.

workers) might be detained five or even six times, as can be seen in Table 6.1. The range of maxima and minima in hospitalization frequency shows great disparity across occupation, although *average* numbers of all commitments by occupation are similar.

The predominance of intellectuals in the subset of involuntary psychiatric hospital residents over 1928–91 reflects their substantial presence in the dissident movement and their salience. Intellectuals account for over

Table 6.3 Total Years Compulsorily Hospitalized, by Occupation

*Occupation**	*Average of all years hospitalized*	*Administrative Average*	*Court Average*
Military	6.8	2.8	8.6
KGB/NKVD	6.6	2.1	5.5
Workers	6.1	2.5	7.5
Students	6.1	1.9	7.7
Religious	5.7	3.8	6.7
Intellectuals	5.0	2.3	5.9
Artists, dancers	5.0	1.4	6.4
White collar	5.0	1.6	5.9
Police	1.0	0.03	1.9
Group means**	5.2	2.7	6.6

* Cases of musicians, peasants, and invalids are omitted from the table because of missing information in one category.
** Includes all cases for which occupation and duration of hospitalization variables are known (390/674).

one and a half times as many detentions in this period as the next most frequently interned group (142/91 = 1.56), and it is notable that the next most frequently interned group is blue collar workers, in the sample of 390/674 for whom occupation information is available, comprising about 58 per cent of the whole sample of detained dissidents. In general, intellectuals make up the largest single occupational category of all dissidents hospitalized, although intellectuals do not comprise the largest group of dissidents. Workers then account for almost one and a half times as many psychiatric hospitalizations as do managers/white collar employees (91/64 = 1.42). Students (29 internments) and priests/other religious vocations[2] (25 internments) provide further occupational clusters among those most often detained. Remaining cases are scattered among artists, musicians, police, military and current or former intelligence officers, and peasants/farmers.

Length of Detention as a Function of Socioeconomic Status

Length of detention also shows some relationship to social strata as indicated by occupation, in Table 6.3. Despite their being hospitalized as frequently as other dissidents on average, police officers were lightly affected by duration of hospitalization. They received minimal administrative detentions of a week or two (0.02–0.03 years) and their court-ordered hospitalizations average under two years. On the other hand, all time hospitalized averages almost seven years for military (6.8) and former or current KGB (Commissariat of State Security) or NKVD (People's Commissariat of Internal Affairs) officers (6.6), followed closely by student and blue collar groups both averaging 6.1 years of total hospitalization time. Intellectuals average five years' total time compulsorily hospitalized, as do artists and white collar workers.

The foregoing observations suggest that not only do somewhat different risks of initial arrest attach to dissidents by virtue of occupation, but once detained, a protester's length of hospitalization could vary notably by occupation. Rule-enforcers such as the military and KGB were held longest, followed by two groups purportedly given a protected status in Soviet society, workers and students. Next longest detained were those with religious vocations. Intellectuals, artists and dancers, and white collar managers were also stringently penalized on average.

The contrast in societal function of judicial v. non-judicial psychiatric confinement which has been hypothesized in other chapters is also illustrated here by the distinct occupational risk profiles of those subject to each type of confinement. The risk of a lengthy administrative or court detention was not evenly distributed across occupation. Artists and dancers on average fell well below the group mean for duration of non-judicial detention, perhaps protected because of local, regional, national or international publicity attending, for example, to ballet dancers, or perceived short-term needs to hospitalize them, for example, to reduce risk of sudden internationally visible emigration. White collar technicians and managers and students were also detained administratively much more briefly than average.[3] Military personnel and priests, ministers, and nuns found themselves hospitalized substantially longer than the group mean for non-court-ordered confinements.

Risking especially lengthy court-ordered commitments were the military (almost nine years on average while the group mean was 6.63), students (7.7 years on average), and blue collar workers (7.5 years). Somewhat shorter than average court-mandated hospitalizations were inflicted on white collar managers and technicians, artists and dancers, and intellectuals.

FREQUENCY AND TYPE OF DETENTION AND DISSIDENT BEHAVIOUR

The nature of the first recorded dissident act appears related to numbers of psychiatric internments experienced by any individual. In these data, records

Table 6.4 First Known Dissident Behaviour

Nature of dissident act	*Frequency*	*Per cent*
Samizdat	59	14.6
Demonstration	58	14.4
Unauthorized border cross	46	11.4
Letter registering new group	37	9.2
Other (e.g. relig.)	29	7.2
Individual petition	28	6.9
Provocative writing	27	6.7
Creation of new group	18	4.5
Mass petition	17	4.2
Joining dissident group	16	4.0
Request for asylum	9	2.2
Hijacking	7	1.7
Rejection of Party guidance	7	1.7
Unauthorized meeting	6	1.5
Refusal to bear arms	6	1.5
News conference	5	1.2
Hunger strike	5	1.2
Riot, other violence	5	1.2
Appeal to foreign power	4	1.0
Unauthorized election acts	4	1.0
Strike	4	1.0
Flag raising/lowering	3	0.7
Renunciation of citizenship	3	0.7
	403	99.7*

* Percentages do not sum exactly to 100 because of rounding error.

exist of type of first dissident act for 403 (60 per cent) of the 674 individuals in the Smith/Oleszczuk data, as per Table 6.4.

As reported in Table 6.4, for 59/403, or 14.6 per cent of protesters for whom this information is known, the first dissident act was samizdat activity such as publishing, composing, duplicating, and distributing self-published materials. As expected since samizdat served as a powerful instrument for mobilization of political opposition, these individuals experienced a distinctly above average number of confinements (1.8 where the group average is 1.17), as seen in Table 6.5. The next most frequent type of first dissident act, demonstrating, characterizes 14.4 per cent of dissidents, who on average also endured more detentions in general (1.95, compared to the group average of 1.17), as well as more court-ordered hospitalizations in particular (0.9 per person as opposed to the whole group average of 0.39). Participation in demonstrations and other dissident

Table 6.5 First Dissident Behaviour and Average Frequency and Duration in Years of Hospitalization per Individual

Dissident Behaviour	*Average Frequency* All	Admin.	Court	*Average Duration** All	Admin.	Court
Samizdat	1.8	1.1	0.70	4.1	1.6	5.7
Provocative writing	1.4	0.4	0.96	6.2	0.8	6.6
Demonstration	1.9	1.1	0.90	5.5	1.7	6.3
Border cross.	1.4	0.7	0.78	6.1	4.8	6.5
Register group	1.5	0.9	0.65	2.4	1.3	2.9
Other**	1.7	1.3	0.44	3.1	0.7	4.9
Petition	1.8	1.3	0.54	4.2	1.6	8.1
Create group	2.2	1.2	1.00	6.9	1.9	8.8
Mass petition	1.6	1.1	0.53	4.4	0.4	11.3
Join group	2.1	0.9	1.10	6.9	4.0	7.2
Request asylum	1.6	1.0	0.56	4.5	4.6	4.2
Hijacking	1.6	0.4	1.14	3.2	0.1	5.2
Reject Party	1.3	1.2	0.17	10.9	7.9	14.0
Unauth. meeting	1.3	0.7	0.67	8.3	4.0	12.5
Refuse arms	2.2	1.0	1.17	4.4	2.3	3.3
News conference	1.2	0.8	0.40	0.9	0.04	1.7
Hunger strike	1.2	0.8	0.40	2.2	2.2	NA
Riot, violence	1.2	0.4	0.80	15.1	25.0	11.8
Appeal to for. nat'l.	1.0	0.3	0.75	7.7	11.0	6.6
Unauth. election behaviour	2.3	1.7	0.67	8.8	2.8	6.0
Strike	1.3	1.0	0.25	3.2	2.8	4.0
Flag raising/lowering	1.0	1.0	0.00	1.5	1.5	NA
Renounce citizenship	2.7	1.7	1.00	2.6	1.1	3.1
Means	1.2	0.8	0.39	5.3	3.3	8.3

* Duration is measured in years.
** 'Other' includes religious processions, appearing at public gatherings near courthouses where politicized trials are under way, etc.

behaviour, including religious processions, and crowd formation outside courthouses while well-publicized trials are under way, as well as prisoners moving into 'forbidden' zones in camps, when taken together as comprising related phenomena, account for the first dissident acts of almost a fourth (21.6 per cent) of this subsample of nonconformists. Groups of individuals for whom this 'other' dissident behaviour were first dissident acts on average were detained disproportionally often as well, 1.3 times administratively and 1.7 times overall respectively.

Among the smaller clusters of other first dissident acts, individual petitioning or 'complaining', accounting for about seven per cent of detainees, was linked to approximately 1.8 hospitalizations (collective petitioning to about 1.6), and on average to 1.3 administrative detentions. Provocative non-samizdat writing, characterizing about 6.7 per cent of psychiatric prisoners, was tied to above-average incidences of all hospitalizations (1.4) as well as a somewhat higher rate of court-ordered commitments (0.96). Creating or joining a new dissident group, involving 4.5 and 4 per cent of detainees respectively, was connected to higher frequencies of hospitalizations in general (2.2 and 2.1 on average) as well as to higher frequencies of both administrative and court-ordered commitments (1.2 and 0.94; 1 and 1.1 respectively).

Creating and joining a new dissident group, rejecting Party guidance and/or returning Party cards, and unauthorized electoral activity were among the riskiest sorts of first dissident behaviour, which yielded the highest numbers of detentions on average (more than two), and the lengthiest average hospitalizations (7–11 years) in these data.

The nature of dissident behaviour may also affect the propensity to receive a judicial – that is, court-ordered and on average longer – detention rather than an administrative confinement when detained. In the set of 403 individuals for whom first dissident act is recorded, the average number of judicial internments in the entire group is under one half. That is, the most typical court-ordered hospitalization experience was one court-mandated detention among two or three dissidents. However, numbers of judicial psychiatric detentions vary by dissident act. The highest average number of these internments by type of dissident act is observed for dissidents who rejected the Soviet state or their responsibilities to it, who participated publicly in political opposition, or who propagated dissident groups. Thus those whose first dissident act was demonstrating, provocative writing, creating or joining an opposition group including religious societies, hijacking planes, refusing to bear arms in the USSR military, or renouncing Soviet citizenship were most often sent to psychiatric hospitals by courts.

For administrative confinements, where type of first dissident act is known, dissent most frequently resulting in administrative detention included much of the same behaviour most likely to result in judicial detention, but also, indicating the versatility of the administrative hospitalization option, included other categories as well. Thus demonstrating, samizdat work, creating opposition groups, and refusing to bear arms were first dissident acts for those whose administrative hospitalizations averaged 1.0 or more. But so were petitioning, as an individual or in a group, rejecting Party guidance, seeking asylum, strikes, and unauthorized electoral activity.

Samizdat behaviour was a real regime irritant catalyzing arrest and forcible confinements.[4] Publishing, composing, duplicating and distributing samizdat materials all appear connected to virtual certainty of administrative detention and substantial odds of a court term.[5]

DURATION AND TYPE OF DETENTION AND PRIOR DISSIDENT BEHAVIOUR

Not only is frequency of detention related to prior dissident acts, length of forced hospitalization and total time incarcerated in camps and prisons are also related to the nature of the first recorded dissident act, even though first dissident acts are not necessarily substantively linked to any subsequent criminal charges. In general[6] for cases in which dissident acts are recorded, total administrative detention time per affected person is about 3.3 years, total court detention time averages about 8.3 years, and total time hospitalized centres on 5.3 years, but some kinds of first nonconforming behaviour attracted heavier sanctions and some were received more leniently.

Surprisingly, in view of the society-wide issue that draft evasion became, refusal to bear arms has been connected with below average *length* – though not *frequencies* – of detentions and incarcerations. Calling an unauthorized news conference was tied to very brief administrative (0.04 year) and court-ordered hospitalizations (1.7 years) as well as to shorter prison and camp time (1.7 years). Letters to register new political groups were also connected with shorter detentions. Unexpectedly, since samizdat activity was a powerful catalyst of prompt arrest, samizdat offences were tied to marginally *shorter* detentions and incarcerations as well. News conferences and letters registering new political organizations may be construed as relatively harmless dissident activity, especially considering state controls on media and the mail. But refusal to bear arms and samizdat refusal to accept the limitations on publication in the USSR are significant acts of defiance of state norms. Future research may establish a theoretical reason for relatively light but not necessarily infrequent penalties exacted in these cases.

Longer than average *administrative* detentions were tied to unauthorized attempts to cross the border (4.8 years), requests for asylum (4.6 years), and rejection of Party guidance (7.9 years). Longer *court* hospitalizations were linked to creation of dissident groups (8.8 years on average), mass petitioning (11.3 years), rejection of Party authority (14 years), and unauthorized meetings (12.5 years). Longer prison and camp incarcerations tend to occur in the same categories for which longer court hospitalizations were ordered.[7]

DEMOGRAPHICS AND FREQUENCY AND TYPE OF DETENTION

If psychiatric detention has been an instrument of rationally pursued state objectives, the two forms of psychiatric repression may have served different functions and may have been targeted against different types of nonconformists. Frequency of use of the two methods might vary, as would the demographic profiles of victims. Extracting from the data those who were only held administratively and those who were only ordered hospitalized as a result of a trial can reveal these contrasts, if they exist.

Total numbers of arrests for court-ordered compulsorily hospitalized dissidents show a mean of nearly 2 (1.8) but a range reaching seven or more. Although the most typical experience is one arrest (61 per cent of cases), persistent activists were arrested three or more times (21 per cent). *Administrative* detainees averaged nearly three arrests per person (2.7), most typically two, and ranged up to eight or more, consistent with their higher average number of recorded dissident acts (4.6 as opposed to 2.7). Seventy-nine per cent of court-ordered psychiatric prisoners were arrested two or fewer times, whereas a comparable proportion (84 per cent) of administrative detainees were arrested four or fewer times.

In occupational profile the two groups of detainees are similar. This similarity implies that both methods have been directed about equally frequently – but not equally lengthily – across socioeconomic status as measured by occupation.

Divergences between the groups emerge when religion and dissident type are considered. In terms of valid or non-missing per cent, substantially more Roman Catholics were hospitalized as a result of court order (9.8/3.4 per cent), as well as more Buddhists and more Jews. Christians without denomination made up 10.3 per cent of administrative detainees but only 1.6 per cent of the court-ordered. Russian Orthodox and Uniates, though victimized in both procedures, also tended to be hospitalized administratively more than by court mandate (20.7 per cent as opposed to 16.4 per cent; 6.9 per cent as against 1.6 per cent respectively).

Administrative and court hospitalizations were targeted against some contrasting varieties of political and religious challengers. More human rights advocates and samizdat enthusiasts were detained administratively only (about 14 per cent compared to about ten per cent; about nine per cent compared to about five per cent respectively). On the other hand, nationalists and anti-Communists tended to be detained by court mandate only (about nine per cent compared to about 3.5 per cent), presumably attracting the more severe and usually longer penalty because of the greater threat to regime values and legitimacy, as well as eventually to the integrity of the Union, posed by this group. These proportions shifted somewhat in the eighties and early nineties, since an analysis of the 1960–81 interval shows not only nationalists and anti-Communists or True Marxists heavily represented among those detained by court order, but also religious practitioners, visa term violators, human rights advocates and samizdat purveyors. The durations and frequencies of terms imposed on nationalists appear to have increased in the eighties.

Some tendency existed to detain women administratively, as we have indicated in other terms, as part of a general pattern of relative clemency towards women dissidents. Women comprised nine per cent of those only hospitalized administratively, while they made up six per cent of those only committed by courts.

These calculations suggest that active Soviet dissidents faced risks of frequent and lengthy detention which varied over time and type of dissenting behaviour as well as by demographic considerations such as the individual's socioeconomic status indicated by occupation. The fact that those hospitalized under court order and those hospitalized administratively had engaged in overlapping varieties of first recorded dissident behaviour suggests that these procedures were not differentially targeted on completely contrasting types of nonconformist behaviour. Instead both were used to address some of the same societal demands for religious and ideological latitude, travel, human rights, nationalist aspirations, and freedom of expression. Administrative measures, being more flexible and prompt than trials, were more widely applied, especially where official intervention would have been time-sensitive, as in a strike, electoral activity, or publicized asylum-seeking.

COMBINATIONS OF RISK FACTORS

Connections between demographic and other attributes of dissidents and forcible commitment have been estimated for one variable at a time in this chapter thus far. But of course dissidents at any point in time can be characterized by several demographic variables and attributes which together may predict their risks of detention. To assess how several such variables taken together may explain political hospitalization when combined in additive linear functions, we have used linear multiple regression (LMR) for preliminary results.

R. Medvedev (1980:15) observed that a dissident's fate depended upon location of residence (Moscow or not), age, prior convictions, behaviour, degree of renown in the USSR and abroad, and social position. Among the possible interpretations of this hypothesis in the variables in our dataset, to which the LMR will add a constant and coefficients for each predictor variable, are:

1. timeinc = metrores + hosp1age + nconvict + sumdsact + occrank

where timeinc is total time incarcerated in any prison, labour camp, place of exile or psychiatric hospital; metrores is a dummy residence variable in which Moscow or Leningrad are assigned the value 1 and all other locations a zero; hosp1age is age at first hospitalization, nconvict is number of convictions; sumdsact is total number of recorded dissident acts; and occrank is occupation given a numerical rank based on reported prestige.

In our data equation 1 yields a multiple R of 0.44, and an R squared of 0.19, at $\alpha = 0.0000$. It represents a small but highly significant relationship, to which age at first hospitalization and number of convictions made the greatest contribution as judged by their respective beta weights of 0.12 and 0.41.

To focus on psychiatric detentions in particular, the same predictor variables are used to estimate total numbers of all detentions per individual:

2. nalldtn = metrores + hosp1age + nconvict + sumdsact + occrank

This equation results in a multiple R of 0.44, R squared of 0.19, and significance level, as above, of 0.0000. It also represents a small but non-accidental relationship, most of which derives from total numbers of dissident acts (beta = 0.27), metro residence (beta = 0.17) and age at first hospitalization (beta = –0.15).

We have shown that in several measures clemency towards women psychiatric detainees existed, and may help explain numbers of detentions. Adding a dummy gender variable to equation 2 produces:

3. nalldtn = metrores + hosp1age + nconvict + sumdsact + occrank + gender

This equation results in an R of 0.44, and an R squared of 0.20, at $\alpha = 0.0000$. Adding gender to the equation produces a slight increase in explained variance, and no appreciable change in the beta weights.

Creating or joining a dissident group has been stringently penalized in a number of indicators of frequency and duration of forced psychiatric hospitalization in our data. Biographical information makes clear that prominent creators of new political and religious associations, as well as publicized members, have been specially targeted for repression at sensitive times. Measures of group membership may then make a contribution to predicting numbers of detentions. Our measure includes membership or leadership in the Helsinki Watch Group, Committee for the Defence of Rights of Believers, independent trade unions, Working Commission on Psychiatric Abuse, Working Commission on the Rights of Invalids, other human rights groups, other political organizations such as nascent parties and anti-Soviet partisans, cultural organizations, and religious associations such as the Society of the Eucharist. Adding this variable (membrshp) to equation 2 yields:

4. nalldtn = metrores + hosp1age + nconvict + sumdsact + occrank + membrshp

In this case again explained variance increases slightly, to R = 0.45 and R squared = 0.20 at $\alpha = 0.0000$. This equation, like the previous ones, also describes a small but statistically meaningful relationship. The beta weight on group memberships is approximately 0.10, or about the same as the weight on number of convictions, indicating that these variables contribute about equally to explaining numbers of detentions in this equation. Sum of dissident acts is the major contributor, with a beta of 0.26, followed by metro residence at 0.16.

Number of interrogations undergone is a reflection of the degree to which a protester may have become conspicuous to the authorities. Adding known interrogations (suminter) to equation 4 produces

5. nalldtn = metrores + hosp1age + nconvict + sumdsact + occrank + membrshp + suminter

This equation yields an R of 0.45 and an R squared of 0.20 also at $\alpha = 0.0000$. The beta weights show that sum of dissident acts continues to make the greatest contribution (0.26), followed by metro residence (0.17), age at first hospitalization (–0.14), number of convictions (0.11) and memberships (0.10). Interrogations is weighted slightly (0.02), and makes little contribution to the relationship, possibly because of missing data in many cases.

We have speculated that psychiatric repression moved out from central cities to smaller ones over time. If so, degree of urbanization may help explain numbers of detentions of individuals. Adding an urbanization of residence variable (urbnum) to equation 5 gives:

6. nalldtn = metrores + hosp1age + nconvict + sumdsact + occrank + membrshp + suminter + urbnum

This form results in an R of 0.45 and an R squared of 0.20, at $\alpha = 0.0000$. Urbanization adds virtually nothing to the equation (beta = –0.01), possibly because a related concept, metropolitan residence, is already included. The major contributors as before remain sums of dissident acts, metro residence, age, number of convictions and memberships.

That these statistical results are essentially unchanged despite alterations in the number of predictor variables supplied and the variety of information available implies that most of the explanatory power lies in the core of variables common to all equations, especially sums of dissident acts, and metro residence. Age, memberships in dissident groups, and number of convictions also make persistent contributions.

These results substantiate Medvedev's views, since they provide evidence of a highly significant relationship among the predictor variables and the outcome, numbers of all detentions. The odds that these relationships are statistical accidents are virtually nil (0.0000). Yet these results leave much unexplained. They account for only about 1/5 of the variation in numbers of detentions.

The small R squared may be due to the use in this preliminary assessment of an additive linear technique in curvilinear data which could be better fit with at least one exponential or interactive term.

However the small relationship may be due at least as much to the influence of omitted variables which do not lend themselves to straightforward meaningful quantification. Among the omitted difficult-to-quantify variables which may be powerful in explaining numbers of detentions for particular nonconformists are the degree of publicity attendant on their causes, the fame of the individual, proximity to major domestic and international events, type of dissident (nationalist, religious, human rights, etc.), ethnicity, and religion.

Finally the modest R squared may be due to the predictor variables providing necessary but not sufficient conditions for detention. This possibility implies the existence of at least one further unspecified catalyst variable, which may be an idiosyncratic one such as dissident conduct when facing arrest, or predispositions of certain judges.

TRIAL CHARGES AND DURATION OF HOSPITALIZATION

Those nonconformists penalized with frequent court trials and formal findings of non-imputability differ in some respects, religion and dissident type but not occupational profile, from dissidents penalized only with administrative – usually shorter – detentions. Those subject to criminal procedures may also differ among themselves. In particular those charged with more serious offences would be expected to be hospitalized longer than those charged with lesser violations.

First charges filed in first trials included treason, terrorism, sabotage, anti-Soviet agitprop, defamation of the Soviet system, insulting authority, resisting the militia, draft evasion, internal passport violations, illegal border crossing, separation of church and state, violations of others' rights by religious practice, prohibited trade, hooliganism, and parasitism. As has been known for some time, this observation means that charges against dissidents were concentrated on 'political' segments of the Criminal Code, in particular in our data on Article 70, anti-Soviet agitation and propaganda (agitprop: 41 valid or non-missing per cent), and Article 190.1, defamation of the Soviet system (24 valid per cent). Other charges brought against several activists in our data were treason (12.5 valid per cent), illegal border crossings (5.5 per cent) and hooliganism (3.2 per cent).

Undeniably more severe and more frequent penalties were exacted from psychiatric detainees who were tried in the first instance under 'political charges', when 'political charges' are defined to include Article 70, Article 190.1, treason, border crossing violations, and hooliganism. In comparison with those charged under other articles or committed without trial, 'political' offenders spent almost twice as long in psychiatric hospitals (7.0 years as opposed to 3.6; $\alpha=0.000$), were detained on average significantly more often (1.6 times versus 1.4 times on average; $\alpha=0.000$), and as previously indicated, were distinctly more likely to be transferred to special regime institutions ($\alpha=0.000$). While their administrative detention time coincided almost exactly with that of other dissidents, the total *court-ordered* hospitalization time considerably exceeded that of other detainees (7.6 years on average, as compared to 4.4; $\alpha=0.000$). The evidence supports a clear finding of disproportionally severe penalties forced on protesters who were burdened with charges of highly politicized offences. Since a wide degree of discretion in choice of criminal charges laid for what appears to be comparable dissident behaviour can be observed, these penalties can be interpreted as evidence of rational state use of court mechanisms to remove particularly obstreperous critics from circulation.

PUNITIVE TRANSFER?

One instrument of compellance of individuals and deterrence and dissuasion of others is punitive transfer to mental institutions of progressively harsher regime. Our transfer data cover one to six transfers between institutions per individual, with a maximum sample size of 428/674 or 64 per cent of all hospitalized dissidents in the Smith–Oleszczuk dataset. In these figures most individuals after their initial hospitalization were transferred once. About a third of known cases were transferred at least twice, and about a fifth were transferred three times. Twelve per cent were transferred four times, and eight per cent five times.

The data do not show a consistent tendency to channel political and religious detainees into strict supervision hospitals. On first hospitalization in our data, protesters were placed almost exactly equally frequently in ordinary standard regime hospitals or in strict supervision hospitals.[8] In transfers to a second institution, the proportion in ordinary hospitals rises to 56.9 per cent. In transfers to a third hospital, the proportion in ordinary hospitals remains roughly stable at 56.1 per cent. Strict observation hospitals do not begin to receive a higher proportion of nonconformists until transfers to a fourth institution, when the proportion of detainees known to be in ordinary regime hospitals falls to 47.1 per cent and the proportion in strict regime detentions rises from 43.9 to 52.9 per cent. But transfers to a fifth institution again are largely to ordinary hospitals, as would be expected since moving to an ordinary observation institution normally precedes release. Remarkably, transfers to a sixth hospital show an increase in commitments to special regime institutions, from 40 to 46.7 per cent, which may imply punitive transfer for those moved most frequently.

The evidence is consistent with reliance on ordinary regime hospitals to confine transferred dissidents, for most known cases in our data. Psychiatric repression in these measures has not been mainly a phenomenon of the strict observation institution, despite some tendency in the literature to define psychiatric abuse as focused on the draconian special regime hospitals. It was instead a systemic phenomenon.[9]

Nevertheless if a punitive purpose is hypothesized, it might be expected that those first confined to special hospitals might continue to be committed to special regime institutions as they were repeatedly transferred, and others who were labelled troublesome or rule-breakers would be moved in from ordinary hospitals. If so, in transfer data the proportions of dissidents confined to special regime hospitals should grow across transfers and tend to concentrate after two or three moves. However a decision tree diagram showing sequential transfers among hospitals does not produce this expected concentration. In fact, tracing strict regime commitments across four placements in institutions shows a tendency for *ordinary* commitments to predominate instead at the second and third hospitalization, although the two groups are split evenly at the fourth hospitalization, which would probably not be the case if the ordinary commitments predominance were only an indication of upcoming release.

Real punitive relationships may be buried in this analysis because we lack idiosyncratic data on psychoprisoner conduct and interactions with hospital staff. Certainly state policy is not the only source of punitive treatment in mental hospitals, and concentration across transfers is not the only measure of state policy. Transfers among wards may be a result of perceived hospital rule infractions or close encounters with guards, and punishing transfers among hospitals may follow from unfortunate interactions with doctors which are essentially personal. Although the data do not support a general finding of punitive transfer based simply on the identification of detainees as political or religious dissidents,[10] specific instances of punitive transfer are known from biographies.

In fact a breakdown of the known transfer data by nationality shows at least one instance of leniency. Latvians are transferred to strict observation psychiatric hospitals significantly less frequently than other nationalities for whom transfer information is available (averaging 1.0 as opposed to 1.4; $\alpha=0.000$). If frequent transfer among ordinary or standard supervision hospitals is also viewed as punitive, the data support a finding of leniency for Belarussians and Estonians as well, since they are transferred significantly fewer times than the whole group (averaging 1.2 and 1.0 respectively, while the group mean is 1.6; $\alpha=0.10$ and 0.000).

A systematic and meaningful difference in transfers does emerge, however, if the data are subdivided by trial charge. Those dissidents whose first charge at first trial was 'political' in that they were charged with violations of the most frequently used political articles in our data, Article 70 (anti-Soviet agitprop), Article 190.1 (defamation of the Soviet system), treason, unauthorized border crossing, or hooliganism, were transferred to strict observation hospitals about three times as often as those committed administratively or not tried under these articles of the criminal code.[11] Transfers to special regime hospitals were signally frequent for those tried under agitation and propaganda charges, defamation, and illegal border crossing. This finding can be interpreted as evidence of punitive treatment of dissenters identified in their records as more 'political' than others. It is not consistent with a medical explanation of need for strict supervision, since those charged with border crossing offences or hooliganism are not necessarily characterized by physicians as 'especially dangerous recidivists' posing a risk to themselves and others and requiring strict observation.

DETERRENCE?

Western criminologists define deterrence as 'the omission of an act as a response to the perceived risk and fear of punishment for contrary behaviour'

(Gibbs, 1975, in Sheley, 1995:342), and they distinguish between general deterrence and specific deterrence. General deterrence dissuades others from undertaking proscribed behaviour which they have not yet carried out, while specific deterrence dissuades particular individuals from repeating prohibited behaviour in which they have already engaged (cf. Sheley, 1995:342).

The Soviet state, faced with the challenges posed by the dissident movement to social order and regime legitimacy, had many sanctions at its disposal to defend state interests against future encroachment, to deter protesters from continuing or initiating political activism or religious observance, and to compel nonconformists to desist, including arrests, interrogations, prison and camp terms, and psychiatric detention. But the effectiveness of such sanctions varied.

The Harvard Project found no effect of arrests on 'generalized political and social attitudes' (Inkeles and Bauer, 1968:37), all the more remarkable since their finding dates from the immediate postwar and Stalin era (1950–51). Although Inkeles and Bauer (1968) show that arrest had no particular effect on political attitude and ideology in the early fifties,[12] implying a surprising systematic failure of massive sanctions and terror to serve deterrence and compellance functions in this context, some research verifies that government sanctions in non-democratic regimes can and do work, in the sense that especially severe sanctions at least temporarily reduce the incidence of deterrable behaviour such as protest demonstrations or casualties from local political group violence (cf. Gupta, Singh and Sprague, 1994, in a study of mainly Latin American countries 1960–80).

However, the relationship between repression-as-deterrent and subsequent dissidence appears sensitive to prior and continuing political, economic and social conditions across nation-states as well as to the status and degree of organization/mobilization and the identity of dissident groups (see Figure 6.1). For example, recorded dissident acts may subside because standards change and formerly prohibited behaviour comes to represent permissible conduct, rather than necessarily only because heavy sanctions work.

Successive Soviet administrations may well have had a special interest in deterring uninvolved or marginally motivated Soviets from joining or increasing their participation in protest movements, not only because of the movement's basic challenge to authority and to societal beliefs but also because of its potential for exponential growth. In our data the average age of dissidents at first arrest tended to decline over the longer term, indicating recruitment of younger people. An increasingly youthful base for the movement is a powerful demographic concern,[13] since it would

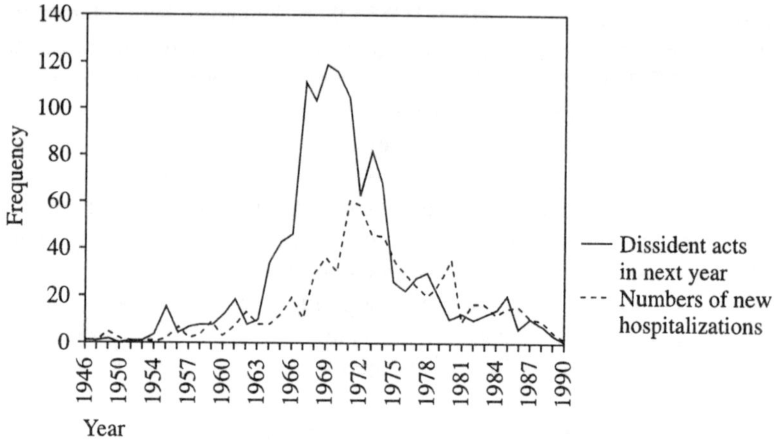

Figure 6.1 New Hospitalizations and Future Dissent

facilitate increasing frequency of dissident activity, possibly increasing intensity, and certainly could lengthen the life of the movement as well as enhance its further growth over time.

One deterrence objective may therefore have been to dissuade others from joining active political protesters, either as new or continuing participants. In retarding the growth of the dissident movement, especially after 1972, the successive Soviet administrations may have succeeded to some extent, since activity levels among this sample of psychiatric detainees dropped off as indicated in the graph of frequency of dissident acts seen in Chapter 5. Nevertheless a slight majority of their recorded dissident acts took place *after* the 1971–72 peak of repression (669/1233 known dated dissident acts or 54.3 per cent). The drop in recorded dissident acts is so precipitous after 1972 as to suggest that new individuals may not have been recruited into the dissident movement. We do not have direct measures of recruitment and can only provide a provisional answer here. However insofar as proportion of first arrests which postdate 1971–72 is an indicator of new participants in political protest and religious practice, our evidence warrants an *increase* and not a decrease potentially attributable to deterrent effects, since about 64 per cent of reported dissident acts took place after 1971–72.[14]

The fact that the average number of dissident acts per detainee is substantially lower for those *not* repeatedly hospitalized may be indirect evidence of a general deterrent effect of multiple detentions of others. Similarly the minute but still significant *negative* relationship at the individual level between all time hospitalized and sums of dissident acts ($r=-0.12$; $\alpha=0.015$) is consistent with a meaningful but quite small general deterrent effect of forced hospitalization.

Soviet governments may also have scored a small and partial success in deterrence at another level, the specific and individual, in that most political protesters and religious observers in our dataset stopped dissident activity after one hospitalization[15] insofar as our records can show, and never averaged more than two or three dissident acts. To what degree this should be attributed to deterrent or compellance policies of the administration is a matter of theory and interpretation. One political hospitalization may represent a threshold beyond which most nonconformists would find intolerably hazardous the combined informal social and official political forces of job loss, housing confiscation, residence permit problems, social stigma, divorce, or rehospitalization and imprisonment.

But if this evidence is consistent with a partial success of general or specific deterrence of dissent, it is in some sense a Pyrrhic victory for the Soviet governments. Specific individual-level deterrence/compellance findings are bimodal. *A core of persistent, highly motivated political challengers emerges from these data,* and in some cases received an embarrassing amount of world press coverage. Repeatedly sanctioned by prison camp or psychiatric hospitalization terms, they actually *increased* their dissident activity after release.

For comparison, in the whole dataset psychiatric detainees averaged only two dissident acts. Including only those dissenters for whom date of at least one dissident act is known, for comparability with the camp and detentions findings, detainees whose activities are reasonably well-documented typically averaged a total of about three (3.36) documented dissident acts over the course of their participation in political protest. But those freed after a second camp term went on to commit *6.4 more* dissident acts on average after their release. Those released from a second court-ordered hospitalization committed on average almost seven (6.8) subsequent dissident acts, and those freed from a second administrative detention committed seven. That is, this core of highly motivated political and religious nonconformists is not deterrable, at least at this level of state sanction or except perhaps by death. A camp sentence is marginally more effective as a dissuader, maybe by virtue of being a debilitator, than either mode of psychiatric repression. These dissidents responded to repeated punishment with even more dissident behaviour. (See Table 6.6: Dissident Acts per Person after Incarceration.)

This finding implies that, as in nuclear deterrence, would-be dissuaders may encounter undeterrable or uncompellable individuals whose political,

Table 6.6 Dissident Acts per Person after Incarceration

Incarceration	*Mean*	*Mode*	*Median*	*Maximum*	*Minimum*
2nd Admin. Detention	7.0	4.0	5.0	16.0	1.0
2nd Court Detention	6.8	2.0	6.0	16.0	2.0
2nd Camp Term	6.4	3.0	4.0	16.0	2.0
All data	2.0	0.0	1.0	16.0	0.0
All data for which dissident acts are known	3.4	1.0	2.0	16.0	1.0

religious or ethical objectives are so highly valued that no conceivable threat is large enough to counterbalance pursuit of their cherished goals. Individuals holding such objectives cannot be dissuaded from seeking to achieve them.[16] It follows that a class of undeterrable acts may exist, which has a prior probability of virtually 1.0 and therefore will not be prevented by application of any state penalty, however monstrous. Some dissident behaviour in the Soviet period may fall into this class.

That hospitalizations were targeted on most persistent dissenters and yet dissident behaviour actually increased after hospitalization demonstrates unambiguous failure of specific deterrence with respect to this subset of all dissidents.[17] This finding is counter-intuitive, but credible on the basis of biographical information. It is relevant to the rationality hypothesis, since it implies application of deliberately calculated state sanctions against a thinking adversary.

Deterrence failure in these data is also supported by correlation analyses which are otherwise unintelligible. Using individuals as cases, number of arrests correlates significantly and *positively* with the sum of all known dissident acts in a linear measure ($r=0.40$; $\alpha=0.000$). If arrests worked as a deterrent, other things such as timing of dissident acts being equal, numbers of arrests should be *negatively* related to sums of dissident acts. Similarly another measure of repression, total numbers of court-ordered incarcerations, correlates weakly but significantly and *positively* with sums of dissident acts ($r=0.22$; $\alpha=0.000$) which would not be expected in deterrence terms unless most dissident acts *preceded* trials, which in these data they do not. In a time series analysis in which a year is a case, frequency of new administrative detentions correlates moderately and again positively ($r=0.63$, $\alpha=0.000$) with dissident acts in the subsequent year, suggesting that administrative hospitalizations stimulate rather than suppress new waves of protest.

Given that administrative detentions are the most typical hospitalization

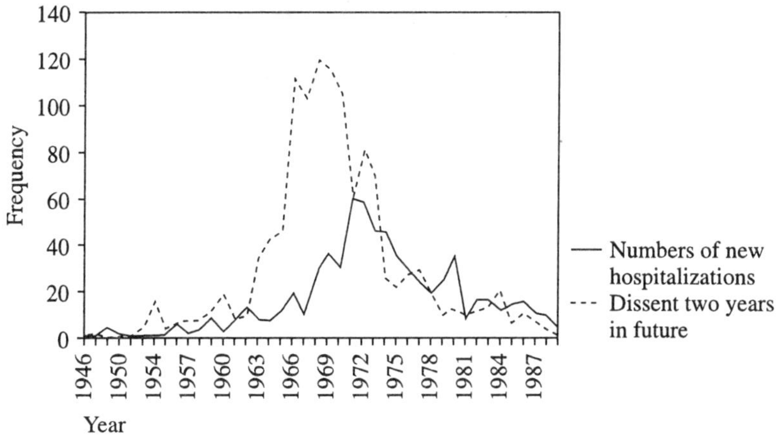

Figure 6.2 New Hospitalizations and Dissent Two Years in Future

for dissidents in these data, and given that administrative commitments lasted on average about two years, a two-year time span might be required for detentions to become widely known as their victims are released, and then to serve as a deterrent to subsequent dissident behaviour. But again, with this lead time incorporated, no deterrent effect is shown in the correlations. Frequency of all hospitalizations correlates significantly and *positively* with numbers of dissident acts two years in future ($r=0.55$; $\alpha=0.000$; see Figure 6.2).

Identical statistical results are obtained from a correlation of frequency of new court detentions per year with frequency of dissident acts in the *following* year (cf. Figure 6.1 above). Frequency of all new hospitalizations is associated even more strongly *positively* with the numbers of dissident acts only one year in future than two years' in future ($r = 0.67$; $\alpha = 0.000$).

If agents of the state are presumed to act rationally, it could be argued that the state resorted to psychiatric methods of deterrence of dissent only after more usual consequences of criminalizing and curtailing nonconformity, such as prison camp terms, failed to reduce dissenting behaviour or activities prompting arrest. We should then find differences in recidivism after hospitalization as opposed to other incarceration. If this hypothesis is correct, on average those who served camp terms should have committed more dissident acts after release than those subject to political hospitalization. In our dataset of Soviet repressed dissidents 1940–81 ($n=2749$), those surviving a prison camp term on average undertook 1.5 dissident acts while those subjected to either administrative or criminal commitment on average had participated in 1.1 dissident acts. These findings are consistent with rational resort to psychiatric detention in some cases after labour camps failed to smother the dissident movement, but would require replication with more detailed time parameters to confirm.

Indications of rational use of sanctions as deterrents can be found in the numbers of prior arrests for those compulsorily hospitalized as opposed to those confined to camps. Systematic differences among numbers of prior arrests for those sent to labour camps, or hospitalized via either criminal trials or administrative procedures, may connote rational selection of appropriate penalties. In the dataset of 2749 Soviet nonconformists, on average those sent to prison camps were arrested 1.22 times before incarceration, roughly as frequently as those hospitalized by the courts at 1.10 arrests before detention. However those subject to administrative detention had been arrested on average 1.55 times before hospitalization. These numbers are coherent with application of administrative hospitalization to protesters whose behaviour is seen as less challenging, hence less damaging if repeated, as well as with use of administrative detention against those who would be difficult to prosecute.

The search for deterrent effects on dissent in several measures of state repression and with one- and two-year time leads yields remarkably little corroboration of any deterrent effects. All of the stronger correlations are in the wrong direction; that is, they denote a reinforcing and not a deterring effect of psychiatric repression.[18]

One explanation could be that deterrence does not work in the short term, if it works at all. The time parameters could function such that repression in the short term ignites increased opposition, as we confirm in several measures here. The newly invigorated movement then may succeed, or may fail to gather appropriate resources to maintain its struggle over time, and is then at risk of being dispersed if heavy sanctions are maintained, the general pattern obtaining in Latin America in Gupta *et al.* In the Soviet case, psychiatric suppression did not crush the movement, which instead experienced a resurgence in the mid-eighties, and was not met with consistently heavy sanctions[19] but with increased scope of free activity and collapse of central authority under glasnost. Instead of squelching nationalist and other political and religious activists, psychiatric repression may actually have propagated dissent along several vectors including from father to son.[20]

SUMMARY

Rational state strategies for defusing dissent are in evidence in this chapter. These strategies, in a number of measures employed here, failed. Deterrence of dissent for the most part failed, both at the specific and general level. Not only do we find that persistent dissenters amplify their activities after repeated hospitalizations, but some evidence suggests that hospitalizations in general may have stimulated new waves of dissident acts. Ordinary regime hospitals were the foundation of deliberate punitive use of psychiatry. Resort to psychiatric hospitalization after prison or camp terms have failed to deter is one indication in these data of rational use of punitive psychiatry. Disproportional penalties, in hospital transfers and in court-ordered detention time, for politicized transgressions is another indication. That the riskiest sorts of dissident behaviour were those challenging state norms and Party values, creating opposition groups, and making unauthorized use of the electoral process also implies rationality on the part of agents of the state, since such behaviour risks the survival of the state.

7 Legal and Political Developments in the Gorbachev and Yeltsin Administrations and After*

> In advanced industrialized societies and in modern, bureaucratic and welfare states, the institutions of violence generally operate more covertly. A whole array of educational, social welfare, medical, psychiatric, and legal experts collaborate in the management and control of sentiments and practices that threaten the stability of the state and the fragile consensus on which it claims to base its legitimacy.
>
> (Scheper-Hughes, 1992:221)

Political use of FSU psychiatric hospitals in the mid-nineties has virtually dropped off the horizon of reported post-Soviet affairs, displaced by more proximal, typically and traumatically Third World public concerns about the exploding inflation rate, bondage to international lending agencies, the growth of the second economy, the resurgent power of organized crime, public safety, disparate risks of outside encroachment, internal war and conflict in the near abroad. These emergency circumstances, with potentially global repercussions in world markets and on immigration, may eclipse the human rights concerns of the calmer seventies and eighties and overshadow the psychiatric reform efforts of the late eighties and nineties. Precisely because the reforms largely failed to redesign the underlying structures which made psychiatric abuse possible, this phenomenon could recur, should it serve the purposes of executive or other governmental agencies. A review of relevant Soviet and Russian law can illustrate why this potential still exists, even after the splintering of the Communist Party and the collapse of the Union.

* The author would like to acknowledge her debt for background information for this chapter to the authors of a number of analyses, summaries and interpretations not publicly released or circulated. Due to the confidential nature of the materials, they cannot be formally cited.

LEGAL DEVELOPMENTS

Evolution of Soviet Mental Health Law and Procedures

The concept of legal responsibility for potentially criminal behaviour, or 'imputability', was codified as early as 1903, in Article 39 of the Penal Code of the Tsarist government (Baker, 1987:60) and later incorporated in Soviet law. As defined negatively, non-imputability encompassed both psychiatric and medical criteria: first, those found non-imputable must have failed to understand the nature of their behaviour and have been unable to control it; and second, their condition must have been brought about by illness, unconsciousness, or mental retardation caused by birth defects or disease.

The 'Instructions on the Certification of the Mentally Ill' issued by the People's Commissariat of Justice in 1918 apparently comprise the first specific Soviet mental health law. A Decree of the Council of People's Commissars created the Peoples Commissariat of Public Health; in May 1918 the special psychiatric commission developed a neuropsychiatric section including the prominent Soviet psychiatrist P.B. Gannushkin (Babayan, 1985:40). At the same time 'Guiding Principles of Criminal Procedure' were issued. These regulations were followed by the 8 May 1919 Statute on Psychiatric Expert Examinations, in which the Peoples Commissariat of Health specified conditions for commitment for evaluation, and related regulations covering psychiatric practice including the 12 December 1919 'Leading Principles of Criminal Law'.

According to these early regulations, non-imputable people not only could not be penalized (article 14 of the 1919 law), a protection which had to be repeated in the 1992 Russian law, but also at that time could not even be formally investigated by the judiciary. Cases were dismissed from the peoples court on this basis (Babayan, 1985:20). Redrafted 'in a matter of a few years', these initial 'Guiding Principles' were so broad that they allowed any perceived mental irregularity to result in hospitalization (Babayan, 1985:21).

New Criminal Codes and Codes of Criminal Procedure reportedly were drafted in 1922 and 1923 respectively (Baker, 1987), amalgamating the 1903 imputability concepts into one blurred notion of non-imputability as mental disturbance. The 1924 Code of Criminal Procedures advanced 'medical measures' for those deemed non-imputable; Article 19 of the 1924 Criminal Code extended vulnerability to compulsory medical measures and other punitive procedures to those as young as 16, formerly not at risk.

In 1926 a new Criminal Code of the RSFSR was published, which was to remain in effect for 34 years. It reiterated that the non-imputable were not subject to criminal penalties, including even those who were sane at the time of commission of some offence but later became ill at the time of sentencing. This latter group could be penalized after recovery, as in the US. No protection applied to those who had acted under the influence of drugs or alcohol (Baker, 1987:62), as is generally also the case in the US.

Article 6 of the Code of Criminal Procedure provides that criminal cases can be dropped if the act in question has 'lost its socially dangerous character' (Baker, 1987:74), or the person in question is no longer 'socially dangerous' (Berman, 1966:254), acknowledging overtly the politically and temporally dependent nature of perceived social danger, and providing a legal basis for large-scale release or amnesty of detainees. It is not accidental that among those detainees examined by the US Delegation to USSR mental hospitals in 1989 was one person whom Soviet psychiatrists evaluated as then exhibiting 'no clinical disorder *now that the political situation in the Soviet Union has changed*' (emphasis added; eds Shore and Keith, 1990:22).

Soviet mental health law included no clear provisions for release from psychiatric hospitals before the 1938 regulations on early discharge by court order. Compulsory treatment and hospitalization were not separately defined until then (Babayan, 1985:21) and were not well dealt with in the law until January 1988. Even at the end of the Soviet era the mechanism of *release* by court order did not function smoothly; some dissenters could not be discharged from special psychiatric hospitals despite their psychiatrists' readiness to do so, because the required court order was not forthcoming.

By 1942 directives on psychiatric examinations had been issued by the Peoples Commissariat of Justice, Internal Affairs, the Procurator's Office, and the Peoples Commissariat of Public Health. These directives specified in Article 8 that although there were no *degrees* of responsibility, not all mental illness necessarily rendered its victims non-responsible. Thus not all disease implied non-imputability or protection from criminal penalties in Soviet law (Babayan, 1985:22). This distinction reopens the option of applying criminal penalties to the mentally ill and helps explain why dissidents found non-imputable have nonetheless been subject to other penalties.

The 1954 Instructions on psychiatric evaluations allowed for *in absentia* examinations (Baker, 1987:462–9, citing Morozov and Kalashnik, 1970:ch. 1:5), but these were to be exceptional, rather than the frequent practice that they had evolved into by the 1960s. *In absentia* examinations did not go the way of the Union, but were still provided for in the 1992 Russian Federation law.

Major changes in Soviet mental health regulations, laws and directives took place in the seventies, late eighties, and early nineties. Serbsky and the Ministry of Health (MoH) rather than the more liberal Academy of Sciences Institute for the State and Law reportedly drafted some of the post-1988 legislation, such as the July 1990 version which appeared in *Meditsinskaya Gazeta* but which failed to be brought to the Supreme Soviet. The 1992 Law of the Russian Federation on Psychiatric Care resulted from revisions of the 1991 draft due to the combined efforts of MoH, Serbsky, IPA or at least the IPA's Yuri Savenko, and other reformers, chief among them Professor S.V. Borodin and Dr S.V. Polubinskaya of the Institute of the State and Law, as well as visiting members of the World Psychiatric Association group. The draft was enacted as law of the Russian Federation, 2 July 1992.

If the reports of Serbsky and MoH influence on mental health regulations are accurate, they imply that in the continuing struggle over the use of law to reform or defend psychiatry, lawmaking in the early nineties was still subject to more conservative forces in the field, which is reflected in the content of the 1992 law.

Some potential milestones in the 1992 law proscribe punitive use of medicine (art. 10(3)) and allow compulsory treatment by court order only. But rights to refuse treatment or to be treated only after written consent to particular measures evidently do not exist for the involuntarily committed (art. 11(1) and art. 12(1) unless art. 29 applies).

The central provisions of these recent laws and guidelines are considered below as they apply to the contemporary procedures of administrative and criminal commitments and as they featured in the larger legal reform of psychiatry before and after the implosion of the Union.

Administrative/Civil Commitment

Emergency hospitalization in ordinary psychiatric hospitals of those not accused of criminal acts was carried out under Article 258 of the Civil Procedure Code of the RSFSR (Bonnie, 1990a:125; Babayan, 1985) and until 1988 'was regulated only by unpublished administrative guidelines' of the Ministry of Health, beyond judicial review or the rule of law (Bonnie, 1990b:326, 335; 1995:10). Such administrative or 'civil' commitments could result if 'family, trade union, public organizations, a procurator, a guardianship agency, or a psychiatric institute' requested a competence examination even of a resisting person (Babayan, 1985:302) – and some commitments resulting from this process were *recorded* as voluntary, thereby restricting opportunities for diagnostic review. As late as the 1992 law on psychiatric care, 'officials' and 'other citizens' could request examinations (art. 25(2)). The same groups and individuals can apply to have findings expunged, though the literature shows little evidence of success in this endeavour. Article 51 of the Code of Civil Procedure stipulated that procedures for examinations be established by the Ministry of Health 'in coordination with the USSR Supreme Court, the Procurator's office, the Ministry of the Interior, and other agencies' (Babayan, 1985:303). This provision created several other lines of influence on findings of insanity from judicial, executive, other governmental, and Party forces, as noted in Chapter 1.

The 1961 Instructions on involuntary civil commitments from the Ministry of Public Health (No. 04-14-32, 9 October 1961) were superseded by the 1971 Instruction of the Ministry of Public Health (No. 06-14-43, 26 August 1971) on Urgent Hospitalization of the Socially Dangerous Mentally Ill. The 1971 Instruction on civil commitment repeated the 1962 definition of 'socially dangerous', making it clear that this term refers to conduct and expressions disturbing to the political and social status quo, including 'incorrect aggressive behaviour towards certain persons, organizations and institutions', cloudy and subjective language virtually identical to that appearing in the Ministry of Public Health Instruction No. 04–14/32 (1962) on forcible commitment. The 'socially dangerous' acts criterion for involuntary commitment is reiterated without definition in Article 13(1) of the 1992 Law of the Russian Federation.

The 1971 Instructions were set aside in 1988 when the Presidium of the USSR Supreme Soviet ratified one of the most significant new laws to date, the previously mentioned 'Statute on Conditions and Procedures for the Provision of Psychiatric Assistance',[1] accompanied and partially undermined by the USSR Ministry of Public Health regulations of 21 March 1988 (Decree 225, Appendix 17 'Provisional Guidelines on the Procedure for Prompt Hospitalization of the Mentally Ill'; cf. Bonnie, 1990b:326–7 fn.). Although the 1988 Provisional Guidelines did not repeat the 1971 language on organizations and institutions, the Statute of 5 January 1988 does include a paragraph permitting involuntary psychiatric assessments of those who 'violate the standards of socialist conduct'. Since this entire phrase constitutes multiple layers of judgments and interpretations defining socialist values, socialist conduct, appropriate standards, and behaviour constituting violations, this language emphasizes the breadth of discretion and the potential scope for abuse granted even in later Soviet law in determining who warrants hospitalization.

The 1988 statute provided that those detained now have a right to an attorney before and during internment. A right of appeal against confinement was also delineated, though individuals may not be informed of these rights. Appeals, however, are forwarded to higher-ranking mental health professionals who presumably are likely to support their subordinates or validate their own prior conclusions (Podrabinek in van Voren, 1989:98).

Criminal Commitments

The Codes of Criminal Law and Procedure of the constituent republics and now the states of the former Union allow involuntary psychiatric evaluation and compulsory criminal commitment to psychiatric institutions. Criminal commitments were regulated by 14 February 1967 'Instruction on Compulsory Treatment of the Mentally Ill Who Have Committed Socially Dangerous Acts', then by 27 October 1970 Ministry of Public Health Instruction 'Forensic Psychiatric Examination in the USSR', and more recently by the already mentioned 21 March 1988 'Provisional Guidelines on the Procedures for Coercive and Other Measures of a Medical Nature in Regard to Persons with Mental Disorders Who Have Committed Especially Socially Dangerous Acts' (Appendix 18, Decree 225, USSR Ministry of Public Health).

The 1967 Instructions did not define social danger, despite the fact that only individuals who 'needed' treatment and posed a societal danger however defined could be hospitalized under Soviet law. The March 1988 Provisional Guidelines from the MoH introduced some memorably equivocal instructions requiring judgment of social danger:

- ordinary or 'standard' psychiatric hospitals were appropriate for those *not socially dangerous* who needed treatment [though it is unclear why outpatient treatment would not suffice for at least some of them];
- intensified or 'reinforced' observation regimes in [selected wards of] ordinary psychiatric hospitals were recommended for those having committed a 'socially dangerous act' but not posing a 'special danger to the community', although such people may be 'nonaggressively dangerous';
- strict observation in special psychiatric hospitals was indicated for those presenting a special danger because of the type of socially dangerous acts carried out.

After hospitalization, for those committed via criminal trial, a judge's order was required for release or transfer to a less restrictive hospital. This is apparently still the case in Russia after the new 1992 law. Thus judges to a degree controlled who was transferred or released, since a psychiatrist's favourable opinion was necessary but not sufficient. Depending on circumstances, judges might be reluctant either to accept or to set aside a medical opinion of a psychiatrist, even though the question of legal responsibility cannot be answered by a psychiatrist and medical testimony does not determine the outcome of the case in law (Bonnie, 1995:14).

Judges may have had political pressures brought to bear on them to reach a particular finding. Since judges were subject to Party discipline in the Soviet period (certainly in higher courts the assessors who heard cases with judges were 'elected' on advice of the relevant Party organization), the Party was a major source of potential political pressures in prominent trials or hearings.

For transfer, a psychiatric opinion that a case should be reviewed sufficed to obtain a court review. Thus, the role psychiatrists played in releases and transfer was pivotal. Yet psychiatrists, as generally state employees, were subject to a variety of political pressures and, like judges, could also be urged to make a positive or negative recommendation.

If the commission of recommending psychiatrists did not reach a straightforward finding on sanity, family members or other interested parties at least in principle could file to have forcible hospitalization ended (Code of Criminal Procedure 412). However neither the 1967 nor the 1988 guidelines created enabling regulations which define procedures for these appeals or protect those petitioning from retaliation, and thereby convert this right into more than a legal fiction. The US Delegation in 1989 unearthed only ten appeals out of 71 000 hospitalizations in Moscow and vicinity during 1988, or approximately 1.4 one-hundredths of one per cent. Two years later the WPA found only two successful appeals against hospitalization or registration in the Moscow region, following a mere 24 cases filed out of more than 80 000 people annually hospitalized or added to the register in the metropolitan area (WPA, 1991:20). Though these figures indicate that the appeal rate doubled in two years, in doubling it reached only 3 one-hundredths of one per cent. Successful appeals were a microscopic 2/80 000 or 2.5 thousandths of one per cent. So at least in the capital in 1989 and 1991 the appeals procedure was not operational (eds Keith and Shore, 1989:6).

In other developments relevant to criminal commitments, the USSR Council of Ministers had composed an apparently competing draft of regulations 'On Psychiatric Care in the USSR' contrasting with the version then under amendment by the Supreme Soviet's Committee on Legislation (Reddaway, 1991:45–6); Reddaway reports that as of 1991 the Council of Ministers draft had not been published. A draft of new legislation on reform of psychiatry circulating in 1991 failed to make two central changes, in that it still did not provide for hearings on request, and could not extend any legal remedy for a false or damaging diagnosis itself.

RECENT DEVELOPMENTS

Draft legislation circulating in 1991 and enacted in 1992 as the Law of the Russian Federation on Psychiatric Care was directed to some of the concerns the 1988 regulations evoked. The 1988 legislation and guidelines may have been hastily composed to be available for the 1989 arrival of the US Delegation visiting mental health institutions and to enhance the probability of readmission of the All-Union Society of Psychiatrists and Neurologists (later Federation of Societies of Psychiatrists and Narcologists) to the WPA, which was achieved conditionally 18 October 1989.

This new Law on Psychiatric Care enacted by the Russian Federation Supreme Soviet in 1992 outlawed punitive medicine, disavowed diagnoses based solely on political or religious opinions (art. 10(1)), reinforced pre-existing rights to legal counsel and to a choice of psychiatrists, provided for forcible treatment solely by court order, and subordinated Russian mental health regulations to the terms of any relevant international agreements Russia signed (art. 2(4)). Any surgical or other irreversible procedures were to be conducted only with the consent of the subject.[2]

Meaningful weaknesses in the 1992 Law of the Russian Federation on Psychiatric Care still make possible political abuse under the terms of the statute. As Bonnie notes in his introduction to the translation of the 1992 law, exactly how to define 'persons suffering from mental disorders' remains a crucial question, since rights are restricted beginning at that point. Definitional discretion[3] remains a vulnerability in psychiatric practice, since the 1992 law allows in some cases for this determination to be reached by as few as one psychiatrist, on the basis of examinations which could be requested for plainly non-medical reasons by officials or other citizens under Article 25(2).

The 1992 law does make appeals to courts more of a reality than previously. Among issues subject to court review are restrictions on type of work (art. 6), and the judge's decision to order commitment (art. 35(3)). However no provision seems to exist for reviews of mental status on request, and no ready remedy for damaging diagnoses, harm to reputation, or personal injury sustained in treatment, and so on, is available.

On close scrutiny, administrative/civil and criminal commitment procedures for dissidents in the Soviet period – as perhaps for everyone committed in the Soviet period – show state design for punishment (Reddaway,

1972; Oleszczuk, 1988a:114) and circumscription of the rights of individuals to defend themselves or extricate themselves from the psychiatric gulag once caught up in it. Oleszczuk (1988a) notes that 'chastisement' is the first of several purposes of sentencing mentioned in Article 20 of the RSFSR Criminal Code as amended to July 1965 (Berman, 1966:151). Arbitrary interpretations of social danger and 'helplessness' have allowed idiosyncratic criminal convictions and administrative detentions. When convenient, both criminal and administrative/civil procedures could be terminated administratively, bypassing provisions for appeals and short-circuiting other legal rights. Mitigating factors liberally provided for in Article 38 of the Criminal Code were often ignored in the case of Soviet dissidents, despite Article 20's final hortatory comment that 'punishment does not have the purpose of causing physical suffering' (*loc.cit.*). Reports of injurious administration of drugs, inadequate access to exercise or sanitation, and other anecdotal evidence make it clear that Article 20 has been widely disregarded in the cases of psychiatric prisoners. The WPA concluded in 1991 that psychiatric practice remained largely 'unreviewed and unreviewable'.

The Law and Psychiatric Measures against Dissidents: Connections between the Procuracy and the Courts

Structural – long-term and functional – connections between the procuracy and the courts were influential in determining the fate of Soviet political and religious activists. These connections existed for a variety of reasons:

1. By law the procuracy serves overlapping, and in some cases, contradictory functions. In interactions with the courts, the procuracy was obligated to prosecute, guard the legality of preliminary investigations, oversee the legality of court decisions and sentencing, and review the propriety of treatment of prisoners.
2. Judges may cooperate with investigators and procurators. In a study of links between the procuracy and the judiciary, Solomon (1987:549) found a decline in acquittals in Soviet criminal cases to about 0.05 per cent or fewer in the late 1980s, which he attributed to cooperation of judges with the perceived needs of investigators and the procurators. From 1940 until at least 1980 acquittals and returns for supplemental evidence were seen as failures for the procuracy.
3. The KGB maintained its own contacts within both the courts and the procuracy (Waller, 1994:283), which could be mobilized for local or more widespread purposes.

These relationships and perceptions are consequential for dissidents prosecuted under the criminal code, since they imply a similar cooperation of the judiciary with the procuracy for court-ordered psychiatric commitments, with an ensuing reduction in the observance of individual rights. There is no necessary reason why new laws on psychiatric commitment would or could undermine this tendency because it follows from a larger structure of personal and professional networks.

The relationship of the procuracy to the courts sets up conditions in which systemic failures of accountability are likely. To indicate only the most obvious, while the procuracy is charged with conducting legal discovery and prosecuting believed law violators, it also bears the responsibility for the legality of the investigation – including the responsibility for supervising *itself* – with attendant conflicts of interest.

Soviet Legality, Law and Practice; Post-Soviet Uncertainty

Of the several divergences between Soviet law and Western law, three are most meaningful for human rights: the place of the individual in the law, the relationship of the individual to the state, and the latitude given to discretion in the two systems. While Western legal systems in general circumscribe or purport to circumscribe official discretion, and do significantly restrict discretion of judges while criticizing arbitrary use of discretion among police officers and prosecutors, Soviet socialist legality relied on discretion at many levels (Baker, 1987).

Soviet socialist legality, focused on the interests of the collective (the state), historically has not conceived of a right of individuals to criticize the regime or the larger society, at least until the Gorbachev administration, and then only within set limits.[4] Despite this focus on the collective rather than the individual, our All-Union data do show a commitment to the ideals of socialist legality as they affect individual dissidents, in that the data illustrate across decades a battle of authority in which the procuracy and lower courts cooperated in some cases to protect dissidents' rights, opposing higher levels of the judiciary (de Boer, 1982 *passim*; Herzen, 1976). In the struggle for dominance some sentences are commuted or quashed, cases dismissed or retried, trials ended, defendants in rare instances acquitted,[5] pardoned or amnestied, and charges thrown out for lack of evidence at all levels (de Boer, 1982).

But the legal system itself is flexible. The appeal mechanism is adaptable and on occasion may have been used to *increase* sentences, as in the case of Revolt Pimenev. Pimenev, a Leningrad physicist, was arrested for distributing anti-Soviet materials, received a heavier sentence on appeal, and paradoxically, was then released early (de Boer *et al.*, 1982; Medvedev, 1980:16). Bonnie (1990a, 1990b:331) found in the 1989 visit of the US Delegation to Soviet mental hospitals that most commonly the requirements of Soviet law had *not* been met in the cases of individuals they interviewed.

The Soviet understanding of individual rights as contingent on the rights of a reified larger society contrasts with the 'natural' rights of individuals as understood in Western law, and results in an interpretation of human rights in which so-called positive rights (or needs, as of housing, food, and so on) have primacy in the USSR while negative rights (which individuals enjoy unless the state intervenes to restrict, for example, the press, or free practice of religion) predominate in the US view. In light of these divergent understandings and priorities in the two states, the many provisions of Soviet and post-Soviet mental health laws and rulings on civil/administrative and criminal commitments which parallel those of the US, if we assume that Soviet administrative commitment is analogous to US civil commitment, may seem startling. This similarity implies that even irregularly industrialized states with disparate economic structures, dissimilar decision-making systems and judiciaries reflecting varying schools of law may draft comparable laws.

It is also noteworthy in East–West comparisons that all mental health regulations which allow involuntary commitment or commitment by others whose interests may not coincide with those of the detainee are prone to deliberate abuse, misapplication, and error. This vulnerability is acute in cases of rules with emergency or time-pressure provisions. As a guarantee against abuse, standards of actual practice are more crucial than the terms of statutes, for at least two reasons: one, information on new statutes may become known only after time lags, or in the case of Soviet administrative hospitalization, may never have been governed by published guidelines until recently (cf. Bonnie); and two, compliance diminishes with effective distance from enforcement agencies, if any. Compliance as a function of enforcement is especially problematical in Russia, Foster concludes, now that 'No concrete mechanisms exist for enforcing laws in the country' (McInerny, 1994).

An authoritarian tradition, evolution of Soviet decision-making systems, and the distribution of power in the USSR, as later in Russia, have stunted the powers of the courts and retarded the growth of separation of powers between the legislature and the executive (cf. Bonnie). No meaningful judicial review of USSR or Russian legislation can be found. Certainly the Soviet Supreme Court has not had the power to review legislation.

With a few stunning exceptions, the judiciary dares not rein in the administration either.[6] Both the legislature and executive can usually circumvent the judiciary; judicial authority over the executive is variable and often easily flouted even in more normal times. As if the institutional environment were not discouraging enough for the prospects for effective legal reform of psychiatry, in the mid-nineties it is not clear which constitutional framework is in effect. Since Boris Yeltsin dissolved the Supreme Soviet in September 1993, ruling thereafter by decree, it is unclear whether the laws promulgated previously by the Supreme Soviet are in effect, or only the decrees of the President (Foster in McInerny, 1994).

While new legal guarantees may be a necessary precondition for the emergence of Western-style human rights of individuals, they will not suffice alone. In some respects the phenomenon of political use of mental hospitals escapes the power of courts to remedy. The courts cannot obviate the fact that psychiatric detention may continue on occasion to satisfy certain executive or other governmental needs. Illustrating the powerlessness of the courts in some circumstances, in periods of crackdowns, compulsory hospitalization and treatment have been allowed under emergency decree,[7] as in May 1969, even in cases of individuals whose original court ruling for 'compulsory measures of a medical nature' had already been *reversed*. The May 1969 decree allowed local idiosyncratic and 'preventive' interpretations of 'social danger' to facilitate psychiatric confinement of anyone detained (US Senate, 1973:24) and seemingly specifies neither medical nor legal rationales for hospitalization (Segal, 1976:269).

POLITICAL DEVELOPMENTS

Soviet human rights observances expanded in the Gorbachev administration. After Gorbachev came to power in 1985, sweeping legal reforms decriminalized some political and religious practices which formerly resulted in arrest and occasional psychiatric hospitalization. The formerly widely employed political Article 190.1 prohibiting defamation of the Soviet system was struck from the Criminal Code of the RSFSR – although Article 64, treason, was not. Article 70, which criminalized anti-Soviet agitation and propaganda, was rewritten to prohibit only advocating the overthrow of the Soviet system. The USSR Supreme Court set aside many convictions for political or religious offences.

The liberalization beginning in 1987 resulted in a sharp reduction in numbers of KGB and Procuracy officers who targeted dissidents. Consequently political arrests and detentions diminished, and political prisoners were freed in large numbers, including one group in the late eighties which comprised the largest single release since the 1950s (Amnesty International, 1989). Systematic waves of new political arrests and psychiatric detentions subsided by the early nineties to vanishingly small levels, though local officials' requests made by phone for hospitalization of 'complainers' and political opponents can be found as late as 1989. In the early nineties, although an occasional new case can be seen, psychiatric detentions were essentially zero. Dramatic changes in the practice of psychiatry entailed releases of large numbers of those incarcerated in psychiatric wards, although expectations of prompt transfers of politicals out of SPHs to OPHs were frustrated. Some sources note many releases from as early as 1983 onwards (Van Voren, 1989:10). By 1989 the Chief Psychiatrist for the USSR Ministry of Health reported 2000 individuals released since 1987 from special psychiatric institutions, after newly created Health Ministry commission reviews of cases from earlier administrations indicated that hospitalization was unnecessary (Amnesty International, 1989:4).

Real liberalization began in the USSR after Gorbachev had been in office less than two years, in January of 1987. At that time political authority was withdrawn from a variety of activities, and thereafter a new and more liberal emigration decree was released. A February 1987 partial amnesty for political prisoners, which did not include psychiatric detainees, was followed in June by a new broader amnesty decreed by the USSR Supreme Soviet.[8] Public opposition to the new regime ceased being equated with anti-Soviet behaviour. New leniency appeared in October, with a continuation of the dual-track policy which was hard on the issue of political prisoners and soft on specifics, as in the Sakharov case (Oleszczuk, 1988b).

An apparently contradictory dual-track policy of increasing latitude for dissent while attempting to maintain societal control was seen as a manifestation of Gorbachev's need for strict legal authority over the bureaucracy, to permit economic development and political modernization. At the same time legal countermeasures against dissent, including use of administrative compulsory hospitalizations, continued to be invoked for citizens inadequately cognizant of their duties to the state (Oleszczuk, 1988b). The government prohibited unauthorized demonstrations and meetings in July 1988 (Knight, 1990:21); and punitive use of psychiatry continued, at low levels, under perestroika. Despite ample evidence, as late as December 1987 the General Secretary denied 'political crime' existed in the USSR, implying it certainly could not have been penalized with hospitalization.

Yet under Gorbachev the tactic of psychiatric detention was used, selectively, to discourage illegal emigration, to influence elections, to add to the flagging efforts to squelch nationalist movements, and to discourage the society-wide creation of new political fronts and parties. The detention of Valeria Novodvorskaya, leader of the Democratic Union, provides an example of instrumental use of psychiatry to attempt assassination of a political movement.

A campaign against corruption in psychiatry, bribery, diagnoses to elude penalties for crime, and so on, can be traced to prominent arrests at Serbsky and elsewhere in 1985. Both these arrests and the subsequent press campaign were limited in that they usually pinpointed specific culpable individuals without necessarily indicting a broader system of psychiatric suppression.

In assessing the significance of alterations in procedure and substance of psychiatric repression, Reddaway concludes 'This [psychiatric] system is in no way essential to the Soviet system of repression' and thus might easily be eliminated without threatening the stability of medical means of control. In fact, he saw the firing of a handful of corrupt psychiatrists in 1987 as a possible start to the process of removing the more visible signs of the mechanism of repression while leaving its function intact (July, 1987 (15–16):7–14). Podrabinek, even less optimistically, held that perestroika bypassed not only the modified and strict regime psychoprisons but also the ordinary regime hospitals as well (Van Voren, 1989).

The Soviet press, subdued for decades on the topic of psychiatric abuse, openly criticized political use of psychiatry from 1987 onwards and began to discuss 'global' values and the ethical values of 'world civilization', admitting the possibility of Western liberal definitions of human rights and Western conventions about the practice of psychiatry in the interests of individuals. The open debate over punitive psychiatry spread through the media, including *Izvestia*, *Kommunist*, *Kommunisticheskaya Pravda*, *Literaturnaya Gazeta*, *Meditsinskaya Gazeta*, *Moscow News*, *Ogonyok*, and *Sobesednik* (Reddaway, 1991:43). As Reddaway observes, among central actors working for reform were the Foreign Ministry under Shevardnadze, the office of Alexander Yakovlev, the Academy of Science's Institute of the State and Law, and even the KGB.

Professional psychiatric associations which for some years had maintained interest in Soviet human rights compliance, including the American Psychiatric Association and the professional societies of the FRG and Great Britain, as well as some individuals in the World Psychiatric Association, participated in this debate and in some cases weighed in with considerable influence because of their perceived importance to the Foreign Ministry's goal of rehabilitating Soviet psychiatry in world public opinion.

The administration of Soviet special regime mental hospitals was transferred to the Ministry of Health from the Ministry of Internal Affairs, with its obvious channel to the KGB and to the regime, and the 1992 Russian Federation Law on psychiatric care provided that compulsory hospitalizations could only take place in MoH facilities. But this administrative change alone, even if finally completely effectuated, does not necessarily imply an end to psychiatric imprisonment because political internment also occurred in Ministry of Health hospitals. Physicians in general remain state employees in significant numbers and to a significant degree. Further, new hires appear to enjoy the option of signing on as MIA employees, with higher salaries than the Ministry of Health can offer. In some institutions, such as the strict supervision hospital at Dvoryanskoye, the same individuals responsible for past abuse appear to remain on the staff with the same operating procedures (Reddaway, 1991:47). Thus physicians remain exposed to a constellation of state as opposed to Party pressures.

Evidence concerning a continuing KGB role in repression is varied and at some levels contradictory. The KGB had maintained a special Fifth Directorate for dealing with dissent and ensuring adherence to Party direction. The Fifth Directorate has undergone some permutations, becoming a chief directorate, and being renamed at least twice: 'Directorate for the Defence of the Soviet Constitutional System' (targeted fruitlessly against the independence movements and ethnic upheaval) and 'Directorate Z'. The Second (Chief) Directorate, of counter-intelligence, also had responsibilities in control of Soviet domestic political life (Knight, 1990; Waller, 1994).

In 1991, before the Gorbachev resignation on 25 December but after the failed coup of 18–21 August, Vadim V. Bakatin was appointed KGB director with the ostensible goal of breaking up the KGB, making it responsive to new legislation, reducing its size, and decentralizing it, at least among the remaining republics (Waller, 1994:65). Waller (1994:111) estimates that the KGB, not including border guards, agents, informers, civilian support, and reservists still amounted to roughly 480000 as of August 1991, while the border guards numbered about 240000 (1994:113). From these numbers we can estimate that pre-reorganization personnel might have amounted to over 720000. The KGB was separated into five autonomous organizations, including a Federal Counter-intelligence Service employing perhaps 75000 people. These organizations reportedly were under Presidential control, and perhaps actually served for a time as allies and potential shields to Gorbachev. KGB personnel fell from 500000 to 400000 in some reports – though Knight (1990:22) saw no net reductions as more forces were directed against organized crime, ethnic violence and other 'mass disorders' including border disputes.

A precise number would be difficult to sort out since large-scale transfers accompanied the KGB's reorganization. Waller's assessment is that Boris Yeltsin's reorganization of 1991 and early 1992 wasted the opportunity to control the KGB, instead leaving the old KGB structure intact. While some observers conclude that the more obtrusive mechanism of KGB officers supervising strict observation mental hospitals has disappeared, Reddaway found a continuing KGB presence in Kazan SPH as late as 1989 (IAPUP, 1989, No. 22:6). It could be argued that the KGB has merely been renamed, while being preserved as a tool for Yeltsin's own purposes, as his decision-making style became less participatory, more personal and increasingly authoritarian. Some commentators saw the 6 April 1995 change in the law governing the Russian Federal Security Service as resurrecting the KGB, enhancing its powers against crime, fascism and corruption but also providing overtly for special forces and interrogation cells.

Preceding the implosion of the Union, the Communist Party fractionated. Functional authority divided, migrated to the republics, after 1991 to autonomous entities within independent states, districts, and cities, and even, following the flight of the gold reserves, abroad. But it is not difficult to imagine that the KGB might be used again to suppress political opposition. While the leadership of the KGB may have found itself temporarily in prison, the domestic functions of the agency appear to proceed albeit with reduced staff and new names.

It may be too early to know whether the reforms constitute enduring structural change. Reformist forces that freed journalism from central censorship had weakened enough by the mid-1990s that new calls for government-assured media accuracy were being heard. Analogously the forces for a liberal attitude towards social criticism and nationalist identity may decay. The fine line between allowing nationalist rights and national political opposition and searching out the instigators of ethnic war may erode. Boris Yeltsin's ferocious over-reaction in Chechnya may indicate how he or a successor would respond to future ethno-national challenges to Moscow rule. The KGB has been occupied as an investigator of crime in ethnic violence as both inter-ethnic and intra-ethnic violence flared and subsided precipitously through the Gorbachev and Yeltsin administrations. To mention only one case, by 1993 Abkhazia separated from Georgia after evidently violating a Russian-brokered truce. An unstable ceasefire prevailed in 1994 in Abkhazia, under UN-sponsored Russian peacekeepers. Another civil conflict in Georgia, incubating in Mingrelia between the followers of the late Zviad Gamsakhurdia and those of Shevardnadze seemed a distinct prospect. Among the contemporary flashpoints raising human rights concerns and presumably interesting the KGB have been Nagorno-Karabakh, Tatarstan, Checheno-Ingushetia, North Ossetia, and Dagestan. Wars of secession and independence, as intensified in Chechnya in 1994–95, and potential separation, as in Tadzhikistan, where the war has taken casualties in six figures, also have marked ethnic dimensions which may interest the security apparatus and Yeltsin advisers apparently preoccupied with security concerns.

Though the KGB had for all practical purposes ceased arresting dissenters and regime critics in 1990, and had showed itself willing to facilitate reform under Gorbachev, four years later in 1994 the KGB officials who had directed and in some cases carried out suppression of dissidents were still in office, as were their lower-ranking staff. KGB practices which facilitated harassment and detention of nonconformists, including keeping files on suspect persons; inserting KGB personnel into religious societies, university groups, and political associations; and maintaining contacts among members of the procuracy and the judiciary, persisted as facts of Russian life in 1994 (Waller, 1994:281–3).

As of this writing, Boris Yeltsin is still in power. Under Yeltsin, the KGB probably has had a continuing role in political and social control functions beyond investigating ethnic violence and the formation of political parties, although this does not necessarily imply central unitary direction of KGB policy. Continuing KGB activities against dissent may reflect the predilections of local officers, which vary from *laissez-faire* to direct and punitive intervention. Historically, anti-dissident arrests could be undertaken on instructions of local Communist Party authorities, as well as national direction from the KGB. Further, national KGB policy on dissent may split, reflecting political rivalry at the highest levels, with effective control over different Directorates in the hands of contending factions, be they Party faithful, modern Westernizers, isolationists, or others.

According to Gelman (1990:107) the General Secretary rather than the Premier has had effective authority over the KGB in the post-Stalin era, although Anatoly Sobchak argued that as a state entity the KGB should legally have been subordinated only to state and not Party authority.[9]

The course of the liberalization in the late eighties was characterized by fluctuations in arrests and trials and by the initial persistence of anti-dissident articles in the media. In addition the first limits of permissible dissent varied markedly geographically, accompanying right-wing opposition to liberalization across the republics in general. The recent period has been distinguished mainly by regime abstention from coercion, at least in the more visible regions. Politically instigated trials decreased detectably from 1986, even in comparison to relatively low levels prevailing previously in 1983–86 (Podrabinek in van Voren, 1989:98). Virtually no trials or consequent psychiatric detentions of dissidents have been witnessed in the mid-nineties, and arrests are infrequent as well as based on less serious charges. Exceptions seem to be of short duration, as in the case of the brief detention (40 days) and examination of Boris Suprunyuk in 1994 on charges of arousing nationalist sentiments in Kazakhstan, after which he received a two-year suspended sentence.

This tolerance of dissent beginning in the late eighties created a fleeting overdue opportunity for discussion and participation within the sinking Soviet system (Oleszczuk, 1988b), illustrated in the unprecedented opportunity to voice divergent views in many sectors of Soviet life, and to abandon the two-track policy in favour of a belated liberalization.

LEGAL REFORM

The legal reform under way not only decriminalized some political and religious behaviour but also defined new rights which bring Soviet and later Russian laws (if not practices) closer to evolving international legal norms. Especially since 1986, changes both in law and practice in Soviet and post-Soviet Russian psychiatric hospitals have resulted in creation of some new standards of accountability, compensation for false hospitalization, and new rights of appeal for those detained. Criminal penalties up to two years in prison or corrective labour have been established for those ordering unjustifiable hospitalization. As already mentioned, in the early campaign against unethical psychiatrists in the spring of 1985, some were arrested at Serbsky and at the All-Union Research Centre for Mental Health.[10] Criminal investigations into specific individuals' psychiatric practices lasted at least into the late eighties.

The Presidium Decree on Conditions and Procedures for Providing Psychiatric Care instituted both patient rights to appeal and to a second opinion. The law now allows those compelled to submit to mental health examinations to choose a psychiatrist not appointed by the court or the procuracy, though whether this right exists in practice is unclear.

The outcomes of the laws enacted in 1988 and 1992 are not yet clear. They gave detainees a right to an attorney at the time of the first investigation, and a right to appeal hospitalization orders. But the impact of the 1988 provisions for appointment of a defence attorney at the preliminary investigation may be trivial, since in 1991 the WPA found those held non-imputable were still being tried *in absentia*, and since the cost of an attorney may be inhibiting. At least potentially meaningful rights to sue psychiatrists for malpractice, or sue police who signed arrest warrants for unjustified arrests, have also been created, but the categories of officials who can be sued remain sparse. (Alexander Kolomna Kuznetsov sued the officer who signed his arrest warrant after his 1971 hospital sentence was overturned and his case closed in 1988; Vladimir Klebanov succeeded in having his several psychiatric diagnoses/sentences at Donetsk Regional Court overturned by the Ukrainian Supreme Court after almost a decade in SPHs.)

This new criminal liability for superfluous hospitalization may be a mirage. How likely plaintiffs are to win such cases when psychiatrists can always claim honest diagnostic error rather than deliberate detention of healthy people is unknown. As noted previously, Soviet citizens in principle have had the right to bring legal complaints against particular officials, and, interestingly for an avowedly collectivist state, evidently *not* groups or collectives, such as, for example, the groups of psychiatrists making up the commissions responsible for compulsory admissions to hospitals. But this protection historically has not inspired much confidence.

An assessment of the January 1988 Statute on psychiatric assistance also yields mixed results. While this law bravely asserted the independence of psychiatrists, professional autonomy cannot be achieved by fiat. The 1988 law is not all that progressive, for at least two reasons. One, this decree conjured up a new category of hospitalizable individuals, in whom mental illness would be inferred, circularly, from nonconforming behaviour which precipitated the initial examination. Second, it still provided for compulsory examination of individuals who may have contravened undefined 'socialist community rules'. Amnesty International reported new detentions in 1989 in which nonconformity alone resulted in hospitalization, and feared that provisions for use of psychiatric imprisonment as a means of social control may actually have been set forth explicitly in the 1988 decree (Amnesty International, 1989:19).

Further, the new laws can be imprecise in their effects, and contain a conflict of interest in that chief psychiatrists, who now have the right to petition the court for releases, bear the obligation both to administer and to assure administrative compliance; that is, to provide their own review of their professional work, an obvious conflict of interest which necessarily yields a failure of accountability. New regulations seem to require chief psychiatrists to account for detentions of individuals, and to receive and process complaints which used to be directed to other officials. But officials have historically applied pressure to the practice of psychiatry via high-ranking psychiatrists, a situation which self-evaluation does nothing to alleviate. The new statutes seem not to have changed this basic structure or to have provided for genuine accountability to a purely professional agency unconnected to the authorities.

In addition the 1988 and later laws and instructions have not been uniformly implemented, not only for bureaucratic reasons including communication delays[11] but also because of perceived contradictions and confusions in the laws. In particular the declaimed policy shifting administrative responsibility for the special supervision hospitals to the Ministry of Health from the Ministry of Internal Affairs has not resulted in the short term in any real policy differences or major personnel changes. Gluzman wrote in 1989 that criminals on parole were substituted for the orderlies serving criminal sentences, and that physicians remained employees of the MVD (IAPUP, 1990, No. 23:20). In 1989 Interior Ministry troops were still deployed at Chernyakhovsk SPH and elsewhere as security guards. Although we were assured by a member of the Moscow Bar Association Presidium in 1989 that the supervisory personnel of the special regime hospitals had already been removed, in 1989 the staffs at Kazan and Chernyakhovsk special psychiatric hospitals remained unchanged (Amnesty International, 1989:18; Podrabinek in van Voren, 1989:100). The persistence of old guard supervisors at Kazan is particularly consequential since numerous reports of serious abuses have originated from Kazan. Two years later, Reddaway (1991:47) indicated that the orderlies at Sychevka (Smolensk) were still convicts despite the 1988 regulations prohibiting the employment of convicted criminals in that capacity.

One explanation for these failures in compliance may be that these institutions were deliberately exempted in the law. The 21 March 1988 law on psychiatric hospitals which provides that reinforced regime hospitals will be considered prisons could be interpreted to mean that in fact such nefarious facilities as Kazan special psychiatric hospital would remain *de facto* and perhaps *de jure* under the control of the Ministry of Internal Affairs. Amnesty International noted that employees of the MVD working in mental hospitals have the option of simply becoming employees of the Ministry of Health as subcontractors or transferred employees, which appears to meet the letter of the law while contravening its manifest intention. Koryagin asserted similarly that few detainees who found themselves in special regime hospitals would be relocated to any Ministry of Health institution which would be less arduous.

So it is not surprising that Podrabinek's information from Tambol Special Mental Hospital as well as from Dnepropetrovsk SPH and Kazan SPH in the late 1980s suggests abominable conditions still existed then, including punitive use of drugs such as aminazine and haloperidol, other chemicals such as sulphazine, and electroshock.[12] Podrabinek found Tambol 'quite typical' of the SPHs at the time. 'Perestroika has not hit them yet' (Podrabinek in van Voren, 1989:103).

On balance the 1988 and 1992 laws and accompanying regulations created many new rights for patients, including the rights to humane and respectful treatment, to information on treatment, to the least restrictive appropriate environment, to minimal time hospitalized,[13] to a psychiatrist selected by the patient on the commission determining the patient's mental health, to an appeal of the commission's findings to the chief psychiatrist, to notice to relatives or to legal counsel, to counsel itself, to confidentiality, and, interestingly, to appeal of the chief psychiatrist's decision to a court. But contradictions and provisions vitiating these rights are also written into the law. The rights to appeal to a court are still circumscribed by the provision that the detainee may have no right to be present (art. 48(2)) if a determination has been made that the detainee's condition does not 'allow' presence in court. The 1992 law seems to have taken a dramatic new step towards allowing patients to refuse treatment in Russia (art. 11(1) and art. 1(1)), which, if true, would be extraordinary since Soviet law had traditionally held that non-imputables do not have this privilege. However both of these articles make an exception for compulsory treatment!

Which of these new rights exist in practice is not yet evident, and scepticism may be indicated since longer established regulations have not been observed. The US Delegation was told in 1989 that virtually none of the political detainees they met with had received copies of the investigator's report or copies of their diagnoses from the evaluator. In addition all had been tried *in absentia*, despite the presumption that most if not all were healthy enough to have appeared at their trials. Further, the required six-month evaluations in criminal commitments were historically 'rarely done' (Segal, 1976:270). The US Delegation found, on interviewing 27 currently or formerly hospitalized dissenters in 1989, that no commission hearing had actually taken place in any of their cases. One report disclosed that even when available, these hearings were so brief as to be meaningless (63 in an hour and a half at one intensified observation hospital, or approximately 86 seconds each on average – 'rarely more than ten' minutes in any case; see Shore and Keith (eds), *Schizophrenia Bulletin* 1989:38, 41).

Perhaps equally or more significantly, efforts to have records of diagnoses struck from public documents such as draft cards were still not effective as late as 1994. Financial and judicial remedies are not available. Despite denials that the registry imposed a 'social tail' of deleterious consequences, the albatross around the neck which registration in fact created had not been perceptibly lightened, even though USSR chief psychiatrist of the Ministry of Health A. Churkin purportedly announced in the late eighties that registrants' occupational, travel and driving restrictions were being 'reconsidered' (Maksimova, 1988).

Unpleasantly, the 1988 law also set out *new* compulsory measures, echoed in the 1992 law, including compulsory outpatient care or (in 1992) examination and involuntary commitment of those whose condition was deemed likely to deteriorate and cause future harm without further treatment, three more levels of judgment calls. Although preventive treatment is also provided for in most US states, it remains particularly vulnerable to misuse in Russia since the projection of a patient's future condition, assessments of whether it would be an improvement or not, and guesses as to whether any change might be likely to prove damaging are all not only inherently subjective but also relative to political climate – particularly, relative to politically determined and mercurial standards of social danger. Procedures defining or providing for preliminary examinations, which can lead to forcible hospitalization, also feature in the 1988 and 1992 laws.

While the new regulations limiting commitment seem at least superficially more liberal, regulations concerning treatment after commitment have not become uniformly more liberal. No time limit on compulsory hospitalization seems to have emerged, though it is usually limited in the US to 90 days. While in 1971, emergency hospitalization by certification required a review within 24 hours, and subsequent reviews every 30 days, the 1988 regulations only mandate reviews at six-month intervals. The 1992 law provides for an assessment within 48 hours of involuntary hospitalization (arts. 29 and 23), and periodic reviews including provisions for release thereafter. Under both sets of pre-1992 regulations, reviews reportedly have been scanty and pro forma. The fact that courts do not supervise reviews may contribute to the lack of serious reconsideration and real accountability (see Bonnie, 1990b:344). Perhaps laws such as that of the Russian Federation providing for financial compensation for unnecessary hospitalization will serve as a constraint in future and provide some remedy for past persecution.

An evaluation of the impact of the regulations set out 21 March 1988 delimiting three types of psychiatric detention (in ordinary psychiatric hospitals (OPHs), in OPHs under intensified observation, and under strict observation in special psychiatric hospitals (SPHs)) conjectures that the 1988 regulations advance patient rights, but perhaps not far. While the guidelines mandate a diagnosis within ten days of arrival, prohibit unauthorized treatment, and grant some restricted correspondence and visiting rights, they do not seem necessarily to extend to equally or more meaningful areas such as the right to refuse treatment, and protections against solitary confinement, restraints, and forced heavy labour. The 1988 Guidelines require complaints to be noted, but do not specify any procedures for settling the issues raised in complaints or for guarding patients against retaliation for complaining.

The procedural guarantees of the new regulations do appear innovative even if perhaps not complete enough to be effective. Yet Soviet lawyers such as B. Protchenko and A. Rudyakov, Soviet dissidents, and Western specialists were sceptical about their actual implications.[14] Soviet lawyers have not found the new regulations an unqualified advance in patient rights (van Voren, 1989:10; *Komsomolskaya Pravda* 16 July 1988.) Some, such as the jurist Dr S.V. Polubinskaya, do not even see the 1988 statute as new. They instead view it as a compendium of pre-existing regulations, such as Article 56 of RSFSR Law on Public Health, and Instruction 3 on Immediate Hospitalization No. 06-14-43, Articles 58 and 59 of the RSFSR Criminal Code on compulsory medical treatment and hospital commitment of the mentally ill, and pre-existing norms, some *sub rosa.*

The 1988 statute preserves, among other anachronisms, the 'disturbance of public order' or infractions of 'rules of the socialist community' as reasons justifying compulsory psychiatric detention (Koryagin in van Voren, 1989:87), much as Brezhnev envisaged violations of the values of the socialist community as a sound rationale for an invasion. The 1988 law still provides for compulsory examination of individuals who may have transgressed 'socialist community rules' or threatened 'moral harm' (revised version of the Law on Psychiatric Care in the USSR), although actual arrests for anti-Soviet behaviour seem to have diminished. And the 1988 decree, which appears progressive in that only physically dangerous individuals could legally be detained, in fact created a new category of those defined as deranged only because they were nonconformists. Among those they were allowed to meet in 1989, the US Delegation found at least four cases presenting no discernible 'social danger' who were still hospitalized despite the new laws of 1988 and 1989 (Shore and Keith (eds), 1989:44), suggesting that the concept of social danger based on the risk of physical violence was not necessarily the dominant one even after the 1988 laws were proclaimed.

Podrabinek (van Voren, 1989:96) found the new statute ominous in that it 'significantly and absolutely increases the possibilities for an arbitrary psychiatric approach'; that is, the law initiates local clinic-level compulsory psychiatric observation without consent of the purported patient, family or lawyer, and without reference to perceived social danger presented by the 'patient'.[15] This power expands the reach of previous laws, which only regulated forcible commitments to residential facilities. The new law was twice fatally flawed in that it did not provide any clear definition of who can be given compulsory psychiatric examinations – thus, almost any person might be at risk – and the law did not limit in practice the duration of the initial examination (Koryagin in van Voren, 1989:87).

The 1988 regulations also expanded the scope of potential abuse of psychiatry since they legalized forcible commitment of those who may have ill-advisedly voluntarily committed themselves at some time, or who were 'voluntarily' committed by family or others.

The 1992 law sets out some improvements over the 1988 regulations, as mentioned above, but substantial defects remain. The 1992 law appears to have resolved conflicts by incorporating contradictory provisions rather than by reaching compromises in its terms. For example, Article 37 extends patient rights to appeal to hospital authorities; to complain to legislative and executive entities, courts, and the procuracy; to meet with counsel or with a priest (but not a rabbi?); and to receive periodicals. But Article 38 guts Article 37 by extending to doctors and hospital administrators the authority to restrict correspondence, patients' access to the telephone, visitors, even detainees' rights 'to have . . . essential items' or wear their own clothes. Article 39 contradicts *itself*, instructing hospital staff to 'facilitate correspondence and forward complaints' but also enjoining them to 'ensure control' of the contents of packages and messages.

As the nearly dialectical provisions of the 1992 law illustrate, the effects of recent changes and additions in Soviet and Russian law are mixed. The psychiatric register, though not dismantled, purportedly protects confidentiality to a higher degree, and reduces the numbers of unwilling patients on the mandatory list of those who must appear at clinics on pain of being followed and forced to appear. However the new legislation does not provide for hearings on request, and diagnoses themselves as a rule cannot be appealed, remaining for the most part outside the purview of the court. Court appeals to have psychiatric evaluations struck from the record only succeed in rare instances where the diagnoses were used as a foundation to obtain a conviction on a criminal charge.

The legal reforms in this area have been extensively evaluated and criticized, both by Western and by Eastern attorneys such as Rudyakov, Protchenko and Polubinskaya. The reforms would have been more powerful and more likely irreversible if the 1988 statute had not been sabotaged by overlapping and constricting regulations from the Ministry of Health. The new laws and guidelines would have been more consequential had they provided some means of significant financial restitution and systematic political rehabilitation for victims of psychiatric imprisonment, or had they provided for revocation of the professional credentials of implicated physicians, including those at the highest levels. While the 1992 law advances protections by requiring that individuals and institutions providing psychiatric care be licensed, no provisions for revoking licences are set out. And of course the licensing process itself would be subject to capture by the same authorities making instrumental use of psychiatry, so that potentially only compliant hospitals and physicians would remain licensed. Further the law finally enacted in 1992 leaves control over hospitals and providers with the very local authorities presumed responsible for many cases of political abuse in recent years (Bonnie, 1990b:336).

Professional structural changes would have been more significant had they allowed for greater diversity in schools of psychiatry being taught, psychiatric methods being practised, and psychiatric theories shaping research, and had they severed connections between the government and the major professional associations. In 1993, the new organization, the Association of Russian Forensic Psychiatrists and Psychologists, like the old All-Union Society, was also dominated by Moscow's Serbsky Institute, with St Petersburg and other major psychiatric centres refusing to participate (Savenko, 1993).

CONCLUSION

In Russia the old infrastructure of psychiatry remains largely in place, although new organizations are coalescing, and traditional practices are challenged. New statutes have conferred an array of new rights and guarantees on those accused, but their real impact remains unknown.

Both civil and criminal cases may be ended administratively – without a trial, without any particular due process or appeal provisions being brought into play. To that extent, some risks of arbitrary detention lie beyond legal remedy unless administrative powers are circumscribed. Some newly proclaimed rights exist only in principle. Implementation in general is equivocal. This is so for several reasons, one of which is that practitioners may not be reliably informed of unpublished guidelines or of new laws and regulations, while patients almost certainly will not be informed, and will lack the resources to locate and retain informed legal counsel. The vast discretion of the authorities to define social danger (or 'imminent' danger and future deterioration, specified in the 1992 law) and to label as socially dangerous, helpless, or likely to deteriorate those who are politically inconvenient or obstreperous has not diminished, and may even have expanded in some contexts. But at least as of this writing, the occasion for the use of discretion against dissidents has subsided.

According to Reddaway in 1991, the establishment forces still maintained control of psychiatry, while liberalizing and reforming influences in the post-Soviet states lacked the power, organizational structures and money necessary to bargain effectively against established agencies and procedures. Political and professional pressures for 'misdiagnosis' of dissidents lingered, while our data show detentions persisted at low levels through the 1980s and intermittently into the early 1990s.[16]

It could be argued that the legal foundation for reform in this sphere remains fragile, not only because the constitutional parameters within which statutory psychiatric reform and enforceable rights of individuals could survive have not been formalized, but also because a tendency to increasing lawlessness can be observed. The mechanisms of enforcement are in disarray and the prevailing legal order is murky. While Yeltsin approved the much amended Draft Constitution in November 1993 which was subsequently supported in referendum, it is unclear whether he now governs by decree.

The 1993 Constitution is phrased in Western terms and contains overtly fanciful provisions (the preamble imaginatively evokes Russia's 'immutable democratic foundations') or idealistic ones, in some instances repeating protections from international human rights law such as the Universal Declaration of Human Rights. Among the judicial provisions in Chapter 1 which might augur for future protection against psychiatric abuse are Article 15's guarantee that unpublished laws are 'not applicable', and that the norms and provisions of international law and treaties, presumably including human rights declarations, form part of the Russian legal system.

The 1993 Constitution advances lengthy, specific citizens rights provisions in Articles 17–64 of Chapter 2. Among the protections advanced which if effected would diminish the odds of arrest for political activists and impede a return to psychiatric repression are prohibitions against torture and harsh treatment (art. 21), guarantees of freedom of movement including exit from the Federation (art. 27), rights of assembly and demonstration (art. 31), prohibitions against forced labour (art. 37), compensation for victims of abuse of state power (arts. 52–3), alternatives to military service for conscientious objectors (art. 59), and adversarial trials and prohibitions against trials *in absentia* (except as federal law may allow (!), art. 123).

However, the 1993 Constitution also lends itself to abrogating newly specified rights in vaguely defined circumstances subject to official discretionary invocation. Thus even if the Constitution is observed, under Articles 55(3) and 56, human rights may be curtailed as required to 'protect the Constitutional system, morality [sic!] . . . defence . . . and security of the state', all of which are fundamentally psychological constructs amenable to idiosyncratic interpretation.

Which provisions in the new Constitution may be put into effect and which will prove consequential and lasting in an environment of Executive dominance is unclear. The failure to reinstate the Comprehensive Law on the Mentally Ill on either of two attempts in 1978 and 1987 may be a historical precedent indicating the fragility and possible evanescence of the current legal reform of psychiatry.

Limits on permissible dissent and on reform efforts vary considerably across time, regions and recently independent states. As of 1995 none of the former republics had passed new laws to supersede the 1988 edict (Bonnie, 1995:12). Whether the outlying republics will in future adopt the new laws and regulations coherent with their own new legal status as independent states, with or without any incremental improvements; set aside earlier hospitalization orders; enact their own new regulations and create new standards of practice; or revert to repressive practices for their own reasons, such as to avoid or mitigate ethnic war, is unknown.

While extensive changes were written into Soviet and later Russian law on psychiatry to mollify the WPA and world public opinion, their practical effect may be minimal. The new guidelines and regulations cannot create the finances, professional independence, incentives or power necessary in the judiciary to serve as a check on punitive psychiatry.

8 Summary of Empirical Findings and Conclusions

> The unprecedented levels of state terror unleashed by the neoliberal military regimes were directly related to the scope and breadth of the social movements: The deeper and more extensive these movements were in civil society, the more extended and savage was the state repression.
>
> James Petras and Morris Morley, *Latin America in the Time of Cholera* (1992:180)

PROXIMAL CAUSES: WHY PSYCHIATRIC REPRESSION?

The Soviet dissident movement from its inception was extraordinarily large, persistent, intricately organized and issue- and class-inclusive. These characteristics alone might have evoked an exceptional state response. Our analyses disclose three other reasons for resort to novel methods of direction and control. On average across administrations, political protest groups and religious societies recruited progressively younger adherents who could maintain a higher level of participation, could remain active longer, and could potentially serve as a base for exponential growth in the size of the movement. The movement was also expanding in two other dimensions: geographically, out from major cities; and substantively, across new issue areas. Issues underlying political protest began to depart from established and internationally acknowledged religious freedom and human rights concerns to venture more often into newer areas such as ecology, antinuclear activism, workplace safety and environmental contamination, and reached overtly anti-Union taboo topics such as anti-Communism and national independence for the republics, or smaller zones, even cities.

While these circumstances do not dictate a state policy response which features primitive reliance on punitive psychiatry, pre-existing structural characteristics of Soviet law, medicine and professional training made the use of psychiatry as a control mechanism a rational, though not inevitable, instrumental choice. To a policymaker interested in preserving Soviet *vlast* (authority), the societal emergency constituted by the dissident movement could have warranted costly counter-measures.

Highlights of our findings and the major explanations advanced for political use of psychiatry substantiate the instrumental use hypothesis. However that is not to say that psychiatric repression succeeded. We argue instead, generating what we conjecture must have been regime objectives, that in some deterrence terms, repression failed.

WAS PSYCHIATRIC ABUSE REAL?

Soviet psychiatric detention without medical justification amounted to nearly 2000 years of human experience in these data. The minimum sum of years of forcible hospitalization equals 1839, counting only the commitments for which durations can be calculated. If calculable prison and camp terms inflicted on those also detained in psychiatric hospitals are counted in detainees' total incarceration time, minimum total detention time in all types of institutions amounts to more than two millennia or 2286 years. Nearly all the time dissidents spent hospitalized, 1326 years, resulted from criminal court commitments, although administrative detentions were more frequent. Among nearly 1000 known detentions, 597 administrative hospitalizations and 400 criminal court-ordered hospitalizations can be documented. At least 345 transfers to strict supervision psychiatric hospitals and 393 transfers to ordinary regime hospitals are known, as well as at least 90 interrogations of psychoprisoners.

The Soviet experience differs from that of other developed societies, in the particular vulnerability of the Soviet mental health care system, judiciary, and investigative agencies to regime and bureaucratic political pressures to select out atypical individuals. While the typical offender in the US classified as mentally unbalanced resembled violators of other societal legal norms (Turk, 1969:148), in the Soviet case (Shatz, 1980; Oleszczuk, 1988), political and religious dissidents who were forcibly hospitalized were *not* similar to violators of other norms. They were, for example, more educated. Such dissimilarities imply state targeting of nonconformists. That is, the usual means of controlling behaviour are not drawing in this group: consequently the state selects special measures.

Our records of arrests and detentions extend back into the late 1920s, and capture psychiatric detentions which began to be methodically employed 1936–38. Some demographic information such as date of birth is available as early as the late nineteenth century. The dataset becomes richer and more detailed in the sixties, and provides continuing information through to the disintegration of the USSR in 1991.[1]

That psychiatric detention for political and religious reasons was real is irrefutable. N. Safronova wrote in *Izvestia* 29 March 1990, 'By now the very dispute about whether there were abuses of psychiatry is a mere exercise in scholasticism. There were; in a totalitarian society it could not have been otherwise. The forcibly imposed totalitarianism made it possible for any form of dissent to be relegated to the realm of psychiatry.'

That unjustified hospitalization was political also is beyond dispute. At the nation-state level the phenomenon is responsive to both internal and external political events. At the individual level, allegations of political violations or religious offences have been regarded by Soviet courts as sufficient evidence of social danger to have dissenters forced into special psychiatric hospitals. Extremely vague psychiatric reviews have sufficed as well. Vladimir Borisov, instructively, was committed for 'incorrect comprehension of the environment' (Antebi, 1977:166). Others, tautologically, after arrest on suspicion of insanity, have been diagnosed as ill for 'inability to live in society without being subject to arrest' (Shore and Keith (eds), 1989:25).

Further, it is clear that psychiatric repression was systemic, centrally directed in its major provisions, and subject to regional and local vagaries in its application. Psychiatric repression not only was *not* limited to the special psychiatric institutions and the Ministry of Internal Affairs, but in several terms was largely a phenomenon of the *ordinary* psychiatric hospitals and the Ministry of Health.

DENIALS FROM SOVIET OFFICIALS AND PSYCHIATRISTS

Despite the evidence, vociferous Soviet denials of Western assertions of political abuse of psychiatry have been heard for decades,[2] without dispelling the original allegations. Soviet accounts of genuinely ill hospitalized people among detained dissidents, while real, and verified by outside observers, rely on a handful of selected and in some cases merely potential counter-examples. They may also rely on a false dichotomy, that one could not be both a genuine dissident and simultaneously or subsequently genuinely mentally ill. This evidence cannot be used to support the contentions either that no healthy Soviets were hospitalized for political reasons or that psychiatric confinement has not been used widely and persistently as a well-focused means of social control.[3] Further, examples of clearly sane individuals arbitrarily detained exceed these counter-examples in the literature by an order of magnitude. Western observers simply do not find substantial numbers of formerly hospitalized dissidents, emigrés or others, to be mentally ill.[4] These denials insofar as they are still heard must then be interpreted as essentially declaratory policy statements without much empirical content, since abuse reports were eventually acknowledged by Soviet authorities and addressed by the Ministry of Health.[5]

EMPIRICAL FINDINGS: CHARACTERISTICS OF PSYCHIATRIC REPRESSION

Repression of dissent via psychiatry was broadly based across time, republics and administrations. Its victims encompassed all major nationalities and religions represented in the USSR, with Jews over-represented, and 'religious extremist' Evangelical Christian Baptists, Reform Adventists, Pentecostalists and Jehovah's Witnesses not consistently most severely sanctioned despite their frequent persecution by the state. Though Russian nationals predominated throughout, in absolute numbers and among those repeatedly detained, the proportion of detainees of this nationality declined after Khrushchev. Occupational profiles of detainees show relative stability over time, featuring large proportions of intellectuals, white collar managers and technicians, and blue collar workers. In contrast, the issue focus of dissidents shifted over time. Across administrations the proportion of dissidents who advocated nationalism and anti-Communism swelled, while the proportion backing broadly defined human rights subsided.

Repression peaked in the early 1970s just after maximal levels of dissident acts were recorded, in terms of frequency of arrests and detentions. In general, protesters were being detained at increasingly early ages, for an expanding array of political causes, but for shorter durations. On average, length of all compulsory hospitalization also declined over the period under study. Administrative detentions show this reduction consistently. In court-ordered commitments, a distinct declining trend does not appear until 1981.

Psychiatric repression was responsive to political pressure from the outside world, especially to needs to achieve larger Soviet foreign policy goals, even at some times at the cost of internal concessions. That concessions were granted in some cases incrementally and cautiously in expectation of a Western response also suggests a rational process directing dissident policy.

While the geographical base of the dissident movement from which psychiatric detainees were drawn expanded, becoming gradually less urban over time, repression remained either under-reported or scarce at the village level in the entire Soviet period.

RISKY ATTRIBUTES OF PROTESTERS

Some demographic attributes and long-term identification with causes are connected to more frequent or lengthy hospitalization terms for Soviet nonconformists, and can therefore be seen as risky attributes. Among the categories revealing differences in frequency and duration of compulsory hospitalization are dissident issue, nationality, occupation, religion and gender. Age, either extreme youth or maturity, has not provided significant protection against forced hospitalization of dissidents, though age at first hospitalization does help predict total number of detentions per individual.

The issue focus of psychoprisoners varied over time. In the whole dataset from the 1920s to 1991, emigration and visa concerns were the most frequent determinant of dissident actions, followed in order of frequency by religious observance; nationalism and anti-Communism; human rights; general anti-system agitation; samizdat propagation; workplace, anti-corruption or environmental complaints; and True Communism. The state appeared especially unforgiving of true Marxists, who averaged an unusually high number of detentions per person. Nationalism and anti-Communism coalesced into the single largest political cause of psychiatric prisoners by the time of Andropov, Chernenko and Gorbachev, displacing the human rights and emigration concerns which had been most salient among their predecessors. Of all causes, nationalism and anti-Communism generated the most frequent criminal commitments. Samizdat work and human rights advocacy provoked the most frequent administrative detentions.

Over time, proportionally fewer Russian nationals were targets of repression, though Russians always predominated without necessarily making up a majority of the sample, and were always among recidivists hospitalized three or more times. Russians and Slavic nationals in general were detained approximately in proportion to the per cent of the Soviet population they comprised. Baltic and Transcaucasian nationals were over-represented in the same terms, partly due to repeated but unusually brief hospitalizations of Balts. Nationality had little effect on frequency of forcible commitments as a rule, but did affect duration. Balts tended to be held more briefly, and Ukrainians, Georgians, Tatars and Dagestanis somewhat longer than average.

Despite utopian ideals of a classless society, the Union exhibited clear divisions by socioeconomic status. In these data a small but significant correlation suggests that in general lower prestige occupations may have been somewhat protected against longer or more frequent compulsory hospitalization for dissidents. This finding is notable since in some individual cases, as would be expected in any country because of the enhanced access to resources and options it implies, higher socioeconomic status insured against maximal penalties.

Because of their large-scale representation in the dissident movement, disproportionally many white collar employees, intellectuals, students, and artists crop up among detainees. But blue collar workers comprised nearly one-fourth of all psychiatric detainees in these data, challenging theoretical views of nonconformist movements as essentially only intellectual and upper-caste, and illustrating the more class-inclusive nature of Soviet repressed dissidents. Among the ideological anomalies revealed here, although workers figured largely in declaratory policy statements and formal justifications for Soviet policy, dissident workers enjoyed no special protection in the workers' state. Blue collar workers were detained especially frequently. Workers, KGB and military personnel were hospitalized longer than other occupational groups on average when all time forcibly committed is measured. Under court order, workers and military spent decidedly longer than other occupational groups in detention. Students, though at risk of long administrative commitments, may have enjoyed some indulgence in that they were at relatively less risk of judicial internment. After detention, though, this leniency vanishes – students were held about as long as intellectuals, and endured especially lengthy court-ordered hospitalizations. Those in religious callings were hospitalized almost as long as students and intellectuals. In these occupational categories some rational reluctance to hospitalize the most vocal or well-connected groups and individuals can be discerned.

While workers received no leniency, some evidence can be found of special dispensations for technocrats, perhaps because they were seen as necessary for the evolution of the Soviet economy. White collar technicians and managers' total hospitalizations were shorter than average, administrative detentions decidedly so (at more than one year less than average for all psychiatric detainees), and court-mandated detentions also were notably shorter (about three-quarters of a year less on average). Intellectuals, artists and dancers were favoured in shorter than average court-ordered hospitalization terms; artists also experienced shorter administrative detentions as a rule. Those in religious professions also benefited from some special consideration, in general being forcibly committed less frequently than other occupational groups, although this consideration evaporated on administrative detention, when they were subject to especially lengthy hospitalizations. It is not coincidental that these groups are also among those most capable of mounting an effective public relations campaign were they to be detained and tried.

Considering other occupational groups, police were interned for the shortest periods, on average. Soldiers were at relatively high risk of non-judicial hospitalizations, and, as might be expected, nonconforming intelligence officers were severely sanctioned.

Religion posed variable risks of frequent and lengthy hospitalization for dissidents. Perhaps the most conspicuous observation is that in several measures Jewish detainees were disproportionally severely penalized. Roman Catholics, Buddhists and Jews were detained more frequently than average by court order. The duration of hospitalization on court order was especially long for Catholics, True Orthodox, Hare Krishna devotees and Uniates. Non-denominational Christians, Russian Orthodox and Uniates were committed more often than average via administrative procedures; after administrative hospitalization Russian and True Orthodox served especially long terms.

An examination of our data by gender reveals a persistent bias favouring women, in a legal environment of some impartiality. Men are over-represented among psychiatrically interned dissidents, as they were among nonconformists in the Soviet Interview Project (Bahry, 1987). Although they may be arrested in comparable circumstances, men are detained longer than women on average, but *not* more frequently in administrative hospitalizations.

This apparent bias in treatment by gender could have resulted from Soviet demographic concerns, though this seems unlikely,[6] or from some lines of mitigation in Soviet law. It might reflect some tendency to charge men with more serious offences for the same types of political or religious behaviour, resulting in lesser charges for women. Our evidence is ambiguous on this point, partly because of the small number of women detainees in the sample. While small sample size militates against controlling for the nature of the behaviour resulting in trial, hence only a partial answer can be hinted at here, Table 8.1 does suggest that lesser charges might be filed against women. As valid (non-missing) percentages in both groups, proportionally fewer women protesters were charged with the most serious crime alleged against both genders, treason, which was a capital offence, and proportionally more women were charged with lesser economic violations, and with hooliganism, penalized by up to a year's imprisonment and/or fines. But in percentage terms *more* women than men were charged with two serious political offences, anti-Soviet agitprop, which carried penalties of up to ten years' imprisonment and five years' exile, and defamation of the Soviet system.

Longer detentions for men may also follow from diagnostic criteria, if diagnosing physicians accept the contention of the Institute of Psychiatry of the USSR Academy of Sciences in Moscow that 'men require longer

Table 8.1 First Charge at First Trial for Men and Women (Charges in approximate order of gravity of penalties)

Charge	*Women* *Valid %*	*Men* *Valid %*
Treason	6.7	11.9
Anti-Soviet Agitprop	46.7	41.0
Defamation of Soviet System	33.3	24.2
Currency and Economic Crimes	6.7	0.9
Hooliganism	6.7	3.1
	100.1*	81.1**

* Does not sum exactly to 100 because of rounding error.
** The data include many more cases of criminal commitments of men than of women, and a wider variety of charges in that subpopulation. The table includes only charges for which entries for men *and* for women are non-zero, which entails omitting charges only preferred against men. Therefore the total per cent for men does not sum to 100.

hospitalization than women, who more frequently respond to outpatient care' (Babayan, 1985:75). This correct 'response' may simply reflect a lower frequency of (and perhaps intensity of) reported interest in politics among Soviet women compared to Soviet men (Bahry, 1987).

RISKY BEHAVIOUR

Some types of dissident messages and varieties of dissident acts have precipitated more frequent or longer psychiatric detentions. Among the most incendiary behaviour in these terms was creating or joining a new dissident group, rejecting Party guidance or returning a Communist Party card publicly, and unauthorized electoral activity, all of which were likely to result in longer and more frequent involuntary hospitalizations. Judicial detentions most often followed rejection of the Soviet state, its symbols, or obligations to it such as military service; public participation in political opposition; and propagation of new dissident groups. Administrative detentions resulted from much the same sorts of nonconformity and agitation such as rejecting Party guidance or annoyingly petitioning, especially if these activities were publicized via demonstrations or samizdat. But in addition administrative hospitalizations tended to be employed promptly where a time-urgent response was required, for instance in dealing with those openly seeking asylum, striking or carrying out other work actions, and undertaking unauthorized electoral activity such as failing to vote for correct candidates, running inappropriate opposition slates, and so on.

Early evidence of the power of the nationalists appears *inter alia* in their presence across the Union from the sixties and even earlier among detained dissidents. Pervasive nationalist agitation and samizdat activity with nationalist messages seem especially risky behaviour for activists.

Samizdat activity and true Marxism[7] presented special risks to dissenters, as did pervasive nationalist agitation. Samizdat were real regime irritants in these data, since samizdat involvement is the single most frequent first dissident act known among those psychiatrically detained in this period, yielding distinctly higher than average numbers of total detentions per individual (1.8 as opposed to 1.2 in the whole sample for which both variables are known). Two other forms of publicizing causes, demonstrations and other provocative writing, resulted unusually frequently in forcible commitments. Targeting of samizdat as well as provocative writing and tacit communicating via demonstrations shows a genuine respect for the political power of the unofficial media. This targeting would be expected if the regime made political use of detention to restrict nonconformist communication, and publicity about it, externally and internally, thereby attempting to limit the diffusion of dissent. The samizdat, demonstrations and provocative writing statistics can then be interpreted as evidence of rational use of forced commitments to attempt to encapsulate the dissident movement.

The most frequent detentions on average were meted out to those repudiating their ties to the state by renouncing Soviet citizenship (2.7 per person). Unauthorized electoral activity was the next most often penalized dissident behaviour (2.3). Also predictably representing a serious regime irritant because it challenges the supremacy of the state, refusal to bear arms for religious reasons was frequently sanctioned, as were creation of a dissident group or party, returning Party cards, and demonstrating, producing among the highest average numbers of detentions (2.1 or 2.2) of any dissident act. *Symbolic opposition to the Union was thus sanctioned more often than violence or hijacking.*

OTHER RISK FACTORS

Timing, as indicated in the administration under which nonconformists began their political activity or religious observance, may have been a risk factor. Consistent with the general pattern of declining penalties for dissent over time,[8] those whose activism began earlier generally suffered longer and more frequent forcible commitments. Those first detained under Stalin were arrested more often, hospitalized administratively more often, and spent more total time incarcerated or hospitalized than those first detained under Khrushchev. Those arrested first under Khrushchev endured more extensive court-ordered commitments and spent more time incarcerated than those first picked up under Brezhnev. The Andropov administration may have been an exception to the trend, since it appears to have imposed more administrative detentions and carried out more arrests proportionally than previously, but small sample size makes any conclusion provisional.

These findings are consistent with the conventional wisdom about the successive administrations, as are the results of the regression analysis indicating, as Medvedev suggested, that dissident behaviour, city of residence, age, and number of convictions are among the risk factors predisposing dissidents to frequent psychiatric penalties.

PROTECTIVE FACTORS

Some types of political and religious dissidents have been consistently less frequently or severely punished for their activities. These protected individuals share some common attributes, which included foreign contacts, extensive networking within the USSR for publicity and mobilization, and some connection to international political issues which were salient for Soviet foreign policy. Perhaps surprisingly, the conspicuousness of their participation in approved social and political activities did not protect the Bahry generations from significant penalties for dissidence.

A WATERSHED IN THE GORBACHEV ADMINISTRATION?

Some evidence for a change in diagnoses of dissidents across administrations can be drawn from the comparisons made by the US Delegation visiting Soviet mental hospitals in 1989 (see eds Shore and Keith, 1989:17). Their Table 2 summarizes three sets of observations on the same hospitalized dissidents: Soviet chart diagnoses made of dissidents on initial confinement, 1989 diagnoses made by Soviet physicians in the presence of Western observers, and US 1989 diagnoses including the views of Soviet-educated physicians among the US delegates. Given that most of the detainees had been hospitalized from three to nine years in 1989, most were first detained before Gorbachev came to power in 1985. Thus their initial diagnoses were made mainly in administrations previous to Gorbachev's. If political use of medicine was a reality and was to some extent centrally determined, and if a real change in outlook occurred with perestroika, the 1989 Soviet diagnoses should have been free to differ from those made on initial hospitalization. And in fact they do. Only seven of 27 cases show agreement between original Soviet chart diagnoses and the 1989 Soviet diagnoses (26 per cent). Nine show a general area of overlap in which the 1989 diagnoses are less severe (33 per cent). Granted, rather than mirroring political liberalization, some of these findings could reflect real improvement in patients' mental health, if it is presumed for the sake of argument that not all these admissions were political cases in the absence of illness. And the presence of the US Delegation may have influenced these findings. But the change which occurs between eras in Soviet diagnoses is not simply an attempt to match US diagnoses for particular people. The 1989 Soviet interpretations match 1989 US diagnoses for only six or possibly seven individuals. The changes in Soviet-made diagnoses of the same individuals may therefore reflect an increased freedom to make informed professional judgments as political pressures shifted.

MEANING OF THE REFORMS

The legal reform of psychiatry under way in the USSR in the late eighties and early nineties foundered with the disintegration of the Union, and then gathered its forces in Russia. Yeltsin in July 1992 signed a new progressive Russian law on psychiatry, but its several guarantees and review mechanisms are not yet implemented (Bonnie, 1995). Conscious of the contribution of a unified attitude towards psychiatric abuse among physicians, the Russian Society of Psychiatrists has since undertaken a draft of a Code of Ethics to govern practice of psychiatry in Russia (Bonnie, 1995) to try to provide some specification of norms of physician conduct, as well as to create a professional basis for opposition to state or other misuse. In the other newly independent states, the 1988 All-Union edict bringing administrative commitments under some legal regulation, albeit with its noted flaws, is the most recent regulation. Bonnie reports (1995:12) that Ukraine and Lithuania have moved forward with their own new draft laws but that they are not yet completed.

Since political use can be made of many articles of criminal codes, the legislation of the early 1990s which specified remedies for those detained under explicitly political articles naturally can extend only partial protection. Simply repealing or rewriting overtly political or anti-religious statutes does not create a solution. Power of the legislature and courts combined also can only provide a partial solution, since abuse originated in administrative units and high level ministries effectively outside the power of the courts or legislature to restrain.

Further, certain structural bottlenecks remain in the partially reformed Russian system. Dissenters confined to strict supervision hospitals because of criminal charges brought against them can only be released by court order or transfer – and the court may refuse, or prior political convictions may have created circumstances in which a release is meaningless. As the case of Adrian Alexandrovich Tarasov illustrates, those forbidden residence in major cities because of previous convictions, but released by court order only to families, who happen to live in Moscow, cannot take advantage of the release because the terms are internally contradictory.

CONCLUSIONS

This study and the relevant literature suggest four explanations of patterns in psychiatric repression of dissidents in the former USSR. We have argued that cultural and historical factors as well as academic biases might create a propensity to resort to hospitalization to restrict dissident behaviour. We have also suggested that punitive, intimidating and issue-neutralizing psychiatry might be a result of public display of natural intergenerational life event conflict, or of conflicts with state norms arising from political socializing events common to certain age cohorts. Many comparatively youthful or elderly dissidents were relatively powerless to escape arrest and detention while they may have presented a real or perceived threat to the regime. Dissenters in politically defined age cohorts may have been more salient, hence more often targeted, because of their higher levels of participation in general, and higher levels of dissident behaviour in particular. It has also been suggested that variations in psychiatric repression rates could be a function of professional socialization in medicine, or of perceived regime needs expressed through various structural arms of the state (procuracy, KGB, Ministry of Internal Affairs' influence in special regime mental hospitals, local officials).

CULTURE AS AN EXPLANATION OF PSYCHIATRIC REPRESSION

Cultural predispositions and historical experience do answer part – even if only a small and invariant part – of the question of why psychiatric measures might be used to squelch dissent although cheaper measures with fewer international repercussions were available, such as expulsion from the university, professional blackballing, and visa denial. Cultural and historical influences may prove in future inquiries to have been factors in the use of psychiatric measures against Eastern and Central European or other dissidents. A relatively low societal tolerance for deviance in general would imply more arrests for dissent and more hospital residence for nonconformists, even without regime-coerced or co-opted psychiatrists. Thus a dissident had relatively higher odds of being diagnosed as schizophrenic or perhaps paranoid for cultural reasons within the USSR (Reich, 1978:36) or some post-Soviet states even without state intervention. Diagnostics of psychiatry appear culture-bound, which by itself may imply a prior probability of political abuse in dissident cases, especially in conformist societies.

Some psychiatric repression may be an artifact of the recent political structure and history of the USSR, and may echo certain long-term themes in the culture. When the USSR fractured, deStalinization of Soviet society was neither complete nor progressing uninterruptedly in all areas, including the academic structure of psychiatry, its journals and graduate institutions, and the Ministry of Internal Affairs hospitals, which perhaps never deStalinized (Reddaway, 1972) until transferred to the Ministry of Health, if at all. The dissident movement itself, in this connection, is seen partly as a response to neo-Stalinist developments in the USSR in 1965–66 (Reddaway, 1972:418; Podrabinek, 1989). The state's identification of the movement as anti-Stalinist and anti-bureaucratic may partially account for the alacrity of state response to dissent.

The fact that small numbers of forced commitments continued to be recorded after Gorbachev came to power, and after massive defections from the Party, may also be an artifact of longer-lived tendencies in Soviet political history and political culture. It is possible to trace the authoritarianism of the Soviet Union to its Marxist-Leninist ideology, with its belief in scientific socialism and claims to political hegemony by the leadership of the Communist Party based on 'scientific knowledge' of the course of human history. The continued use to 1991 and the end of the Union – albeit at very low levels – of psychiatric hospitals to confine political and religious dissidents, and the continuing risk that the Russian government may attempt to capture psychiatry for instrumental purposes again, is more difficult to explain in these terms. Perhaps some forms of authoritarianism survive the abandonment of the ideology in which they were embedded. More generally this observation suggests the possibility that the source of authoritarianism in the Soviet Union and across many of the newly independent states is older and more enduring than the 1917 October

Revolution, older than the political philosophy which precipitated the Revolution, and perhaps older than tsarism.

Political culture, authoritarian traditions, and centralized political structures make a contribution to explaining an underlying propensity to resort to repressive measures against dissidents. But like arguments relying solely on totalitarian or authoritarian political structure, these factors cannot provide a full explanation since they cannot account for failure of systematic psychiatric repression to appear in cultures like Poland, which closely resembles the Soviet one, with analogous political structures. Similarly the political culture argument cannot account for the emergence of sporadic cases of psychiatric repression in contrasting cultures such as Latin American ones.

Since culture is approximately constant for the purposes of short-term studies, a cultural predisposition argument also cannot explain fluctuations in levels and lengths of psychiatric detention. If only cultural factors were responsible, they would explain an approximately stable level of psychiatric hospitalization of dissidents.[9] While this rate might be relatively high compared to underlying rates in Western industrialized countries,[10] it could not by itself account for the variability observed over time in psychiatric detentions. Although dramatic historical changes began in the USSR with Gorbachev in 1985, it is unclear that they were cultural, and in any case the Gorbachev administration cannot have shaped most of our findings based on data from the late 1920s onwards.

While authoritarian political cultural factors have abstract explanatory power, they constitute elements of a general explanation of any state behaviour undervaluing individual rights. They do not provide a precise argument specifying which aspects of history, political structure or culture imply that disproportionally more Soviets labelled as dissidents would be confined to psychiatric hospitals than in non-authoritarian societies, much less why in some cases they resided in Soviet hospitals for decades. Cultural and historical predispositions then provide at most a partial explanation of a more general phenomenon – the abrogation of individual rights of which psychiatric repression is one example. Therefore despite their intrinsic power and interest, historical and cultural factors cannot by themselves fully explain the dramatic patterns in psychiatric repression of dissent which are indicated here.

PROFESSIONAL TRAINING AND SOCIALIZATION IN MEDICINE AS AN EXPLANATION OF PSYCHIATRIC REPRESSION

Some measure of psychiatric repression of dissidents follows from the nature of academic training given psychiatrists in some countries and within some schools of the old USSR (Fireside, 1979: *Soviet Psychoprisons*). Soviet psychiatry, like all Soviet medicine, has been handicapped by lack of resources, restricted access to world research, forbidden lines of inquiry, and deficiencies in formal training, curricula, and certification standards. As a discipline psychiatry has been a battlefield of opposing orientations. However, the Moscow Snezhnevsky school imposed itself, even for a time on the radically different school in Leningrad.

This paradigmatic conflict factor, like culture, is largely invariant over most of the period under study, even granted the proliferation of new institutes of psychology after 1985. Therefore, like culture, academic perspective should not account for much of the variability observed in these data over time, although it may help shape variations across location depending on where local doctors were trained. Treatments for mental maladies are reported to be roughly comparable in East–West comparisons since the mid-sixties or mid-seventies (Miller, 1985:22), except that the Soviets may have prescribed somewhat higher doses of drugs. Neither does there appear to have been an upsurge in the power of the Snezhnevsky school within the USSR which would precede or correspond with the peaks in these data, or a decline in it which would coincide with the drop in the late eighties to virtually nil by the early nineties, although Russian psychiatry including the Moscow school is undergoing some reorganization.

If academic training factors comprised the chief explanation of internment of dissidents, psychiatric detentions should be concentrated in Moscow, the site of the MVD-directed and Snezhnevsky school-dominated Serbsky Institute, or in regions where most psychiatrists are Moscow-trained. This in fact appears to have been the case in the period studied by Bloch and Reddaway. But in our data overall they are concentrated in Leningrad. Leningrad's Bekhterev Institute, which never adopted the Snezhnevsky school's views and criticized vehemently the adverse and potentially long-term consequences of arbitrary findings of incompetence, was itself a less likely source of a finding of incompetence for political activists than Moscow, Kazan and other centres. Nevertheless Leningrad predominated in Soviet-era political use of psychiatry. At least in the aggregate Podrabinek is correct in observing that 'psychiatric repression was practiced in Leningrad to no less a degree than in Moscow' (Van Voren, 1989:104). This would probably not be the case if academic training bias were the central explanation of political use of psychiatry. Population size of the two cities does not seem to provide an answer since Leningrad/St Petersburg is only about half the size of Moscow, and on that basis alone is unlikely to have been home to substantially more nonconformists than Moscow. Our data also fail to support the idea that more detainees were Leningrad residents. For cases in which city of residence is known, when hospitalized, exactly twice as many detainees were Moscow residents as Leningrad residents. Presumably, since suspect individuals can be brought in to any city to be examined and hospitalized, Leningrad predominates in these data because of transfers.[11]

If professional socialization were the central source of unjustifiable hospitalizations of dissidents, the Soviet-trained emigré psychiatrists accompanying the US Delegation in 1989 would not have had a basis in professional judgment for failing to corroborate the findings of their Soviet colleagues. The fact that American-resident Soviet-trained psychiatrists did disagree with their Soviet-resident Soviet-trained counterparts on the diagnoses made of hospitalized dissenters implies that professional training cannot be the sole explanation for political use of psychiatry. Similarly, if professional training and socialization rather than political factors were the main explanation of psychiatric abuse, it would not have been possible for Soviet-resident Soviet-trained psychiatrists, re-examining the same patients, and relying on their own previous training and diagnostic criteria, to find, as they also did, excessive reliance on schizophrenia diagnoses (20/5 cases or perhaps 400 per cent overuse).

While socialization presumably has a non-zero effect on diagnosis, if professional socialization of mental health professionals were the main determinant of political hospitalization, the evidence should not show variations over short time periods. However it might show variations by occupation and socioeconomic status, if professional socialization inculcated deference to some classes or professions. The Soviet paternal attitude towards patients does not seem to have featured deference to any particular type of patient, however, or even towards other psychiatrists.

Professional socialization in any case would most likely result in relatively uniform hospitalization rates, rather than the significant differences observed here based on nature of dissident behaviour and other divergences among detainees. The professional socialization explanation, for example, advances no particular reason for religious belief to result in a classification of insanity, let alone why certain religious beliefs were penalized more heavily than others. In an avowedly atheist state, professional socialization might simply imply training physicians to classify religious belief as superstition, rather than delusion. Certainly psychiatry worldwide does not usually define adherence to religious or ethical belief systems as demented unless they are particularly colourful or involve automatic weapons.

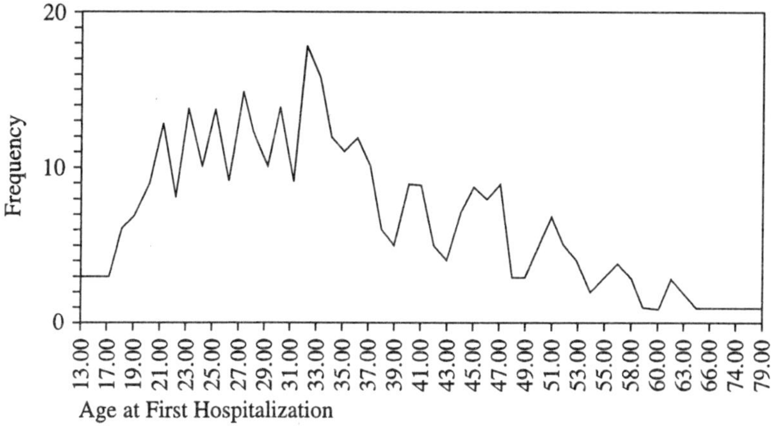

Includes only cases for whom date of birth and date of first hospitalization are known.

Figure 8.1 Age at First Hospitalization

INTERGENERATIONAL CONFLICT EXPLANATIONS OF PSYCHIATRIC REPRESSION

Intergenerational conflicts over the meaning of societal norms arise continuously. Normal life-cycle generational conflict implies links among dissident behaviour defined as criminal, age, and relative powerlessness *vis-à-vis* enforcers. Generational identity may interact with occupation, education and other status-related indicators in producing nonconforming behaviour. As a matter of observation of empirical evidence, if intergenerational conflict as a result of life cycle patterns were the central reason for compulsory hospitalization of Soviet nonconformists, targets for hospitalization would be mainly conspicuous elderly people or obstreperous juveniles, and family conflicts would bulk large as reasons for attracting the attention of the mental health authorities. But neither of these conditions holds in these data. The age profile of psychoprisoner dissidents does not follow a U-shaped curve but, just the opposite, it is generally concave downward, given some irregularities.

As Figure 8.1 shows, forcibly confined dissidents in this sample were for the most part adults,[12] though many were relatively young. They were certainly not predominantly over 65, and were not usually juveniles, although nine were under 18. Their average age at first hospitalization was 34.7, with a median of 33, a minimum of 13 and maximum of 79. If a life cycle event interpretation of the intergenerational conflict hypothesis were the primary explanation for psychiatric repression, most detainees should come from target populations of vulnerable individuals in major life transitions, and perceived conspicuous misfits; that is, juveniles and the elderly or perhaps in some cases the recently or badly married. Changes in frequency of commitments should follow demographic patterns, especially among juveniles and cohorts of older people.

As Reddaway notes in the introduction to *The Case of Leonid Plyushch* (Sapiets, 1976:iv) and elsewhere, allegations of insanity and potential social danger tended in the USSR to originate with the *prosecutor* rather than with family or local community members. (The prosecution directed psychiatric evaluation in the USSR, and examination protocols were authorized by the Ministry of Health, either alone or in collaboration with the procuracy, the Supreme Court of the USSR, and/or the Ministry of Internal Affairs.) One Independent Psychiatric Association summary for 1989 to 1990, listing reasons that individuals consulting the IPA had encountered conflicts with psychiatrists, reported that family conflict accounted for only 9.6 per cent of the cases (IAPUP, 1990, No. 24:12). Although the predictable venal exceptions can be found of family members submitting their kin to mental examination because of disputes over living space,[13] marriage and divorce, or conflict over childrearing and child custody, most cases of detentions in these data do not originate with family complaints. Where evidence of family involvement can be obtained, one finds mainly examples of families *preventing* the internment of their members, as did Fyodor Petrovich Edamenko's in the Mercer data. Neither do most cases arise from attorneys or physicians acting for the dissidents. The point of origin of the bulk of complaints – in the prosecutor's office – diminishes support for the argument that psychiatric commitments of Soviet dissidents result from normal intergenerational conflict, since life cycle intergenerational conflicts should instead result mainly in family[14] and community complaints.

The dynamics discovered here do not appear to echo demographic change in the erstwhile USSR. For example, the Soviet population was ageing in general, not becoming younger. Those stigmatized by hospitalization are not mainly in the predicted target groups of adolescents or elderly. Neither do life cycle generational patterns of dissidence characterize the Soviet demographic or political experience. Close encounters with the KGB are not 'mainly a function of youth' and inexperience (Bahry, 1987:86), and major life cycle events seem to exert no particular impact on unorthodox behaviour. For these reasons we discount the life-cycle interpretation of the intergenerational conflict argument as a general explanation here.

However, a different interpretation of generational effects, the formative political event age cohort explanation as advanced by Bahry in Soviet Interview Project data, does shed some light on the phenomenon of psychiatric repression. In this view, major worldview-forming political experiences and not a demographer's standard score of years are the delimiters of 'generations'. Not surprisingly, Bahry finds the purge generation born 1910–18 distinctly more conformist than those without direct experience of mass terror. The post-Stalin cohort of Soviets with higher educations, on the other hand, is 'significantly more unorthodox than any other age or occupational group' (1987:85) in political behaviour. They would therefore be more likely than other age and educational groups to be subject to arrest and subsequent hospitalization. Thus the post-Stalin cohorts that Bahry defines, the most active conforming and nonconforming behaviour groups with dates of birth between 1925–40 and 1941–60, could be expected to be disproportionally represented among the inmates of psychiatric prisons.

In our data these politically engaged generations were more heavily sanctioned in that the durations of their detentions were remarkably long. Their higher levels of participation in approved social activism such as Komsomol work did not insure them against the lengthy hospitalizations occasioned by their political protest.

Bahry also finds that in some respects material success does not affect political nonconformity, an observation of great relevance for a theory of state control and coercion of its nationals. In her study, those with the security of *nomenklatura* positions did not show a reduced tendency towards various politically deviant behaviours compared to others (1987:87), and perceived inequities in material goods remained causes of protest among them. This asymmetry suggests that in the SIP data, sharp differences in material conditions gave rise to political deviance but even a substantial degree of economic security was not enough to prevent political nonconformity from arising from this or other causes.

INSTRUMENTAL REGIME USE AS AN EXPLANATION OF PSYCHIATRIC REPRESSION

Our results bring together evidence in several forms of an adaptive, selective, intelligent and time-sensitive application of psychiatric measures against political protesters and religious activists. Drawn from the internment and release data, background substantive information, and theoretical insights in the literature, these results are best explained as depicting a rational pattern of repression and relaxation coherent with instrumental regime use of psychiatric hospitalization as a versatile, responsive means of social control.[15]

The close statistical relationship between numbers of known dissident acts and numbers of arrests or new hospitalizations is evidence of rationality, if the state's goal is to use arrest and psychiatric detention as a punitive and/or deterring response to nonconforming behaviour. Frequency of detention tracks numbers of dissident acts, not only in the aggregate but also at the individual level, at the All-Union level and at the republic level. Further, it reappears in political-event generations, since the cohorts defined by Bahry are significantly more heavily sanctioned than later age cohorts, consistent with their higher average levels of dissident acts. This consistency in frequency of hospitalizations suggests a uniform, centrally directed process of repression which monitors and responds to levels of dissident acts. At the same time *length* of detentions varies sufficiently across republic to argue for ample discretion in application of this penalty at the republic level.

Except for some differential targeting by socioeconomic status, and the tendency for length of detention to decline, little quantitative indication of general differences in regime policy towards dissent across administrations appears here.[16] Average time hospitalized does vary across administration but would seem at least in the post-Stalin period to be responding largely to changes in levels of dissident acts rather than well-articulated differences in policy.

The hypothesis that rational assessment of regime needs determines policy towards dissent implies not only that the state attempts to repress dissident behaviour at some times, as when dissent threatens state legitimacy or invites secession, but also that the state may enhance the opportunities for dissident behaviour and relax sanctions against nonconformity at other times, such as during liberalization drives or for public relations reasons, be these internal, external, long- or short-term. This hypothesis also implies that in periods of crackdowns some classes of dissidents may be selectively targeted and others deliberately exempted, or, conversely, that in periods of liberalization some individuals, classes of people, or less visible regions may still be victimized.

The state may clamp down on nonconformists, or it may relax enforcement of norms, to use dissent as a mobilizer or as a communication medium with the exterior world. In this context the 1980s' moderation in numbers of arrests, resort to detentions in smaller less visible cities, and the dramatic declining trend in length of administrative detentions can be viewed as at least partially due to the Soviet desire, now largely accomplished since 1989, to re-establish its links to the world psychiatric community and other international professional, political and economic organizations. This Foreign Ministry objective was achieved despite the selection in the late 1980s of 'new' leadership for the Soviet All-Union (Scientific) Society of Psychiatrists from among the same cohort directing the Society during periods of marked abuse. The appearance of a draft code of professional ethics from the Russian Society of Psychiatrists in the mid-nineties would seem a more progressive sign.

Compulsory commitments of obstreperous individuals subsided and virtually disappeared by the early nineties. This dwindling would be expected for several reasons, including the decreased importance of conformity to discredited Soviet values, and higher priority given by the Russian and the newly independent states' governments to emergency measures directed towards salvaging something of value from an eroding political structure, ebbing authority, and the deteriorating economy under overwhelming pressure of inflation.

Among the reasons for tolerating dissent which Spechler sets out in a study of Soviet arts and culture (1982:264–5) are three particularly relevant to the early and mid-1990s:

- Concern for the economy or social unrest increases;
- A major change of any kind is perceived as necessary by the leadership;
- Instrumental use of dissidents appears (appeared) feasible; as, in our case, first to show compliance with human rights regulations, to clear the way for rejoining the World Psychiatric Association, and to mobilize the populace or the bureaucracy for change in policy.

Further, if the state is rational, or those acting in its name are rational, it may deliberately try to maximize the returns and minimize the losses of any resources generated or expended by Soviet policy towards dissent. Maximizing returns on resources generated by political use of psychiatry can be defined as an example of rational instrumental regime use of mental hospitalization to squelch dissent or further other state objectives. In this context, the exchange of allegedly insane nonconformists such as Natan Shcharansky for intangible political assets such as world public opinion, or for valued espionage agents or politically prominent individuals held abroad shows instrumental use. Vladimir Bukovsky, traded in December of 1976 for Luis Corvalan Lepe, general secretary of the Chilean Communist Party, is an example. In another case, Valentin Moroz, Alexander Ginzburg and three other political prisoners were exchanged for two Soviet officials previously working in the US.

Punitive Use, and Selective Rewards

Punitive use of psychiatry presumes rationality, or rather, rationality presumes both the ability to reward and to punish, as means to achieve a stable set of ranked objectives. Not surprisingly, evidence of both selective leniency and punitive use of sanctions comes to light in these data.

Punitive use of drugs for violation of psychiatric institution rules – even on juveniles – has been reported by many credible sources (Bonnie, 1990:326; Kozheurov and Mikhalych, 1992). If deliberate induction of side effects via administration to dissidents of drugs and other chemicals is defined as torture, this practice survived in the USSR/FSU through the 1980s and in a few cases into the early 1990s, although state torture as an overtly declared adjunct to the legal system was abolished in the West in the eighteenth and nineteenth centuries. Among well-confirmed cases our data show at least two individuals who reported being tortured in detention, and others who were subjected to violence. At least four were beaten, at least three committed suicide in incarceration, and at least a dozen died in dubious circumstances which could not be unravelled.

The context in which this information should be judged is unclear. The practice of ordinary Soviet medicine[17] and ordinary Soviet psychiatry was perceived as punitive against Western standards, even taking into consideration the lamentable state of Western public psychiatric hospitals before the reforms of the last 20 years.

While a pattern of punitive transfer of dissidents from ordinary to strict supervision psychiatric institutions is not documented here in general, punitive use of transfers becomes evident in these data when the detainee population is divided by charges pressed at first trial. That those charged with political offences were transferred into special regime hospitals at a significantly higher rate than those charged with other violations of the criminal code or those hospitalized administratively, can be interpreted as deliberate punitive application of harsh conditions. These punitive measures may have had compellance functions, to force dissidents to stop prohibited behaviour by for example incapacitating them, or they may have had deterrence functions, specific or general, to encourage individuals to choose not to dissent.

State penalties exacted from psychiatrists opposing the perversion of mental health techniques to state purposes also give evidence of punitive use, where state penalties cannot be attributed to incompetence or other infractions. These penalties imply a policy of optional instrumental use of psychiatry. Prominent examples of physicians censured, imprisoned, sent to labour camps, exiled or detained for their views are the psychiatrists

Anatoly Koryagin and Semyon Gluzman. Similarly Vitaly Petrovich Romanenko lost his job as a result of unwillingness to facilitate instrumental use of psychiatry (IAPUP, 1988, 19:35). Conversely, Dr A.V. Snezhnevsky, CPSU member, 'for services to the Soviet state' received the Hero of Socialist Labour title, the Order of Lenin, and other prizes and medals (*Meditsinskaya Gazeta*, 17 July 1987:3).

The mere existence at least as late as 1985 of an array of 'therapy-and-labour rehabilitation centres . . . and corrective labour colonies' (Yastrebov, 1985) under the Ministry of Internal Affairs offers mute testimony to punitive purpose.

Selective Leniency Variations in frequency and duration of court-mandated hospitalizations versus administrative ones applied to the former republics show some higher tolerance in the Baltics than elsewhere,[18] along with repeated selective penalties. Political and religious nonconformists resident in the Baltic republics tended to be detained for shorter periods, but more often than the psychoprisoner population in general. They were also somewhat over-represented among detainees, considering the proportion of the USSR population they comprised. All time hospitalized is significantly shorter in Latvia and Lithuania; dissidents in Lithuania and Estonia experienced shorter administrative detentions; but in Estonia court detentions of protesters averaged above the norm. Latvians also experienced fewer transfers to special psychiatric hospitals. In the case of the Baltic republics their economic importance to the Union may have provided some insurance against lengthy hospitalizations, especially of white collar managers and technocrats. (Relative leniency found at the All-Union level towards white collar managers and technocrats compared with those in other occupations can be interpreted as a reasonable consequence of the need to develop the Soviet economy.) The Baltic independence movements were well advanced, which may have been one reason for close attention and repeated but comparatively light sanctions in this region.

Relatively brief but frequent detentions, especially administrative detentions, suggest adaptability and selective use of sanctions where other goals besides control of the protest movement must be met simultaneously. This pattern can be interpreted as evidence of a rational search for a time-urgent response to multiple goals.

Does Deterrence Deter?

The presence of several cases in our data of individuals who were freed from hospitals after recanting political or religious beliefs, and of others whose commitments were lengthened after their refusal to recant,[19] clearly shows instrumental imposition of a deterrence/compellance relationship between some Soviet state employees and dissenters. One interpretation is that the state's objective was to deter other actual or potential rabble-rousers by compelling detained nonconformists to abdicate closely held values, and to reward recanting. This is rational, goal-oriented behaviour, although it is not necessarily effective, especially without specification of time parameters.

If the instrumental use hypothesis is the best supported explanation in these data, the question arises whether larger-scale psychiatric repression via arrests and hospitalizations actually *worked* in the FSU to deter dissident activity, presuming deterrence was at least one of its purposes. Although our evidence is consistent with a state policy of applied psychiatric sanctions to attempt to suppress the dissident movement, our measures of deterrence success are quite limited.

Some deterrence success may be evident in the fact that most compulsorily hospitalized Soviet nonconformists were subject to only one arrest and one hospitalization. A threshold effect may exist at that level, beyond which the combined perils of job loss, divorce, and further risk of arrest or hospitalization are sufficient to dissuade many dissidents from continuing activity. But those repeatedly hospitalized are recidivists in the sense that they *increase* dissident behaviour after multiple involuntary commitments. Thus for strongly motivated protesters, deterrence fails at the individual level.

Deterrence also fails over time in the aggregate, in that most recorded instances of dated dissident acts took place *after* the peak in compulsory hospitalizations. Further, the stronger statistical associations between measures of forced hospitalizations and numbers of dissident acts in subsequent years all proffer evidence of reinforcing rather than deterring effects.

The lack of evident support for successful deterrence of dissent via forced hospitalization may derive from some peculiarities in the hypothesized relationship. The association between repression, in both its deterrence and compellance aspects, and dissent may be curvilinear over time.[20] While repression may work in the short term, it may also generate increased resistance and reduced legitimacy, attracting more individuals to the cause, and thus repression may fail, in the medium or longer term, to curtail the size or activity level of the opposition group, even if particular individuals are dissuaded from continuing participation.

Like the death penalty in the US, whose popular support is ideological and is not based on evidence that capital punishment actually serves general deterrence functions, psychiatric repression may have been supported across several Soviet administrations for reasons which had little to do with any actual success of psychiatric suppression as a short-term specific deterrent. In fact the relationship may have operated in the other direction: the dissidents may have deterred the Soviet authorities. On some occasions visible dissident activity well-publicized in the West may have deterred the regime from imposing the most extreme penalties on prominent advocates of political and religious causes.

Our results can most coherently be interpreted as deliberate regime use of psychiatric medicine to attempt to deter, dissuade, defuse and generally discredit dissent. Data clearly show a correspondence between dissident behaviour levels and subsequent hospitalizations. However the expected negative relationship between incidence of hospitalizations and later dissent, which would exist if general deterrence worked, is elusive in these data. Patterns of psychiatric repression are consistent with other varying needs of the regime across the period under study.

The most frequent method of detention of dissidents, locally ordered administrative detention without trial, was and apparently in Russia still is especially amenable to short-term instrumental political use. Rational use of forcible commitments is evident in the fact that although both administrative and court-ordered detentions were visited on those undertaking similar dissident acts, the more prompt and flexible administrative detention procedure was employed against those whose behaviour presented time-urgent problems. The regime must also have appreciated the value of indefinite postponement of trial, and the diversion of any consequent domestic publicity for dissident causes which discreet administrative hospitalization or quick emigration might offer.

NO ASYLUM

Unhappily the potential for the perversion of psychiatry to instrumental use by any state remains a continuing concern relevant in the 1990s. In the early 1990s, press reports identified current or former political prisoners in psychiatric wards as far-flung as those of Kenya, Angola, Zaire, Turkey, Cuba, Argentina, Chile, Hong Kong, the Czech Republic, Slovakia, Bulgaria, Hungary, Poland, Romania, Germany, and what was then Yugoslavia. Whilc a Geneva Initiative-affiliated group is working with Eastern and Central European national psychiatrists to develop new standards of professional ethics as an obstacle to renewed or continuing abuses in that region, other areas are not so fortunate.

Soviet forced hospitalizations were ended because of essentially unstable alterations in the political terrain, and consequent changes in political priorities, which could shift again along any of a variety of societal fault lines. Thus while it may seem appropriate to write a post-mortem of Soviet psychiatric abuse, it would be premature. The risk still exists of a resurrection of psychiatric hospitalization in Russia and the independent states as a deterrent to political action, at least below some threshold of civil violence and some level of cost. That the secret police have become interested in the environmentalists is one indication of a potential target population. The possibility of renewed political use of mental hospitals remains even though it is unclear to what extent the expense of psychiatric incarceration can be tolerated in an environment of hyperinflation and implosion of the currency.

Soviet political, social and professional structures which facilitated regime use of this medical instrument of deterrence, compellance and defence in many cases still exist, and the old structural features which allowed mitigation, appeal and lawsuits for damages had been underused or even largely fictitious,[21] while the new ones are not yet fully implemented. In Russia, even though the national power of the Party was destroyed by the early 1990s, local Party officials were still able to order detentions. Bonnie (1995:16) cites two incidents as late as 1995 in which the Russian lower house, the Duma, tried but failed to enlist the power of psychiatry in political control over religious 'cults' and organizations and in procedures to certify Russian officials competent to hold office. Most of the erstwhile Union republics have not enacted their own laws regulating psychiatric detentions after 1988, and in any case legal reform alone would provide inadequate protections.

The ambiguity of various hospital administration changes, a sparse handful of prominent firings, financial exigencies which exacerbate the underlying poverty of the health care system, and the superficiality and frailty of legal remedies previous to the 1992 Russian law together imply that the mechanism of punitive psychiatry in Russia has thus far been only partially restructured and – however dusty – remains available or reconstitutable for future use as an instrument of official societal control, whether officials call themselves Marxist-Leninists, 'authoritarian reformers', as Nursultan Nazarbayev has so glibly identified himself in Kazakhstan, or something even more imaginative.

Some amount of psychiatric confinement of political dissidents or religious nonconformists in future may follow from idiosyncratically perceived domestic political needs of the moment or the short-term future, and may begin in ways which pass muster as legitimate. It might, for example, be desirable in the interests of public safety to restrain and render harmless followers of apocalyptic, purportedly religious cults who happen to know how to manufacture poisons or who hold nuclear weapons. The recent Russian instances of appeal to psychiatrists for aid with problems of state, which failed, show how easily political use of psychiatry could be justified unless new professional conduct standards bar the way and alternative professional career paths can be pursued which are not controlled by the government, Party agencies or similar authorities.

FUTURE RESEARCH

The greater permeability of post-Soviet society gives grounds for some expectation that access to detailed Party, governmental and security records might expand and may eventually yield a more complete portrait of social trends in the Soviet era. Still much must have been destroyed, stolen, rendered fanciful in the original, or falsified later. Lebedev (1992) claims that some of the destruction began before the fall of the Union; for example, that Krychkov issued orders in late 1989 for the KGB to begin obliterating their records of 'current operations'. On balance, the records which survive the pandemonium of the disintegration of the Union and the continuing economic emergency will present a complex information source even more difficult to decipher and interpret in future than standard Kremlinological materials whose set phrases and publication parameters were more or less understood.

Any future research in the archives of the Communist Party of the Soviet Union Central Committee, which are now available for example on microfilm at the Hoover Institute in the USA, may shed more light on historic regime policy at the highest levels towards punitive medicine as a tactic against dissenters. Although at the end of the Soviet period reports of new hospitalizations dropped to zero or near-zero, probably not all detainees who would be considered political or religious dissidents in the terms used here have yet been identified or released. The possibility that arrest reports and initial investigative reports on political and religious nonconformists could eventually become available means that directives and action policy statements on state control of dissent via psychiatric sanctions may be unearthed. These could substantiate the instrumental use hypothesis directly.

Other relevant information might become available as specific records from former Soviet archives are declassified, including those of the Centre for the Preservation of Contemporary Documents, the Russian Centre of Conservation and Study of Records of Modern History, Russian State

Archives, the Russian Foreign Policy Archives, the Russian Presidential Archives, the KGB Archives, the GRU Archives, and the military archives of the CIS *inter alia*. Further inquiry may answer what accounts for the timing of major political and legal events such as the release of Instructions on Urgent Hospitalization of the Socially Dangerous Mentally Ill in 1961, and their re-release in 1971. Countless questions will remain unanswered.

> We cannot wash ourselves clean of the past if there is no soap.
> (Ye. A. Yevtushenko, Secretary of the Board of the USSR Writers Union, at the Congress of Peoples Deputies, 1989)

Appendixes

Table A.1 Articles Used in Soviet Dissidents' Trials: Russian Soviet Federal Socialist Republic Code of Criminal Law (Sources: H.J. Berman, 1966, Code as amended 1965; V. Sokolov, 1983)

Article Number	*Substance*
15	Preparation and attempted crime
17	Complicity in a crime
36	Deprivation of rank, medals, honours and titles
43	Mitigation of sentence
58	Compulsory hospitalization ('measures of medical character') in general (ordinary) and special (strict supervision) psychiatric hospitals
59	Special psychiatric hospitalization when socially dangerous act creates special danger for society
64 (Old 58)	Treason
(Old 58.10)	Subversion of Soviet government
(Old 58.11)	Organization for subversion of Soviet government
65	Espionage (including transfer of non-secret information)
66	Terrorist act (assassination or assault)
67	Terrorist act (assassination or assault) against representative of foreign state
68	Sabotage, mass poisoning, propagation of epidemics
69	Wrecking state, economy, social organizations, infrastructure
70	Anti-Soviet agitation and propaganda
72	Organizational activity related to articles 64–70, especially dangerous crimes against the state, including participating in 'anti-Soviet organizations'
74	Violation of rights of nationalities or agitprop to do so
75	Releasing state secret without treason or espionage
77	Banditry
77.1	Violation of prison camp discipline, incl. terrorizing inmates
78	Smuggling, incl. weapons, drugs, poisons, biological agents
80	Draft evasion
83	Illegal border crossing (exit or entry, except to seek asylum in USSR)
88	Currency speculation, violation of rules of fiscal transactions
88.1	Failure to report a crime against the state, including those 'in preparation' or related to an anti-Soviet organization
88.2	Concealing a crime against the state
89	Theft of state property
90	Openly stealing state property
91	Assault with intent to steal state property

Table A.1 (cont.)

Article Number	*Substance*
92	Embezzlement of state property, abuse of position
93	Stealing state property by swindling
93.1	Large-scale theft of state property
96	Petty theft of state property
98	Intentional destruction of state property
102	Intentional homicide under aggravating circumstances
107	Incitement to suicide, including by insults to one's dignity
117	Rape
122	Non-payment of child support
130.2	Defamation
142	Separation of church and state, church and school
153	Private enterprise (including co-ops)
154	Speculation
162	Participating in a prohibited trade
173	Bribe-taking by officials
174	Bribe-giving
180.2	False report of crime
181	Perjury, including known false translations
182	Refusal to testify
186	Escape from internal exile
189	Concealing crime
190	Failure to report crime, including those 'being prepared'
(190.1)	Defamation of Soviet system
(190.2)	Defamation of the flag or other national symbols
(190.3)	Collective activity against the social order
191	Resisting authority
191.1	Resisting policeman or people's guard (*druzhinnik*)
191.2	Endangering policeman or people's guard
(191.6)	False report against the police or guard
192	Insulting authority or a public official
192.1	Insulting police or guard
(193.13)	Evasion of military service
196	Forgery of documents, stamps, certificates; Counterfeiting
198	Violation of internal passport rules
198.1	Evasion of military training or registration
206	Hooliganism
208	Receiving stolen property
209	Vagrancy and begging
210	Corrupting minors, including by parasitism
218	Illegal possession, manufacture, carrying, etc., of firearms and explosives
224	Making or supplying illegal drugs or poisons
227	Violation of rights of others by religious observance, including drawing minors into religious groups
228	Making or purveying pornography
249	Draft evasion by maiming or other method

Criminal Codes of the Union Republics (Sources: De Boer, Driessen and Verhaar, 1982; H.J. Berman, 1966; V. Sokolov, 1983)

RSFSR UK	*15*	*17*	*43*	*64*	*68*	*70*	*72*	*80*	*83*	*88*
SSRs										
Armenian				59	63	65	67	75	78	83
Azeri				57	61	63	65	73	76	81
Byelorussian				61	65	67	69	77	80	85
Estonian				62	66	68	70	78	81	86
Georgian				65	69	71	73	81	84	89
Kazakh			39	50	54	56	58	66	69	74
Kirghiz				58	62	64	66	74	77	82
Latvian				59	63	65	67	75	78	83
Lithuanian	16			62	66	68	70	79	82	87
Moldavian		17		61	65	67	69	77	80	85
Tadzhik				61	65	67	69	78	81	86
Turkmen				62	66	68	70	79	82	87
Ukrainian		19		56	60	62	64	72	75	80
Uzbek				54	58	60	62	70	73	78

RSFSR UK	*89*	*92*	*93*	*93.1*	*96*	*98*	*117*	*142*	*153*	*154*
SSRs										
Armenian	86	90	89	90.1	92	96	112	141	154	156
Azeri	83	96	85	88.1	87	91	109	141	152	153
Byelorussian	87	91	90	91.1	94	96	115	139	150	151
Estonian	88	93	91	93.1	94	97	115	137	146	152
Georgian	91	94	93	96.1	95	100	117	148	164	165
Kazakh	76	76.4	76.3	76.5	77	82	101	130	165	168
Kirghiz	84	87	86	88.1	89	90	108	141	155	156
Latvian	85	88	89	89.1	90	95	121	137	148	142
Lithuanian	90	94	93	95	98	99?	118	143	161	164–5
Moldavian	119	123	122	123.1	124	127	102	142	163	161
Tadzhik	89	92	93	96	97	99	121	151	166	167
Turkmen	90	93	94	95	96	101	122	153	169	171
Ukrainian	81	84	83	86.1	85	89	117	138	150	154
Uzbek	114	117	119	119.1	141.1	122	94	145	174	175

Table A.2 (cont.)

RSFSR UK	*162*	*173*	*174*	*190.1*	*190.2*	*190.3*	*191*	*191.1*	*191.2*	*196*
SSRs										
Armenian	162	185	186	206.1	206.2	206.3	207	207.1	209.1	213
Azeri	158	170	171	188.1	188.2	188.3	189	189.1	191.1	194
Byelorussian	160	169	170	186.1	186.2	186.3	187	187.1	189.1	192
Estonian	148	164	165	194.1	194.2	194.3	182	182.1	184.1	
Georgian	172	189	190	206.1	206.2	206.3	207	207.1	209.1	215
Kazakh	164	146	147	170.1	170.2	170.3	171	171.1	173.1	178
Kirghiz	165	180	181	196.1	196.2	196.3	197	197.1	199.1	202
Latvian	151	164	165	183.1	183.2	183.3	184	184.1	186.1	190
Lithuanian	162	180	181	199.1	199.2	199.3	201	201.1	203.1	208
Moldavian	164	187	188	203.1	203.2	203.3	204	204.1	206.1	209
Tadzhik	175	186	187	203.1	203.2	203.3	204	204.1	206.1	210
Turkmen	181	194	196	214.1	214.2	214.3	215	216.1	220	223
Ukrainian	148	168	170	187.1	187.2	187.3	188	188.1	190.1	194
Uzbek	179	152	153	191.4	191.5	191.6	192	192.1	194.1	197

RSFSR UK	*198.1*	*206*	*208*	*209*	*210*	*218*	*224*	*227*	*228*	*249*
SSRs										
Armenian	214	222	224	225	231	232	229	244	228	257
Azeri	196.1	207	214		215	220	225–6	142.1	228	244
Byelorussian	199	201	203	204	205	213	219	222	223	238
Estonian	189.1	195	203	201.2	202	207	210	201	200	224
Georgian	218	228	229	234	236	238	252	233	232	267
Kazakh	182	200	78, 139	201.1	201	202	214	200.1	215	236
Kirghiz	206	215	217	239	218	229	235, 235.1	136.1	240	255
Latvian	194	204	93, 145	211	210	218	222	212	209	238
Lithuanian	211	225	228	240	241	234, 235	232	144	242	263
Moldavian	213	218	220	221	224	227	225	143	223	250
Tadzhik	215	220	222	223	224	234	240	243	244	259
Turkmen	228	236	100, 162	238	239	249	256, 257	263	264	279
Ukrainian	192	206	213	214	280	222	229	209	211	192, 243
Uzbek	199.1	204	121, 132	220	218	210	216	147.1	221	237

Table A.3 Confirmed Cases of Soviet Psychiatric Detainees

The Table lists political and religious activists known by name who were forcibly hospitalized while believed to be victims of punitive medicine.

Bloch and Reddaway (1984:253–62) *Coverage*: 1977–83	**Koppers (1990:74–176)** *Coverage*: 1920s to 1990	**Mercer (1991a and b; 1992)** *Coverage*: through 1991	**Podrabinek (1981:158–83** *et al.*) *Coverage*: late 1950s(?) through late 1970s	**Smith and Oleszczuk (1988a; 1989)** *Coverage*: 1960–81 before additions
Agapova, A.R.				
		Agayev, N.A.		
			Aikhenvald, V.A.	
	Akhmetov, N. Sh.			
Akinkin, I.				Akinkin, I.V.
Alekseyenko, S.S.	Alekseyenko, S.S.		Alekseyenko, S.S.	Alekseyenko, Se. S.
	Aleksandrov, G.M.	Aleksandrov, G.M.		
	Alekseyev, V.I.			
				Amalrik, A.A.
	Andreyev, A.		Andreyev, A.	Andreyev, A.
			Andreyev, A.S.	
				Andreyev, V.N.
Anisimov, A.			Anisimov, A.A.	
Antipov, I.	Antipov, I.	Antipov, I.		Antipov, I.
				Antonov, I.Y.
			Antonov, M.F.	Antonov, M.F.
	Argentov, A.A.			Argentov, A.L.
Artsimovich, V.V.				
				Artyushchenko, B.T.
Arutyunyan, E.B.				Arutyunyan, E.B.

Table A.3 (cont.)

Bloch and Reddaway (1984:253–62) *Coverage*: 1977–83	**Koppers (1990:74–176)** *Coverage*: 1920s to 1990	**Mercer (1991a and b; 1992)** *Coverage*: through 1991	**Podrabinek (1981:158–83** *et al.*) *Coverage*: late 1950s(?) through late 1970s	**Smith and Oleszczuk (1988a; 1989)** *Coverage*: 1960–81 before additions
Asselbaums, T.T.	Asselbaums, T.T.			Asselbaums, T.
		Avakyan, S.A.		
	Avgustov, R.T.			Avgustov, R.T.
Avramenko, V.I.	Avramenko, V.		Avramenko, V.I.	Avramenko, V.I.
		Bablik, V.		
	Baiduk, Io.			Baiduk, I.
		Bakunin, Yu.		
	Balakhonov, V.F.			Balakhonov V.F.
Baranov, N.I.	Baranov, N.I.		Baranov, N.I.	Baranov, N.I.
Barats, V.M.				
Batovrin, S.Y.				
	Batshev, V.S.			Batshev, V.S.
	Batulin			
Baturov, Y.				
	Bazdyrov, V.P.			
Bebko, V.V.				
				Bedrylo, S.
	Belau, I.			Belau, I.
				Beletskii, V.I.
Belikova, L.I.				
Beloborodov, L.	Beloborodov, L.		Beloborodov, L.	Beloborodov, L.E.
	Belov, E.			Belov, E.
		Belov, S.I.		

Belov, S.P.	Belov, S.P.			
Belov, Y.S.	Belov, Yu. S.		Belov, Y.S.	Belov, Yu. S.
		Benzo, V.G.		
				Bernadsky, S.
	Bernshtam, M.S.		Bernshtam, M.S.	Bernshtam, M.S.
Berozashvili, M.I.				
Besov, A.				
Bezzubov			Bezzubov	
Biletsky, V.				
				Bogdanas
				Bogu, I.
Bondarenko, A.T.	Bondarenko, A.T.	Bondarenko A.		
Bondarev, Y.; P.Y.			Bondarev, Y.	Bondarev, Y.
			Bopolov	Bopolov
	Borisov, V.			
			Borisov, V.I.	Borisov, V.I.
Borisov, V. Ev.	Borisov, V. Ev.		Borisov, V. Yev.	Borisov, V. Ev.
Borisov, V.S.	Borisov, V.S.		Borisov, V.S.	Borisov, V.S.
Borodin, N.I.	Borodin, N.I.	Borodin		
Borovik, P.I.	Borovik, P.I.		Borovik, P.	
		Borovikov, V.A. (?)		
Borovsky, A.N.	Borovsky, A.N.	Borovsky, A.N.		Borovsky, A.
Borovsky, V.				
Boss, D.Y.	Boss, D. Ya.		Boss, D.Y.	Boss, D.
Bragunets, E.				Bragunets, E.
Breslavsky, N.I.	Breslavsky, N.I.		Breslavsky, N.I.	Breslavsky, N.I.
				Brind, Yu.
				Brodsky, I.A.
				Broslavsky, V.
				Brovko, Yu. P.
Bublik, V.K.	Bublik, V.K.		Bublik, V.K.	Bublik, V.K.

Table A.3 (cont.)

Bloch and Reddaway (1984:253–62) *Coverage*: 1977–83	**Koppers (1990:74–176)** *Coverage*: 1920s to 1990	**Mercer (1991a and b; 1992)** *Coverage*: through 1991	**Podrabinek (1981:158–83** *et al.*) *Coverage*: late 1950s(?) through late 1970s	**Smith and Oleszczuk (1988a; 1989)** *Coverage*: 1960–81 before additions
	Bukovsky, V.K.		Bukovsky, V.K.	Bukovsky, V.K.
Bulakh, E.P.				
	Bulev, A.K.	Bulev, A.	Bulev, A.	
		Bushenko, S.		
Bushin, V.P.				Bushin, V.P.
Buterus, G.T.	Buterus, G.T.			
Butko, A.A.				
	Butkus, D. Ju.			Butkus, D.J.
	Buyakov			
	Bychkov, G.A.		Bychkov, G.A.	Bychkov, G.A.
Bykov, A.N.				
		Bykov, O.		
Bykov, S.			Bykov, S.	
			Bykov, V.	Bykov, V.
				Bykov, V.I.
Bykovsky, I.A.				
	Cebanu, V.V.	Cebanu, V.V.		
Cekanavicius, A.	Cekanavicius, A.	Chekanavicius, A.	Cechanavicius, A.	Cehanavicius, A.
				Celykh, A.L.
	Chepula, A.G.		Chepula, A.G.	Chepula, A.N.
	Cherep, A.I.			
	Cherkashin, V.			
Cherkasov, A.A.		Cherkasov, A.A.		

				Chernogorov, A.Y.
Chernyshov, V.I.	Chernyshov, V.I.		Chernychov, V.I.	Chernyshov, V.I.
Cherpakov, G.G.				Cherpakov, G.G.
Chertkova, A.V.	Chertkova, A.V.	Chertkova, A.V.		Chertkova, A.V.
	Chinnov, A.F.		Chinnov, A.F.	Chinnov, A.F.
			Chudakov, N.	
Chudakov, V.S.				
Cidzikas, P.	Cidzikas, P.		Cidzikas, P.	Cidzikas, P.
				Cilinskov
				Cypin, L.B.
	Dagys, S.L.			
Danchev, V.				
	Danilov, N.N.		Danilov, N.N.	Danilov, N.N.
			Danilov, O.	
				Danne, E.E.
			Davarashvili, B.	Davarashvili, B.O.
		David, G.		
				Davidovich E.A.
Davletov, R.S.	Davletov, K.S.		Davletov, K.S.	Davletov, K.S.
Davydov (Ryzhov), V.V.	Davydov (Ryzhov), V.V.			Davydov, V.V.
				Degtyarev, V.N.
Demyanov, N.I.				
Demyanov, N.I.			Demyanov, N.I.	Demyanov, N.I.
Denisov, A.I.			Denisov, A.	Denisov, A.
		Denisov, Ye.		
				Deonisiadi, G.V.
Dmitrienko, V.				
Dobromyslov, V.V.			Dobromyslov V.V.	Dobromyslov, V.V.
	Dobrovolsky A.A.			Dobrovolsky, A.A.
		Dobrov, L.F.		

Table A.3 (cont.)

Bloch and Reddaway (1984:253–62) *Coverage*: 1977–83	**Koppers (1990:74–176)** *Coverage*: 1920s to 1990	**Mercer (1991a and b; 1992)** *Coverage*: through 1991	**Podrabinek (1981:158–83** *et al.*) *Coverage*: late 1950s(?) through late 1970s	**Smith and Oleszczuk (1988a; 1989)** *Coverage*: 1960–81 before additions
		Dogilis, V.		
	Dolgy, P.V.			
Domnitsa, A.				Domnitsa, A.
				Dremlyug(-a), V.A.
				Dubrov, A.V.
	Dubrov, A.V.			
				Dubrovik
Dubrovin, V.				
Duvanov, A.				
Dvoretsky, F.P.	Dvoretsky, F.P.	Dvoretsky, F.P.		Dvoretskii F.P.
				Dvoretskii I.G.
		Dzhanashvili, R.M.		
Dzibalov, V.A.	Dzibalov, V.A.		Dzibalov, V.A.	Dzibalov, V.A.
				Dzyuba, Yu. V.
		Edamenko, F.P.		
Efimov, A. (not L.)				Efimov, A.
			Yefimov, L.	Efimov, L.
	Egides, P.M.		Yegides, P.M.	Egides, P.M.
Ekimov, A.A.				Ekimov, A.A.
				Eikhvald, V.
				Ershov, V.M.
Erygina, E.N.				Erygina, E.N.
Evdokimov, B.D.	Evdokimov, B.D.		Yevdokimov, B.D.	Evdokimov, B.D.

Fadayev, N.	Fadayev, N.	Fadayev, N.		
	Fainberg, V.I.			Fainberg, V.
Fedorenko, I.G.				Fedorenko, I.G.
			Fedorov, L.K.	
Fedorov, V.				
Fedotov, G.A.	Fedotov, G.A.		Fedotov, G.A.	Fedotov, G.A.
				Fedotov, G.A.
				Fedotov, I.P.
Fedyanin, V.				
	Feigin, G.I.			Feigin, G.I.
			Feinberg, V.I.	Fainberg, V.I.
				Fetisov, A.A.
Fin, R.T.	Fin, R.T.			
Finkel, F.	Finkel, F. Ya.			
	Forpostov, G.		Forpostov, G.	Forpostov, G.
			Frolkin, I.L.	Frolkin, I.L.
				Gaidar, N.
			Galanskov, Y.T.	Galanskov, Yu. T.
			Galashov, N.P.	
Galko, K.A.				Galko, K.A.
			Galler, L.M.	
Gallyamov, S.				
Ganyushkin, A.J.			Ganyushkin	Ganiushkin, A.J.
Gavrilenko, A.G.				
Genke, N.S.			Genke	
Gershkanu, N.	Gershkanu, N.			Gershkanu, N.
Gershuni, V.L.	Gershuni, V.L.	Gershuni, V.L.	Gershuni, V.L.	Gershuni, V.L.
				Gilev, N.F.
				Gimbutas, Ju.
			Gitelman, Y.N.	

Table A.3 (cont.)

Bloch and Reddaway (1984:253–62) *Coverage*: 1977–83	**Koppers (1990:74–176)** *Coverage*: 1920s to 1990	**Mercer (1991a and b; 1992)** *Coverage*: through 1991	**Podrabinek (1981:158–83** *et al.*) *Coverage*: late 1950s(?) through late 1970s	**Smith and Oleszczuk (1988a; 1989)** *Coverage*: 1960–81 before additions
Glebov, K.				
Glukhov, A.L.				Glukhov, A.
Glukhova, A.M.				
		Glukhov, Yu. V.		
		Gogiashvili, G.		
	Golikov, V.M.			Golikov, V.M.
				Golovanov
				Goncharov, V.M.
				Konin, L.S.
Gonin, V.M. (not 'Konin')				
	Gorbanevskaya, N.E.			Gorbanevskaya, N.E.
		Gordgiyan, A.		
			Grachev	Grachev
				Greshchuk, I.A.
		Gridasov, V.K.		
	Grigas, V.E.			Grigas, V.E.
	Grigorenko, P.G.		Grigorenko, P.G.	Grigorenko, P.G.
			Grigoryev, D.	
Grishakov, A.T.				Grishakov, A.T.
Grishchenko, O.G.			Grishchenko, O.	
Grishchuk, I.A.		Grishchuk, I.A.		
Gritskov, I.S.				
		Gromov, V.C.		

Gu (Goux), R.				
				Gubanov, L.E.
	Gudilin, V.			Gudilin, V.
		Gura, S.		
Gusarov, V.N.	Gusarov, V.N.		Gusarov, V.N.	Gusarov, V.N.
	Gusyakova			Gusyakova
		Gyurdzhan, A.I.		
		Hasanov, A.Y.		
	Igrunov, V.V.		Igrunov, V.V.	Igrunov, V.V.
	Ilchenko, A.	Ilchenko, A.M.		
				Ilyakov, V.V.
Ilin, A.	Ilyin, A.I.	Ilin, A.I.	Ilyin, A.	Ilyin, A.
	Iofe, O. Ye.		Iofe, O. Yu.	Iofe, O. Yu.
				Iosif, Ja.V.
Isachkin, A.I.				Isachkin, A.I.
Ivanitsky, A.				Ivanitsky, A.
Ivankov-Nikolov, M.V.	Ivankov-Nikolov, M.V.		Ivankov-Nikolov, M.V.	Ivankov-Nikolov, M.
				Ivanov, A.M.
Ivanov, V.I.				
	Ivanov, Yu. E.			Ivanov, Yu. E.
Ivanova, R.	Ivanova, R.			Ivanova, R.
				Jacenko, V.A.
				Jacishin, M.
			Yakhimovich, I.A.	Jakhimovich, I.A.
				Jakimov, P.I.
	Jankauskas, A.			Jankauskas, A.
	Jasulevicius, K.			
	Jirkov, G.K.			
Jogesma, H.	Jogesma, H.		Jogesma, H.	Jogesma, H.
				Jonaitis, E.G.

Table A.3 (cont.)

Bloch and Reddaway (1984:253–62) *Coverage*: 1977–83	**Koppers (1990:74–176)** *Coverage*: 1920s to 1990	**Mercer (1991a and b; 1992)** *Coverage*: through 1991	**Podrabinek (1981:158–83** *et al.*) *Coverage*: late 1950s(?) through late 1970s	**Smith and Oleszczuk (1988a; 1989)** *Coverage*: 1960–81 before additions
	Kalanta, R.			
Kalinichenko, V.V.	Kalinichenko, V.V.			
	Kalinin, Yu.			Kalinin, Yu.
	Kalishin, A.	Kalishin, A.S.		
Kalkutin, M.				
			Kallas, T.	Kallas, T.
				Kalosh, H.V.
				Kalosh, H.V.
Kalugin, A.		Kalugin, A.I.		
Kalyuzhny, V.D.	Kalyuzhny, V.D.			Kalyuzhnii V.D.
Kamardin, V.				
Kamensky, N.S.			Kamensky, N.S.	Kamensky, N.S. H?
	Kanafiev, A.	Kanafiev, A.M.		
Kapishin, A.S.				
				Kaplun, I.M.
Karaliunas, V.	Karaliunas, V.			Karaliunas, V.
	Karapetyan, S.	Karapetyan, S.		
			Karasev, V.	Karasev, Ul. H?
Karibzhan-Uly, K.	Karibzhan-Uly, Kh.			
Karmanov, A.			Karmanov, A.	
	Karmanov, K. Yu.	Karmanov, K. Yu.		
				Karmonov, V.
				Karoliunas, V.

				Karymov, I.
Kashin, V.	Kashin, V.			Kashin, V.
Kashkov, Yu. A.				Kashkov, Yu. A.
	Kasyan, S.M.			
Kazakevicius, L.				
		Kazhdan, V.V.		
Keisin, Yu.				
				Kekilova, A.
Khailo, V.P.	Khailo, V.P.			Khailo, V.P.
	Kharitonov, V.N.			Kharitonov, V.N.
		Khasanov, A.		
Khomyak, I.G.	Khomyak, I.G.			Khomyak, I.G.
				Khramisov, V.
Khudyakov, Yu. V.				
Khutorskoi, Ya. A.				
	Kindeyev, L.			Kindeev, L.
Kirsnauskaite, Z.S.				Kirsnauskaite, Z.
Kislik, V.S.				Kislik, V.S.
Klebanov, V.A.	Klebanov, V.	Klebanov, V.		Klebanov, V.A.
				Kleimenova, A.N.
Klimasauskas, G.				Klimasauskas, H.
Klishch, M.			Klishch, M.	Klisch-Klesch, M.
		Kochan, R.		
			Kochkin, A.V.	Kochkin, A.V.
Kochubei, A.			Kochubey, A.	Kochubei, A.N.
Kolchugin, S.	Kochugin, S.			
	Kolesnik, V.P.			Kolesnik, V.P.
Kolesov, I.N.				Kolesov, I.N.
Kolishenko, V.A.	Kolishenko, V.A.			Kolishenko, V.A.
Kolomiets, V.	Kolimiets, V.			Kolomiets, V.

Table A.3 (cont.)

Bloch and Reddaway (1984:253–62) *Coverage*: 1977–83	**Koppers (1990:74–176)** *Coverage*: 1920s to 1990	**Mercer (1991a and b; 1992)** *Coverage*: through 1991	**Podrabinek (1981:158–83** *et al.*) *Coverage*: late 1950s(?) through late 1970s	**Smith and Oleszczuk (1988a; 1989)** *Coverage*: 1960–81 before additions
Kolyshev, M.A.				
Komarov, A.E. (Yev.)	Komarov, A.E.			
	Komarov, E.E.		Komarov, Y.Y.	Komarov, E.E.
	Komarova, F.N.			Komarova, F.N.
	Komarovsky, V.			Komarovsky, V.
			Komissarov	
	Konevalov/Konovalov, Yu.I.	Konevalov, Yu.I.		
Konin, L.S.				Konin, L.S.
Konovalikhin, V.I.				Konovalikhin, V.
Kopeiko, N.				Kopeiko, N.
Kopytin, P.N.	Kopytin, P.		Kopytin, P.	Kopytin, P.
	Korablev, N.			Korablev, N.
Korchak, V.				
Koreisha, I.T.				
Korfidov, V.N.		Korfidov, V.N.		
				Korneichuk
Korol, V.N.				
	Korsakov, K.A.	Korsakov, K.A.		
Kotov, A.N.	Kotov, A.N.		Kotov, A.N.	Kotov, A.N.
				Koval, I.T.
				Kovalenko, N.I.
Kovalev, A.S.	Kovalyov, A.S.			

Kovgar, B.	Kovhar, B.		Kovgar, B.	Kovgar, B.F.
		Kozhevnikov, Yu. A.		
		Kozhin, V.V.		
			Kozlov	Kozlov
	Kozlov, A.P.		Kozlov, A.P.	
	Kozlov, A.		Kozlov, A.	
		Kozlov O.V.		
Kozlov, V.		Kozlov, V.		Kozlov, V.
Krasivsky, Z.M.	Krasivsky, Z.M.		Krasivsky, Z.M.	Krasivsky, Z.M.
	Krasnyak, V.I.		Krasnyak, V.	Krasnyak, V.I.
Kravchuk, Ya. Yakovlevich				
			Kravchuk, Ya. Yaroslavovich	
Kravtsov, K.N.				
				Kravtsov, L.E.
	Kreek, S.K.		Kreek, S.K.	Kreek, S.K.
				Kristi, I.G.
				Krulsky, Ya. Y.
Krylov, B.	Krylov, B.			Krylov, B.
	Krylsky, Ya. Yu.		Krylsky, Ya. Yu.	Krylsky, Ya. Y.
	Kryuchkov, N.N.			Kryuchkov, N.N.
				Kryuzhkov
	Kubyshkin, V.P.	Kubyshkin, V.P.		Kubyshkin
Kucherenko, V.I.				
				Kudiene, V.
Kudryatsev, E.	Kudryatsev, E.			Kudryatsev, E.
Kukarskikh, G.V.				
Kukobaka, M.I.	Kukobaka, M.I.		Kukobaka, M.I.	Kukobaka, M.I.
Kulish, N.				

Table A.3 (cont.)

Bloch and Reddaway (1984:253–62) *Coverage*: 1977–83	**Koppers (1990:74–176)** *Coverage*: 1920s to 1990	**Mercer (1991a and b; 1992)** *Coverage*: through 1991	**Podrabinek (1981:158–83** *et al.*) *Coverage*: late 1950s(?) through late 1970s	**Smith and Oleszczuk (1988a; 1989)** *Coverage*: 1960–81 before additions
Kuma, T.	Kuma, T.E.	Kuma, T.		
Kume, A.	Kume, A.			
		Kurbatov, V.V.		
				Kushev, E.I.
Kushnirenko, I.				
Kusidis, A.				
Kutsil, D.D.	Kutsil, D.D.			
	Kutyavin, A.F.			
	Kutyavina, Z.P.			
Kuzkin, A.	Kuzkin, A.			Kuzkin, A.
Kuzmin, I.				Kuzmin, I.
	Kuznetsov, A.K.			
Kuznetsov, G.		Kuznetsov, G.	Kuznetsov, G.	Kuznetsov, G.
	Kuznetsov, S.			
			Kuznetsov, V.V.	Kuznetsov, V.
				Kuznetsova, E.F.
Lapmann, J.R.				
Larin, I.K.				
	Larin, I.M.		Larin, I.M.	Larin, I.M.
				Larov, Yu. K.
	Lashkevich, N.	Lashkevich, N.		
				Latyshev
				Laucius, J.

	Lavrov, Yu. K.			Lavrov, Yu. K.
				Lavut, A.P.
Lazda, P. Ya.	Lazda, P. Ya.			
Lazinskas, V.				Lazhinskas, V.
	Lazuta, I.V.		Lazuta, I.V.	Lazuta, I.V.
			Leivond, J.	Leiwand, J.
		Leonov		
Lesnov, B.V.	Lesnov, B.V.			Lesnov
Levenkov, N.V.	Levenkov, N.V.			
				Levin, Yu. L.
Lipinskaya, V.A.		Lipinskaya, V.		Lipinskaya, V.A.
	Lipinskaya, V.O.			
		Lishchenko, O.E.		
				Lisitsky
	Litvinov, I.M.			
				Litvinov, P.M.
		Lomakin, P.P.		
				Lonchakov, M.
				Losik, P.V.
	Lubentsov, A.	Lubentsov, A.		
				Luchkiv, V.
				Luchkiv, V.S.
	Lukanin, V.		Lukanin, V.	Lukanin, V.
Lukosevicius, P.	Lukosevicius, P.			
				Lukyanchuk, G.Y.
	Lukyanenko, L.G.			Lukyanenko, L.G.
Lukyanov, A.A.				
Lukyanov, E.				
Lupinos, A.I.	Lupinos, A.I.	Lupinos, A.	Lupinos, A.I.	Lupynis, A.I.
Lutsik, M.P.	Lutsyk, M.P.		Lutsik, M.P.	Lutsyk, M.P.

Table A.3 (cont.)

Bloch and Reddaway (1984:253–62) *Coverage*: 1977–83	**Koppers (1990:74–176)** *Coverage*: 1920s to 1990	**Mercer (1991a and b; 1992)** *Coverage*: through 1991	**Podrabinek (1981:158–83** *et al.*) *Coverage*: late 1950s(?) through late 1970s	**Smith and Oleszczuk (1988a; 1989)** *Coverage*: 1960–81 before additions
Lutskiv, V.S.	Lutskiv, V.S.			
Lvov, S.R.	Lvov, S.K.		Lvov, S.	Lvov, S.
Lyapin, A.S.	Lyapin, A.S.			Lyapin, A.S.
Lysak, P.A.	Lysak, P.A.		Lysak, P.A.	Lysak, P.A.
				Lysenko, A.L.
				Lysenko, P.L.
Lysov, V.F.				Lysov, V.F.
			Machko, V.	
		Mahinya (Mohinya), A.A.		
		Mahmodov, K.		Makhmudov, K.
			Mamutov, Z.	
				Maiauskas, I.
			Majauskas, V.	
	Makarenko, M.Y.			Makarenko, M.Y.
		Makarova, O.V.		
Makeyeva, V.Z.				Makeyeva, V.Z.
Makhayev, O.			Makhayev, I.	
Makhayev, O.				Makhayev, O.
Makhrov, E.S.				Makhrov, E.S.
Maksimov, V.S.	Maksimov, V.S.			Maksimov, V.S.
				Malkhasyan, A.
	Malkhazyan, A.			Malkhazyan, A.
	Maltsev		Maltsev, V.	Maltsev, V.I.

	Maltsev, Yu.V.		Maltsev, Yu.V.	Maltsev, Yu.V.
Malyarevsky, S.V.				
Malyshev, K.P.	Malyshev, K.P.		Malyshev, K.P.	Malyshev, K.P.
				Malyshev, V.M.
Manko, A.G. (not Matko)	Manko, A.		Matko, A.	Matko, A.
Maresh, A.	Maresh, A.			Maresh, A.
	Maresin, V.M.			Mareshin, V.M
	Margorin, N.			.
Marikov, V.G.				
		Marinjuk, A.W.		
				Markaitis
				Markevich
				Markovich, A.
			Martyahov, V.	
Martynov, Y.P.				
Mashkovtsuv, V.A.	Maszkowcow, W.A.			
Maslennikov, N.				
Mastrosov				
	Matykin, V.I.	Matykin, V.I.		
			Maximov, V.S.	
				Maziliauskas, E.
Medvedev, I.V.	Medvedev, I.V.			Medvedev, I.V.
	Medvedev, Zh.A.		Medvedev, Zh.A.	Medvedev, Zh.A.
Meleshko, V.P.	Meleshko		Meleshko, V.P.	Meleshko
	Melngailis, G.	Mengailis, G.		
Melnikov, L.I.				Melnikov, L.I.
Merkushev, V.I.				Merkushev, V.I.
Meshko, O.Ya.				Meshko, O.Ya.

Table A.3 (cont.)

Bloch and Reddaway (1984:253–62) *Coverage*: 1977–83	**Koppers (1990:74–176)** *Coverage*: 1920s to 1990	**Mercer (1991a and b; 1992)** *Coverage*: through 1991	**Podrabinek (1981:158–83** *et al.*) *Coverage*: late 1950s(?) through late 1970s	**Smith and Oleszczuk (1988a; 1989)** *Coverage*: 1960–81 before additions
Mikhailenko, A.V.	Mikhailenko, A.V.	Mikhailenko, A.V.		
Mikhailov, I.I.	Mikhailov, I.I.			
		Milyukhin, V.N.		
				Milyutin, O.
				Mirchuk
	Mirkushov, V.I.		Mirkushov, V.I.	Mirkushov, V.I.
Moiseyev, V.M.	Moiseyev, V.M.	Moiseev	Moiseev, V.M.	Moiseyev, V.M.
		Molokanov, Ye.		
Monakhov, A.	Monakhov, A.	Monakhov, A.	Monakhov, A.	
	Montlevich, V.M.			Montlevich, V.M.
			Morkovnikov	Morkovnikov
				Moroz, V.Y.
			Morozov, N.	
		Morozov, S.		
	Morozov, V.F.	Morozov, V.F.		
Moskvin, O.N.				Moskvin, O.N.
	Mucenieks, J.A.			
	Mukhamedyarov, R.G.		Mukhamedyarov, R.G.	Mukhamedyarov, R.G.
	Mukyan, I.A.	Mukyan, I.A.		
	Mumichak, I.	Mumichak, I.		
Muraviev, P.M.				
		Musatov, A.		
				Musatov, G.A.

Musatov, S.V.	Musatov, S.		Musatov, S.V.	Musatov, S.V.
			Musienko, M.S.	Musienko, M.S.
		Nabokin		
Naletov, V.M.				
	Naritsa, M.A.		Naritsa, M.A.	Naritsa, M.A.
		Naskovets, M.D.		
Nastavin, A.A.				
	Nastushenko, L.			Nastusenko, L.
	Naudziunas, B.			Naudzhyiunas, B.
		Nazarovets, N.		
		Nedelin, Ye.		
				Nekipelov, V.A.
	Neznanov, V.T.			Neznanov, V.T.
		Nikiforchuk, A.		
Nikitenkov, V.N.	Nikitenkov, V.N.		Nikitenkov, V.N.	Nikitenkov, V.N.
				Nikitenkova, L.P.
Nikitin, A.V.	Nikitin, A.V.			Nikitin, A.V.
Nikolayev, E.B.	Nikolayev, E.N.		Nikolayev, Ye.B.	Nikolayev, E.N.
Nikolayev, V.D.	Nikolayev, V.			Nikolayev, V.D.
				Nikolsky
	Nikretin/Nekredin, Yu.			
	Nizhinskiy, A.P.			
		Novikov, A.B.		
		Novikov, V.I.		
Novodvorskaya, V.	Novodvorskaya, V.	Novodvorskaya, V.	Novodvorskaya, V.	Novodvorskaya, Ya.
Nozhak, O.	Nozhak, O.			Nozhak, O.
Ochimov				
	Oganesyan, V.S.	Oganesyan, V.S.		Oganesyan
	Ogurtsov, I.V.			Ogurtsov, I.V.
	Ojekov, P.			

Table A.3 (cont.)

Bloch and Reddaway (1984:253–62) *Coverage*: 1977–83	**Koppers (1990:74–176)** *Coverage*: 1920s to 1990	**Mercer (1991a and b; 1992)** *Coverage*: through 1991	**Podrabinek (1981:158–83** *et al.*) *Coverage*: late 1950s(?) through late 1970s	**Smith and Oleszczuk (1988a; 1989)** *Coverage*: 1960–81 before additions
Okinin, E.	Okinin, E.		Okinin, Y.	Okinin, E.R.
			Okunev, V.I.	
		Oleynikov, Yu.		
	Oreshkin, P.			Oreshkin, P.
			Orlov, A.	
Osadchuk, I.				
Oshchepkov, V.G.				Oshchepkov, V.G.
				Osipov, V.N.
		Osmanov, Yu.		
			Ovechkin, V.V.	Ovechkin, V.V.
Ozhegov, R.N.	Ozhegov, R.N.	Ozhegov, R.N.	Ozhegov	
				Ozhelov, A.
			Palchevsky	
		Palchikov, A.N.		
Panasyuk, I.				
			Panov	Panov
	Pankov, N.A.			
	Pankova, N.			
		Pankratova, I.		
			Panteleev, V.	Panteleev, V.I.
	Pantin, V.			Pantin, V.
	Paramonov, G.K.		Paramonov, G.C.	Paramonov, G.K.
Parasenkov, F.	Parasenko (?), F.			Parasenkov, F.

Pargamunik, E.				
Parkhunov, V.G.				
Paskauskiene, A.			Paskauskiene, A.	Paskauskiene, A.
				Paulov, B.P.
				Pavlenkov, V.K.
	Pavlov, A.			
	Pavlov, B.P.		Pavlov, B.P.	Pavlov, B.P.
Pavlyuk, V.K.	Pavlyuk, V.B.			
				Pennanen, A.
Pervushin, V.K.	Pervushin, V.K.	Pervushin, V.K.		
		Petrashov, I.F.		
				Petrov, V.V.
Petrov, Yu.				
				Petrovna, L.A.
Pihelgas, J.A.	Piheljas, J.			
				Pimenov, R.I.
	Pintan			Pintan
	Pinyayev, A.F.	Pinyayev, A.		
	Prigov, S.K.			Pirogov, S.K.
			Pisarev, S.P.	Pisarev, S.P.
		Pivovarov, A.		
Plakhotnyuk, M.G.	Plakhotnyuk, M.H.	Plakhotnyuk, M.	Plakhotnyuk, N.G.	Plakhotnyuk, M.G.
	Plenainen, A.			Plenainen, A.
	Plyushch, L.I.		Plyushch, L.I.	Plyushch, L.I.
Pochinok, P.M.				
				Podyapolsky
Polezhayev, A.V.				Polezhayev, A.V.
Polynek, V.S.	Polynek, V.S.	Polinek, V.S.		
				Polylitsin-Potse
	Ponomarenko, A.			

Table A.3 (cont.)

Bloch and Reddaway (1984:253–62) *Coverage*: 1977–83	**Koppers (1990:74–176)** *Coverage*: 1920s to 1990	**Mercer (1991a and b; 1992)** *Coverage*: through 1991	**Podrabinek (1981:158–83** *et al.*) *Coverage*: late 1950s(?) through late 1970s	**Smith and Oleszczuk (1988a; 1989)** *Coverage*: 1960–81 before additions
Ponomaryov, A.D.	Ponomaryov, A.D.		Ponomarev, A.D.	Ponomaryov, A.D.
		Ponomaryov, M.		
				Popov
				Popov
			Popov, B.	Popov, B.
		Popov, K.		
				Popov, V.T.
Popov, V.V.	Popov, V.V.		Popov, V.V.	Popov, V.V.
Popov, V.	Popov, V.	Popov, V.		Popov, V.
	Poskiene, B.			Poskiene, B.
				Postapov
	Potapov			Potapov
Potylitzyn, S.A.	Potylitzyn, S.		Potylitsyn, S.A.	Potylitsyn, S.A.
Pozdnyakov, A.N.				Pozdnyakov, A.N.
		Pozharskiy		
Pribytkov, L.S.				
Pridyba, I.				
		Prigov, D.		
Prilepko, A.A.			Prilepko, A.A.	Prilepko, A.A.
	Prisacaru, N.G.			Prisacaru, N.
Pruzhanovsky				Pruzhanovsky
		Pskov, A.K.		
Puntusov, A.P.			Puntusov, A.P.	Puntusov, A.P.

Purtov, I.			Purtov, I.	Purtov, I.V.
Purtov, S.	Purtov, S.	Purtov, S.	Purtov, S.	Purtov, S.
				Pushkin, A.
Rabinovich, V.N.				Rabinovich, V.N.
Radikov, I.F.			Radikov, I.F.	
Rafalsky, V.P.	Rafalsky, V.P.	Rafalsky, V.	Rafalsky, V.P.	Rafalsky, V.P.
		Ravins, M.		
				Rementsov, V.I.
		Reshetov, V.		
				Revnyuk, M.K.
		Revyakin, M.		
Reznikov, Yu.V.				Reznikov, Yu.V.
	Riga, A.S.	Riga, A.		
	Rinkevich, I.V.	Rinkevich, I.V.		Rinkevich, I.V.
	Rips, I.A.		Rips, I.A.	Rips, I.A.
		Rodinov, I.		
				Roshiyan
Roshiyanu, I.				
Roslan, A.A.				
			Rotshtein, Yu.	
Rozhdestvov, V.P.	Rozhdestvov, V.P.			Rozhdestvov, V.P.
Ruban, V.F.	Ruban, V.F.		Ruban, V.	Ruban, V.F.
			Rudenko, I.	
		Rukosuev, A.I.		
Runov, A.F.	Runov, A.F.			Runov, A.F.
	Rustan, I.			Rustan, I.
	Ryabokon, V.			
Rybak, G.	Rybak, G.			
	Rybak, V.V.			
	Rybakov, A.		Rybakov, A.	Rybakov, A.
				Ryss, I.

Table A.3 (cont.)

Bloch and Reddaway (1984:253–62) *Coverage*: 1977–83	**Koppers (1990:74–176)** *Coverage*: 1920s to 1990	**Mercer (1991a and b; 1992)** *Coverage*: through 1991	**Podrabinek (1981:158–83** *et al.*) *Coverage*: late 1950s(?) through late 1970s	**Smith and Oleszczuk (1988a; 1989)** *Coverage*: 1960–81 before additions
	Saakyan, A.			
	Saakyan, K.			
Sadunas, J.				
	Safronov, N.V.			
	Safronov, P.			Safronov, P.I.
				Sakulsky
Salaseviciute, Z.				
	Salaty, V.			Salaty
Salum, V.				
Samkharadze, N.M.				Samkharadze, B.M.
Samoilov, E.V.	Samoilov, E.V.		Samoylov, E.V.	Samoilov, E.V.
	Samsonov, N.N.		Samsonov, N.N.	Samsonov, N.
			Samsonov, V.	
	Sapezhko, Yu.P.		Sapezhko, Yu.P.	Sapezhko, Yu.P.
Sarbayev, A.A.				
Sarpania, R.				Sarpania, R.
	Sarkisyan, A.			
Saveleva, N.				
			Savin, V.	
Savurenko, Yu.				
	Scurybin, M.P.			
Sebelev, P.M.			Sebelev, P.M.	
Semenov				Semyonev

	Senin, A.			
	Serebrennikov, N.V.			
		Serebrov, F.		
Sergeyev, M.S.	Sergeyev, M.S.			Sergeyev, M.S.
Sery, V.I.				Serii, V.I.
Selev (?), D.				
				Sevalneva, O.I.
	Sevelyev, D.			
	Sevruk, V.L.			Sevruk, V.L.
Shabura, N.				
	Shaburov, N.A.			
	Shakina, V.I.	Shakina, V.I.		
Shaporenko, D.				Shaporenko, D.
	Shashenkov, E.V.		Shashenkov, Y.V.	Shashenkov, E.V.
Shatalova, T.N.				
Shatravka, A.I.	Shatravka, A.I.			Shatravka, A.I.
Shatravka, M.I.	Shatravka, M.			Shatravka, M.I.
Shavrov, V.M.				Shavrov, V.M.
Shef, G.				
		Sheludkov, A.L.		
		Shetinskiy, V.G.		
Shevchenko	Shevchenko			Shevchenko
	Shikhanovich, Yu.A.			Shikanovich, Yu.A.
				Shilkrot, B.L.
	Shimanov, G.M.		Shimanov, G.M.	Shimanov, G.M.
Shimko, A.				
Shipilov, V.G.	Shipilov, V.G.	Shipilov, V.		
			Shipilov, V.I.	Shipilov, V.I.
			Shklovsky, V.L.	
	Shlepnyov, V.		Shlepnev, V.	Shlepnyov, V.

Table A.3 (cont.)

Bloch and Reddaway (1984:253–62) *Coverage*: 1977–83	**Koppers (1990:74–176)** *Coverage*: 1920s to 1990	**Mercer (1991a and b; 1992)** *Coverage*: through 1991	**Podrabinek (1981:158–83** *et al.*) *Coverage*: late 1950s(?) through late 1970s	**Smith and Oleszczuk (1988a; 1989)** *Coverage*: 1960–81 before additions
Shtein, L.Ya.	Shtein, L.Ya.		Shtein, L.	Shtein, L.
Shushenkov V.N. (not Shunenkov)	Shunenkov, V.		Shushenko, V.N.	Shunenkov, V.N.
				Shutkin, A.F.
				Shuvalov, V.L.
Shvachko, N.T.			Shvachko, N.	
Shvedov, L.I.			Shvedov	
				Shvoruk
Sichko, V.P.				
Sidenko, F.A.	Sidenko, F.A.			Sidenko, F.A.
		Sidorchenko, A.I.		
		Sidorov, V.		
				Silmale, M.A.
Simkin, A.A.	Simkin, A.A.			
Sinigovsky, V.V.				
Skobov, A.V.	Skobov, A.V.	Skobov, A.V.		Skobov, A.L.
Skochok, P.	Skochok, P.I.			Skochok, P.I.
	Skrebets, O.F.			Skrebets, O.F.
				Sleshnev, V.
				Slishevskii, I.I.
Slobodenyuk, E.P.				
	Smirnov, O.		Smirnov, O.	Smirnov, O.
		Smirnov, V.		

Smirnov, V.P.				Smirnov, V.P.
				Smirnov, V.S.
	Smirnova, V.S.			
	Sokolov, A.			
Sokolov, V.P.				Sokolov, V.P.
				Sokulsky, I.G.
	Sokurenko, A.P.	Sokurenko, A.		
				Soldatov, S.I.
Solomeinikov, B.V.	Solomeinikov, B.V.			
	Solovyov, O.G.			Solovyov, O.G.
				Solovyov, V.
Sopoyev	Sopoyev			
Sorokin, N.A.	Sorokin, N.A.			Sorokin, N.A.
				Spashchenko, V.A.
Spinenko, V.N.	Spinenko, V.V.	Spinenko, V.N.	Spinenko, V.	Spinenko, V.
	Starchik, P.P.			Starchik, P.
		Stashenko, G.		
Statkevicius, A.	Statkevicius, A.		Statkevicius, A.	Statkevicius, A.
Steba, I.M.				Steba
Stepanchuk, A.				
	Stepanov, A.		Stepanov, A.	Stepanov, A.
	Stetsenko, G.N.			
Stolper, V.I.				
Stolyar, Ya.M.				Stolyar, Ya.M.
	Storozhevoi, P.N.			Storozhevoi, P.A.
				Stroeva, E.
Stroganov, S.M.			Stroganov, S.M.	Stroganov, S.M.
	Stroyeva, A.		Stroyeva, Y.V.	Stroyeva, E.
				Stus, V.S.
		Styshchuk or Stetsyuk, K.N.		

Table A.3 (cont.)

Bloch and Reddaway (1984:253–62) *Coverage*: 1977–83	**Koppers (1990:74–176)** *Coverage*: 1920s to 1990	**Mercer (1991a and b; 1992)** *Coverage*: through 1991	**Podrabinek (1981:158–83** *et al.*) *Coverage*: late 1950s(?) through late 1970s	**Smith and Oleszczuk (1988a; 1989)** *Coverage*: 1960–81 before additions
Sudakov, S.				
Sukharev, D.F.				
	Sukharevich, F.	Sukharevich, F.F.		
Sulimov, V.				Sulimov, V.
	Suprunyuk, G.			Suprunyuk, G.
	Suslensky, Ya.			
Suslin, V.				
		Suvorov, L.M.		
	Sytinsky, V.	Sytinsky, V.I.		
		Tabelev, L.L.		
	Tamonis, M.			Tamonis, M.
	Tamoshevich, S.			Tamoshevich, S.
	Tarakanov, Yu.P.			Tarakanov, Yu.P.
	Tarasov, A.A.			Tarasov, A.A.
		Tarasyavicius, G.		
		Tarasyavicius, M.		
	Tarsis, V.Y.			Tarsis, V.Y.
Terelya, I.M.	Terelya, I.M.		Terelya, I.M.	Terelya, I.M.
			Tereznikov, G.	
				Terleckas, A.N.
Ternopolsky, Yu.				
		Ternovsky, L.		

		Timchuk, A.P.		
Timokhin, V.K.	Timokhin, V.S.	Timokhin, V.S.		Timokhin, V.S.
	Timonin, I.		Timonin, I.	Timonin, I.
Titov, V.G.	Titov, V.G.			Titov, V.
	Titov, Yu.		Titov, Yu.	Titov, Yu.V.
Tovstenko, V.N.				Tovstenko, V.N.
	Trifonov, G.N.			Trifonov, G.N.
Trifonov, V.I.	Trifonov, V.I.		Trifonov, V.I.	Trifonov, V.
Trish, V.G.				Trish, V.
Trotsyuk, P.M.			Trotsyuk-Nozlyuk, P.	
Tselykh, A. (not V.)	Tselykh, V.		Tselykh, A.	Tselykh, V.
Tsurikov, V.A.	Tsurikov, V.A.			
	Tsygankova, L.			Tsygankova, L.
	Tumerman, A.L.			Tumerman
Tursunov, V.A.	Tursunov, V.A.			
				Tustsevich, S.I.
	Tystsevich, S.I.			Tystsevich, S.I.
Tyurichev, V.V.	Tyurichev, V.V.	Tyurichev, V.		
Ubozhko, L.G.	Ubozhko, L.G.	Ubozhko, L.G.	Ubozhko, L.G.	Ubozhko, L.G.
				Udovenko, G.
			Ugnachev, A.K.	Ugnachev, A.K.
				Ukolov, N.
				Ukovenko, G.
			Uletsky, I.	
Ulyanchenko, L.S.				Ulyanchenko, L.S.
Usans, R.				
Utemov, M.Yu.				
Valendo, L.A.				Valendo, L.A.
Valkov, N.A.	Valkov, N.A.	Valkov, M.		
				Valkova, N.A. H?

Table A.3 (cont.)

Bloch and Reddaway (1984:253–62) *Coverage*: 1977–83	**Koppers (1990:74–176)** *Coverage*: 1920s to 1990	**Mercer (1991a and b; 1992)** *Coverage*: through 1991	**Podrabinek (1981:158–83** *et al.*) *Coverage*: late 1950s(?) through late 1970s	**Smith and Oleszczuk (1988a; 1989)** *Coverage*: 1960–81 before additions
Valov, Yu.Z.				
			Varennikov, I.S.	
		Varfolomejev, M.	Varganov, K.P.	
Varnavsky, V.V.				
Vasilev		Vasilev, V.V.		Vasilev
	Vasilev, V.V.			
				Vedernikov, V.
				Velichkovsky, V.
				Verba
Veretennikov, V.A.				
Vetrov, N.				
Vinkh, M.				
	Vinokurov, B.D.			Vinokurov, B.D.
	Vishnevskaya, Yu.		Vishnevskaya, Yu.	Vishnevskaya, Ju.
			Vishnyarsky, D.	
Vitokhin, Yu.A. (not Vetokhin)			Vetokhin, Yu.A.	Vetokhin, Yu.A.
Vivtash, Yu.S.				
				Vladykin, N.I.
	Vladykina, P.R.			Vladykina, P.R.
Vodochkoria, M.P.				
Volik, I.V.				

	Volkov			Volkov
Volkov, E.E.	Volkov, Y.Y.			
Volobuyev				Volobuyev
Voloshchuk, A.A.				
				Volpin, A.S.
	Vorobyov, O.I.			Vorobyev, O.I.
Vorona, A.P.	Vorona, A.P.			
Voronov, N.P.	Voronov, N.P.	Voronov, N.P.		
	Vorav, I.			
Vorozhbit, M.P.				
	Yagodin, V.	Vostrikov, Yu.G.		
		Vyushkov		
	Yakhimovich, I.A.	Yakimenko, P.D.	Yakhimovich, I.A.	Yakhimovich, I.
	Yakovlev			Yakovlev
Yakubenko, N.I.				Yakubenko, N.I.
Yanin, V.G.		Yamikov		
Yankov, G.T.				Yankov, G.
Yankovich, A.I.	Yankovich, A.I.			Yankovich, A.I.
				Yanshin
Yasako, R.	Yasakov, R.			
		Yastrebtsov, Y.		
Yatsenko, V.A.	Yatsenko, V.A.			Yatsenko, V.
Yavorsky, A.	Yavorsky, A.			
			Yematinov, Y.	
	Esenin-Volpin, A.S.		Yesinin-Volpin, A.S.	Yesinin, A.S.
	Yevsyukov, S.D.			
				Yudin, V.A.

Table A.3 (cont.)

Bloch and Reddaway (1984:253–62) *Coverage*: 1977–83	**Koppers (1990:74–176)** *Coverage*: 1920s to 1990	**Mercer (1991a and b; 1992)** *Coverage*: through 1991	**Podrabinek (1981:158–83** *et al.*) *Coverage*: late 1950s(?) through late 1970s	**Smith and Oleszczuk (1988a; 1989)** *Coverage*: 1960–81 before additions
	Yufimets, S.			
Yurlov, D.				
				Yurlov, O.
		Yuzhkov or Vyushkov, V.A.		
Zabolotny, A.A.			Zabolotny, A.	Zabolotny, A.
Zadkov, G.N.			Zadkov, G.	Zadkov, G.
Zaitsev, N.				
Zaitsev, V.K.				Zaitsev, V.K.
Zakirov, Sh.				
Zaks, V.	Zaks, V.			
			Zalessky-Enelin, I.A.	
Zavalnyuk, V.M.				
				Zdorovets, B.M.
	Zhamkochyan			
Zharov, Yu.S.				
	Zheleznov, A.I.			Zheleznov, A.I.
				Zhigalkin, V.
				Zhikharev, E.
Zhikharev, M.N.	Zhikharev, M.N.	Zhikharev, M.		Zhikharev, M.
		Zhirkov, G.		
				Zhuk, V.
			Zilbermovich, B.Y.	

Zotov, M.V.				
Zotova, V.V.	Zotova, V.V.			
Zuyev, B.			Zuyev, B.	
Zverev, M.S.			Zverev, M.S.	Zverev, M.S.
Zypre, A.P. (not Zipre)				Zhipre, A.P.
				Zyryanova, A.D.

H? = individual appears in the Smith–Oleszczuk data as a dissident but no record of psychiatric hospitalization was found.

(?) = researcher has reserved judgment that individual may not be a political or religious dissident.

No judgment is made or implied concerning correct transliteration or spelling of names, since unlike the authors of the other compendia, we have not interviewed the individuals concerned and have no basis on which to resolve divergent spellings.

Sources:

Sidney Bloch and Peter Reddaway, *Soviet Psychiatric Abuse: The Shadow over World Psychiatry* (London: Victor Gollancz, 1984), pp. 253–62. For Bloch and Reddaway original sources, consult Bloch and Reddaway, 1977, 1978, 1984, 1985. Their compilation includes some 346 victims. We gratefully acknowledge their permission to reprint this list of names.

Koppers' sources are described and further information provided in *A Biographical Dictionary on the Political Abuse of Psychiatry in the USSR* (Amsterdam: Geneva Initiative/International Association on the Political Use of Psychiatry, 1990), esp. pp. 177–9. Unlike Smith–Oleszczuk data, the Koppers information includes non-Soviet nationals. We much appreciate Koppers' permission to reprint his list of names.

Mercer cases are comprised of all individuals mentioned under internments or releases in the American Psychiatric Association revised lists dated 6/10/91, kept up to date until 1991 by the APA Office of International Affairs. Records of non-Soviet nationals are included. See also our discussion of the incidence of mental illness among dissidents. Ellen Mercer, a member of the US Delegation sent to USSR mental hospitals in 1989, found genuine mental disorders among individuals whom the US Delegation had requested to interview. She emphasizes that among all data from any source may appear individuals who were genuinely ill at some time or who became mentally ill while detained. We thank Ellen Mercer for her permission to reprint the APA list of detainees here.

Podrabinek's cases appear in *Punitive Medicine* (New York: Khronika, 1979) and (Ann Arbor: Karoma, 1980), pp. 158–83. He reports that his sources include a network of 'former fellow inmates' (Podrabinek, 1989:99) as well as the Moscow weekly *Express Khronika* which he now edits. We are grateful for A.P. Podrabinek's kind permission to reprint this data.

For a discussion of the sources of the Smith–Oleszczuk data, see the chapter on the database. Only individuals believed to be Soviet nationals and known to have engaged in dissident behaviour prior to their hospitalization are included.

Notes

1 POLITICAL HOSPITALIZATION: CONCEPTION, CONCEPTUALIZATION AND CONDUCT

1. For example, Ekaterina Panova was hospitalized for praying too loudly that Poland would win its independence; Kologrivov was committed for participating in the 1830 revolution in France; a cadet, Zhukov, was interned for composing a poem on freedom during the time of Alexander I (Antebi, 1977:89). (Faced with detention in the Soviet period, Maria Spiridonova eluded hospitalization, as did Angelika Balabanova, who found herself instead in Turkestan.)
2. Data for the 1950s are less rich than those for the 1960s, and our original data, described in Chapter 2, ended in 1981. For this study the original data have been supplemented with the data graciously provided by the Director of the Office of International Affairs of the American Psychiatric Association Ellen Mercer, and by Dr Andre Koppers of the International Association on the Political Use of Psychiatry (Amsterdam), extending the analysis from the late twenties to 1991.
3. For example, in *Vesti iz SSSR* (*USSR News Briefs*), 30 Oct. 1990, the editor Cronid Lubarsky shows 97 political prisoners for the whole USSR, of whom 13 were political detainees still hospitalized, some of whom may have suffered mental illness while coercively confined.
4. See for ex. *Hufvudstadsbladet* from Helsinki, in Swedish, 13 March 1991:22, in FBIS *Daily Reports* WEU-91-058 of 26 March 1991:1–2.
5. Fictitiously, as it was subject to massive inflation, the ruble remained pegged at its official value of R1=$1.70 US until April of 1991. In April 1991, Gorbachev floated the ruble to 7=$1.00 US. In January of 1992, R100=$1.00 US, and by 1995, rubles were exchanged at over 4800 to a US dollar. In the summer of 1995 travellers to Russia reported exchange rates of 4900–5000 to a dollar. In the 1991–92 period alone, prices increased a hundredfold while wages increased only tenfold.
6. Foreign Broadcast Information *Daily Reports* for various regions in the early 1990s chronicle recent psychiatric detentions for political reasons in Sub-Saharan Africa (Kenya and apparently Angola), Hong Kong, and a number of East/Central European countries including the Czech Republic, Slovakia and Poland. The International Association on the Political Use of Psychiatry notes at least some sporadic cases in Bulgaria, Cuba, Germany (GDR), Hungary, Romania, Turkey and Zaire. Other cases from the 1970s and 1980s can be documented in the former Yugoslavia, Chile and Argentina. Although systematic psychiatric suppression was not used in Argentina during the generals' 'war against all' (1976–83), or in Chile under General Pinochet, allegations have been brought against particular psychiatrists in these societies.
7. US statistics on overtly political offences can be elusive in the standard sources. Since political crimes tend to result in arrests by federal officers,

they have not been reprinted in the *Uniform Crime Report* and do not appear clearly in the *Sourcebook of Criminal Justice Statistics*, although 'terrorism' is listed. Some account of US political crime statistics can be derived from the *Sourcebook*, despite political crimes not being well indexed. In the 1987 volume (published 1988), the effects of ethnicity, gender, and socioeconomic status can be identified, and reports of the following political crimes can be found:

- 'international terrorist incidents involving U.S. citizens or property' (US Department of Justice, 1988:361);
- passports, visas, and entry permit violations (1988:458: Tables 5.42 and 5.43) as well as immigration and nationality crimes (1992:551);
- deportations 1908–86. In each decade covered, the category 'subversive or anarchistic' accounts for the single largest number of deportations (1988:410, Table 4.34); the 1992 source covers 1983–92 and shows criminal/narcotic charges and 'entered without inspection' as the main reasons for deportation in the 1980s, noting that those with pre-existing mental illnesses are excludable aliens (1992:472, Table 4.48).
- national security and selective service violations as well as immigration charges resulting in prison (1988:516, Table 6.53); national security charges usually result in a small number of imprisonments, only one in fiscal 1986;
- various vague charges whose opportunistic political use is possible, such as vagrancy, curfew violations, loitering, 'suspicion', and so on.

The same source in 1992, while obscuring most political crimes under the heading 'all other offenses except traffic' also reports bombings and abuse of public office.

8. The American Psychiatric Association's authoritative reference, the *Diagnostic and Statistical Manual of Mental Disorders* (*DSM-IV*, 4th edn, 1994:91), defines a syndrome of 'negativistic, defiant, disobedient, and hostile behavior toward authority figures' not dissimilar to the observations on some detained dissidents. *DSM-IV* notes (1994:92) 'transient oppositional behavior is very common in preschool children and in adolescents . . .'.
9. In the report of the US Delegation which visited Soviet psychiatric hospitals in 1989, both Westerners and Soviets interviewed a Ukrainian nationalist detainee concurrently. When no psychotic symptom appeared, the Soviet interviewer merely changed the diagnosis from schizophrenia to psychopathy (Shore and Keith, 1989:18–19).
10. East/West perceptions of issues as social or medical problems may also contrast: for example, though alcoholism is increasingly perceived in the West as a chemical addiction subject to medical treatment, it remains viewed essentially as a social problem in post-Soviet society.
11. The *DSM-IV* also recognizes classifications of schizophrenic conditions based on expected development over time, including episodic and continuous forms (1994:286). In contrast to Soviet practice, the *DSM-IV* clearly states that these labels *cannot* be applied when symptoms first appear, but only after at least a year has elapsed.
12. See G.E. Sukhareva's *Clinical Schizophrenia Among Children and Adolescents* (Kharkov, 1937) for a discussion of the symptomless stage of

'sluggish schizophrenia'. Soviet apologists such as P. Morozov and A. Tiganov trace the concept of asymptomatic schizophrenia to the West, to a Swiss psychiatrist E. Bleuler writing in 1911 about 'latent schizophrenia', and subsequently to American psychiatrists Hoch and Palatin on 'pseudoneurotic schizophrenia' (IAPUP:1990, No. 23:365–7; 24:3. See the Soviet response appended to the report of the US Delegation visiting USSR mental hospitals in 1989, eds Shore and Keith, 1989.) O. Vilensky (Prof. and MD) attributes sluggish schizophrenia ('langour') to the Soviet psychiatrists L. Rozenstein and A. Kronfeld working in 1932 (Vilensky, 'Psychiatry and Politics', *Argumenty i Fakty* 7–13 April 1990 (14):7, in FBIS-SOV-90-073, 16 April 1990:68–9).

13. A psychiatric diagnosis form reprinted in Baker from *Forensic Psychiatry* (G. Morozov and Ia. Kalashnik, 1970) lists eight forms of schizophrenia.
14. At the national level, in Moscow, the Institute of Psychiatry in the USSR Academy of Medical Sciences has collected files of 10000 or more family members and relatives of those diagnosed as schizophrenic (Babayan, 1984). According to Koppers (1990:139), L.I. Plyushch's psychiatrist believed schizophrenia ran in the Plyushch family because his son was interested in bees . . .
15. Koppers (1990:34) indicates that Dr Morozov also held the rank of General in the KGB 1977–80, co-edited the *Korsakov Journal* and co-edited the best established Soviet text on forensic psychiatry.
16. Cases exist in which prominent Soviet psychiatrists have reported the 'impossible' disappearance of schizophrenia, as well as remission in non-periodic forms. The report of the US Delegation's visit to Soviet psychiatric hospitals in 1989 (*Schizophrenia Bulletin* supp. to Vol. 15, No. 4, 1989) notes that even in cases where in principle Soviet diagnostic criteria allowed for disconfirmation of schizophrenia over time, because the disease did not progress as predicted, because symptoms disappeared, or because the individual concerned failed to deteriorate, this evidence to the contrary did not cause diagnoses to be altered.
17. The diagnosis of 'sluggish schizophrenia' was evidently in clinical use until at least the late 1980s (Podrabinek in Van Voren, 1989). In defence of Soviet practice, E.A. Babayan countered that the World Health nomenclature includes a related 'latent schizophrenia' (1985:60–1). Eduard Armenakovich Babayan, Cand. Med., a psychiatrist and Department Head in the USSR Ministry of Public Health in the 1970s and early 1980s, and prominent defender of Soviet psychiatry, appears to have been discredited in 1986, blamed for the failure of the anti-alcohol campaign. However he seems not to have suffered permanent harm; in 1990 he was a board member of the All-Union Society of Psychiatrists.

    Note that if a protester is committed in an asymptomatic condition, what condition s/he should show to be discharged is difficult to define.
18. See Koppers for other cases such as those of A.V. Chertkova, O.Y. Iofe, K.Y. Karmanov, V. Klebanov, A.E. Komarov, V.V. Spinenko, and Yu. Vineshnevskaya. The US delegation in 1989 found 24 of the 27 internees they interviewed (89 per cent) had been initially hospitalized with diagnoses of schizophrenia and seven (26 per cent) with some aspects of psychopathy.
19. Samizdat are self-published, often surreptitiously circulated materials which allowed censorship to be circumvented and taboo topics to be publicized.

20. Anatoly Ivanovich Koryagin was arrested after criticizing punitive use of drugs in psychiatry; he was rearrested in 1981 and sentenced in June to the standard seven years in a labour camp and five years of exile commonly meted out to nonconformists. The 1981 arrest followed his activities on behalf of the Working Commission to Investigate the Use of Psychiatry for Political Purposes, whose entire staff eventually was imprisoned. When released in 1987 Dr Koryagin emigrated to Switzerland. He was nominated for a Nobel Peace Prize in 1987. (Cf. many sources, incl. van Voren, 1987; Radio Liberty *USSR This Week*, 29 Aug. 1986:10.)
21. See Elena Salina, 'Ripples in the Water', *Stolitsa* (Moscow) (3), March 1991:53–5, in Reddaway 1991:46 and fn.
22. V. Korneev, 'Indefinite Stay in Lunatic Asylum', 23 Dec. 1990 *Izvestia* (Union edn) in Russian:6, in FBIS-SOV-91-002, 3 Jan. 1991. This article does not reveal whether those detained would be classified as dissidents according to our criteria set out in Ch. 2 on the database. See Reddaway, 1991:47.
23. In a Moscow news service interview with Tatyana Kuropayeva on 5 April 1990, R.A. Medvedev describes his brother Zhores' arrest, and attributes to Y.V. Andropov the remark '"It's probably the boys from the [KGB's] directorate of excessive zeal who are responsible for this one."' (Tatyana Kuropayeva, 'Psychiatry and Politics – What Has Changed?', Moscow news in Russian, 1745 GMT 5 April 1990 in FBIS-SOV-90-068, 9 April 1990:45.) (The KGB maintained a special Fifth Directorate for dealing with dissent and ensuring adherence to Party direction. The Fifth Directorate has since undergone some permutations, becoming a chief directorate, and being renamed at least twice: 'Directorate for the Defence of the Soviet Constitutional System' (directed fruitlessly against the independence movements and ethnic upheaval) and 'Directorate Z'. The Second (Chief) Directorate, of counter-intelligence, also had responsibilities in control of Soviet domestic political life. (Cf. Knight, 1990; Waller, 1994.)) Some commentators saw the 6 April 1995 change in the law governing the Russian Federal Security Bureau as resurrecting the KGB, enhancing its powers against crime, fascism and corruption and providing overtly for special forces and interrogation cells.
24. Moscow domestic news service in Russian, 1745 GMT 5 April 1990, in FBIS-SOV-90-068 9 April 1990:45, Tatyana Kuropayeva, 'Psychiatry and Politics – What Has Changed?'
25. Feldshers are comparable to paramedics or physician's assistants in the US. Some are midwives.

    The ambulance service carries out civil commitments by force. Thus, attendants witness detentions.
26. See *Moscow New Times International*, English, No. 50, December 1992:32, in FBIS-USR (not SOV)-93-006, 15 Jan. 1993:55–6.
27. Citing the *Sunday Times*, 21 May 1972, Bloch and Reddaway report that these women were found 'morally defective' following the births, and were hospitalized for no other reason.
28. Evidence shows unnecessary and potentially political hospitalizations in the US over the 1960–91 interval under study here. Some individuals 'not requiring hospitalization' may be kept in mental institutions for some months or longer, since these categories show non-zero entries for first admissions

and also for individuals in residence at the end of the year in US Department of Health sources. US Department of Health (1963), *Patients in Mental Hospitals 1960: Part I: Public Institutions for the Retarded* lists admissions of individuals without mental retardation who are not shown in residence at the end of the year. USDOH, *Patients in Mental Hospitals 1960: Part II: Public Hospitals for the Mentally Ill* shows a variety of politically manipulable categories of admission, including 'diseases of unknown cause' (loc.cit.1963:II-26), 'antisocial reactions' (1963:II-26), and **admissions without mental disorder** both to public prolonged care mental hospitals (1963:II-27) and to psychopathic hospitals (1963:II-43). Those admitted without mental illness to prolonged care and psychopathic institutions do appear to remain in residence at the end of the year in the sixties.

29. For the entire USA, Atay *et al.* (1993:2) report 4431 'additions' to state and county mental hospitals in the category 'no mental disorder', or approximately 0.016 per cent of a total of 277 813 individuals in data which include estimates for states failing to report, for fiscal year 1990. Hospital residents showing ***no mental disorder*** across the country amounted to 967 of 92 059, or about 0.011 per cent (1993:48). The proportions of healthy people detained compared to the total population hospitalized decline by age in the Atay data (see 1993:2 and 48). Thus some aspects of US detention may be generational and focused on youth, though this observation is uncertain due to dissimilar size of the age groupings. In these tables 'total' refers to the total number of people hospitalized irrespective of mental health status.

Table 1.2 Sane Persons Committed to US State and County Mental Hospitals in 1990

# years in range	n=17	n=7	n=20	n=20	n=?
Age range	<18	18 to 24	25 to 44	45 to 64	65, >65
Number sane	412	700	2483	698	138
Total	21 022	38 196	159 337	47 421	11 837
Per cent sane	0.020	0.018	0.016	0.015	0.012

Table 1.3 Sane Residents in US State and County Mental Hospitals in 1990

# years in range	n=17	n=7	n=20	n=20	n=?
Age range	<18	18 to 24	25 to 44	45 to 64	65, >65
Number sane	96	127	484	188	72
Total	5273	7108	43 445	21 420	14 813
Per cent sane	0.018	0.018	0.011	0.009	0.005

30. For example, the emigré orthopaedist Dr Vladimir Golyakhovsky (Zak) reports attempting to protect his son from the Army by having him declared an outpatient schizophrenic (Golyakhovsky, 1984).
31. The US Delegation designed their own diagnostic interview on the basis of the DSM-III-R Structured Clinical Interview Psychiatric Disorders Version (SCID-PD), the International Personality Disorders Exam (IPDE), the DSM-III-R Checklist, and detailed information on legal history (see ed. Shore and Keith, 1989:13).
32. In addition they interviewed 20 others informally.
33. One was committed following a dispute with his work supervisor which may or may not have concerned political issues; another, during a disintegrating marriage.
34. Disingenuously, some commentators blame the new Independent Psychiatric Associations for the misdiagnosis problem, an interpretation which can be rejected out of hand since the misdiagnoses for the most part precede the creation of the new professional bodies.
35. According to a team of physicians, prevailing conditions in the Dvoryanskoye SPH in Volgograd Oblast were such as to bring about mental collapse (*Izvestia* report of December 1990).
36. For example, among known dissidents is a student named Dmitriev, a member of the Union of Communists, who was arrested for nonconformist behaviour. He is not included among the psychiatric detainees, although he was hospitalized, because we found credible information that he was ill. For the same reason we have omitted the case of Y.V. Glukhov from the analyses.
37. See coverage on the creation of a commission to review malpractice claims and contested diagnoses, Moscow World Service in English, 410 GMT 4 Feb. 1989 in FBIS-SOV-89-025, 8 Feb. 1989:68–9.
38. A 1990 public opinion survey in Moscow and an outlying town reports that most respondents agreed people 'rarely go to a psychiatric clinic voluntarily'. See Elena Salina, 'Ripples in the Water', *Stolitsa* (Moscow) No. 3, March 1991:53–5, in Reddaway, 1991:46 fn.
39. It is also worth noting in this context that in 1994 the Ministry of Health (Russian) maintained a confidential 'Second Department' comprised of four divisions named by ordinal numbers and one 'special' division (Oleynik, 1994:210).
40. Ordinary regime prison camps and hospitals differed from special regime or 'strict observation' or 'supervision' counterparts in a variety of ways including the greater severity of conditions in special regime camps and the overt role of the KGB in administering special regime maximum-security forensic hospitals.
41. This practice evidently did not result in routine six-month commission hearings for psychiatric detainees.
42. Interestingly, Vartanyan served from 1977–83 on the WPA Ethics Committee.
43. IAPUP reports that after the All-Union Society advised the World Psychiatric Association in 1988 that the AUSNP would seek readmission, the organization changed its name at its October 1988 meeting to the All-Union Society of Psychiatrists and Narcologists. The name change reflected the neuropathologists' creation of their own association and the narcologists'

affiliation with the psychiatrists to redefine the old organization, pointing to an interesting focus on drugs and/or alcohol (IAPUP, 1989, No. 21:2–3). (Reddaway (1990:1, 1991) showed 'All-Union Scientific Society of Psychiatrists' or AUSSP in 1990 and 1991.)

44. According to the *Korsakov Journal* No. 6, 1989, reprinted in IAPUP, 1989, No. 22:41–2, in 1989 20 of the 23 or about 87 per cent of the members of the 'All-Union' Society presidium were from Moscow.

45. See M. Ryan's translation in the *British Medical Journal*, Sept. 1979.

46. See V. Rozboynikov, 'Instructions to Put Him Away', Moscow edition of *Izvestia* in Russian, morning edition, 29 June 1989:3; in FBIS-SOV-89-133 13 July 1989:83–4.

47. The 24-hour certification rule was in effect both before, and according to, the 1988 regulations.

48. A. Novikov (1987) quotes detainee V. Davydov as saying 'Soviet law does not provide for life imprisonment . . . But for many psychiatric prisoners, it's a real threat.'

49. Bloch and Reddaway (1977:265) and Koppers (1990:137–8) indicated that Mykola Plakhotnyuk, a physician arrested in 1972 after samizdat work, was held 'periodically not responsible'.

50. 'There are a great many schools and hundreds of disagreements. Thus, one and the same person may be adjudged a schizophrenic in Moscow, a psychopath in Leningrad, and healthy in Kharkov' (A. Novikov and others, 'A Closed Subject', *Komsomolskaya Pravda* 11 Nov. 1987:11, in *Current Digest of the Soviet Press* 39(46):1–3; cf. discussion on diagnostic variability, *supra*).

51. (2+5)/(12+11) or 7/23=0.3043.

52. *Instruction on the Procedure for Applying Compulsory Treatment and Other Medical Measures to Mentally Ill Persons Who Have Committed Socially Dangerous Acts*, 14 Feb. 1967, part D, section 18 as translated in Morozov and Kalashnik, 1970.

53. For further comment and analysis on inappropriate and inconsistent use of insanity findings among a specific nationality, Lithuanian dissidents, see Oleszczuk, 1988:116–18.

54. General Edwin Walker provides a notable counter-example to the trend in the US to find dubious individuals legally competent to stand trial. The General, after his arrest in 1963 in Mississippi in the US Deep South for opposition to desegregation, to which his vivid comments on 'the anti-Christ conspirators of the Supreme Court' (Turk, 1982:53) had drawn attention, was sent for psychological evaluation even before the Federal Court had been asked to order a mental examination. The alacrity of this manœuvre may have been designed to avoid legitimizing opposition to federal troops desegregating the South. The example of Ezra Pound often cited to show US political abuse of psychiatry is more difficult to interpret because his purported offences took place in wartime while he was in Italy.

55. A number of those arrested for unauthorized attempted border crossing have been found sane. Although Rubenstein and others report that most dissidents assessed at the Serbsky Institute are found insane (1980, 1985:140), clearly not all regime critics are automatically thought to be mentally ill, and thus the phenomenon is somewhat more complex to explain.

56. Thomas Szasz, *Psychiatric Justice* (New York: Macmillan, 1965).

57. Basaglia, Franco, 'Institutions of Violence', in Nancy Scheper-Hughes and Anne M. Lovel (eds), *Psychiatry Inside Out: Selected Writings of Franco Basaglia*: 59–86 (New York: Columbia University Press, 1987a).
58. Press accounts in the late 1980s reveal a connection operating in the other direction, in an anti-corruption campaign against a small number of Soviet psychiatrists who would provide an insanity finding for a price to career criminals otherwise likely to be imprisoned. This campaign viewed in context appears to have been part of the Foreign Ministry's efforts to rehabilitate the image of Soviet psychiatry abroad. (See Reddaway, various.)
59. The 1992 law is ambiguous on this point, providing for legal counsel at several junctures but not clearly allowing consultation before diagnosis.
60. Even though a police officer can order one.
61. See paragraph 31 of the 1967 *Instruction Pertaining to Compulsory Treatment of the Mentally Ill Who Have Committed Socially Dangerous Acts* and paragraphs 4b, 10c, 11c of the 21 March 1988 'Provisional Guidelines on the Procedures for Coercive and other Measures of a Medical Nature in Regard to Persons with Mental Disorders Who Have Committed Socially Dangerous Acts'.
62. 1954 Instruction, Ch. IV, section 26, although WPA 1991:17 indicates 30- to 90-day exams at Serbsky as a matter of fact if not of law.
63. See Article 59 of the Criminal Code of the RSFSR, which noted, paragraph 3, 'Persons committed to a special psychiatric hospital shall be kept in conditions of a reinforced supervision that excludes the possibility of their commission of a new socially dangerous act.' (Berman, 1966:175)); that is, in psychiatric prisons, with barbed wire and guard dogs.
64. Bloch and Reddaway (1977:102) note that psychiatrists employed ratings of social danger from 1–5, while security officials composed their own scale(s).
65. The US Supreme Court's recent fixation on due process, including rights of appeal, places a higher value on procedure than on guaranteeing an opportunity to present evidence of innocence.
66. Not all of these hospitalizations are necessarily political.
67. That inappropriately high levels of drugs and use of non-indicated drugs could still be encountered in a group of pre-selected hospital residents and those recently released in several cities, by a visiting group of US specialists in the USSR on invitation of the Soviet government in 1989, well after many discharges, suggests that abnormalities in practice were widespread, or that inappropriate drug treatment represented standard practice. That at least 10 of the 27 interviewees (37 per cent) were affected may imply that excessive drug use was not only geographically widespread but severe in that where it took place the proportion of those affected was substantial.

    Among the implicated pharmaceuticals are antipsychotic drugs such as the phenothiazines chlorpromazine, moditen, stelazine and flupromazine, butyrophenones such as haloperidol (haldol), and thioxanthenes such as chlorprothixene; antidepressants such as the tricyclical imipramine; and idiosyncratic treatments such as insulin with a shot of vodka. (See Babayan, 1985:132, Mercer and Koppers.) Reports of potentially fatal insulin subcoma 'treatment' and atropine used as a punishment have also been published (see eds Shore and Klein, 1989).
68. See *Voprosy Narkologii* (Moscow), No. 1, 1990, cited in Reddaway, 1991:47

fn. Sulfazine has also been reportedly used on children. What could possibly account for the use of sulfazine in children, who are usually regarded by definition as incapable of giving informed consent, is difficult to imagine.

69. As we will show in Chapter 4, the most typical pre-hospitalization experience for dissidents detained in psychiatric institutions is one administrative detention. A slight majority in our data experienced no court-ordered detention; about 43 per cent were held once on court order.

2 CHARACTERISTICS OF THE EVIDENCE: THE DATABASE OF PSYCHIATRIC HOSPITAL DETAINEES

1. An anti-Ukrainian ethnic aspersion.
2. Military tribunals and NKVD hearings were coded as trials.
3. Dr Andre Koppers of the Geneva Initiative on Psychiatry, P.O. Box 3754, 1001 AN Amsterdam, The Netherlands, indicates that he also has collected records on psychiatric repression in the 1940s and 1950s in the USSR. However, he has not yet had the opportunity to publish a study on this period.
4. Religions coded encompass Adventist, Armenian Apostolic, Evangelical Christian and Baptists (ECB), registered ECB, Roman Catholic, Islamic (Shiia), Islamic (Sunni), Jehovah's Witness, Jewish, Orthodox (Russian), Orthodox (True, TUC), Pentecostalist, and Uniate. Some individuals were reported as participating in 'Buddhist activities' without an unambiguous statement that they were Buddhist; these are not coded Buddhist. Later in the Soviet period some Hare Krishna members were arrested and evidently detained.
5. Numbering among the nationalities coded at various levels of specificity for this project are Armenian, Assyrian, Azeri, Bashkir, Bulgarian, Byelorussian, Chinese, Chuvash, Crimean or other Tatar, Estonian, Finnish, Georgian, German, Greek, Kazakh, Kirghiz, Latvian, Lithuanian, Meskhetian, Moldovan, Mordovian, Ossetian, Polish, Russian, Tadzhik, Turkmen, Ukrainian and Uzbek. Nationalities are coded by self-identification or assigned by given name, patronymic and/or surname. Although the latter pattern of nationality assignment understates the influence of maternal nationality in mixed marriages, thereby for example potentially underestimating the numbers of matrilineally determined nationalities such as Jews, any resulting inaccuracy is probably small since most detainees are Russian nationals in the Russian Republic, where the intermarriage rates are relatively low. From *Narodnoe khozyaistvo SSR*, Ryan (1993:63) reports the 1988 and 1989 intermarriage rates for Russian men in the RSFSR at 9.7 and 9.8 per cent and 11.1 per cent for Russian women.
6. Occupations recorded include student, intellectual (researcher, author, poet, professor, diplomat if mainly academic), peasant (and/or farmer), blue collar worker (mason, dispatcher, truck driver, mechanic, other skilled trades), white collar worker (technician, nurse, journalist, engineer, doctor's assistant; most physicians unless also academics or politicians), artist/dancer, musician, government official (not including intelligence officers or police), KGB or NKVD, police, officially invalid, priest, minister or other religious.

7. We gratefully acknowledge the editors' kind permission to consult their data to expand and enrich our information on cases of political or religious dissidents who were forcibly hospitalized without apparent medical need. De Boer, Driessen and Verhaar request that additions and emendations be forwarded to:

   The Institute of Eastern European Studies
   Oude Hoogstraat 24
   P.O. Box 19101
   1000 GC Amsterdam
   The Netherlands

8. Centre for the Study of Religion and Communism, Heathfield Road, Keston, Kent BR2 6BA, England.

9. We acknowledge with gratitude the permission to Dr Andre Koppers to use his data. Dr Koppers is a researcher for the Geneva Initiative on Psychiatry (International Association for the Abolishment and Prevention of Political Psychiatry), formerly the International Association on the Political Use of Psychiatry, in Amsterdam. The Geneva Initiative, while continuing to oppose political use of psychiatry wherever this practice is encountered, has widened its objectives to include promoting professional autonomy and the structures making it possible in psychiatry globally.

   Interested readers may inquire about the ongoing Research Project on Psychiatric Abuse in the Former Soviet Union, conducted by the Geneva Initiative on Psychiatry, P.O. Box 3754, 1001 AN Amsterdam, the Netherlands.

10. Radio Liberty reports that its publications reflect information from 600 Soviet, Western and emigré periodicals as well as Soviet and East European broadcasts and global media. The Radio Liberty Samizdat Archive compiles what is believed to be the largest collection of samizdat material in the West, organized by political issue, dissent type, authors and signatories. Radio Liberty published approximately 45 issues annually of annotated samizdat in their bulletin *Materialy Samizdata.*

11. Reddaway (1977:348; 1977: Appendix I) counted about 365, leading to estimates that the number held annually must be at least two or three hundred, with variable releases and replacements.

12. We include earlier information for descriptive purposes but suspect that the small available sample size in the Stalin era results in unstable estimates from that period.

13. In his study of repression of Lithuanian dissent Oleszczuk shows that representative data can be collected for 1970–81 from the *Chronicles of Current Events* and any one of a specialized source concentrating on the group under study, an emigré source publishing in the West, or the records of a major human rights agency interested in the fate of the group (1988:210).

14. While the inclusiveness question is intrinsically unanswerable, some clues can be found that the Western and Soviet sources relied on here have accounted for a high proportion of *all* cases. The World Psychiatric Association noted on its visit to Moscow, Kiev and Dnepropetrovsk in 1991 that among the ten current or former detainees they met with, seven were already known among Western human rights groups while the remaining three had become known through unofficial Soviet channels to Yu. Savenko's

Independent Psychiatric Association. Since we have drawn upon both Western and unofficial Soviet sources to construct our sample, the 1991 observation suggests that at least under conditions prevailing in the early nineties we would have captured a high percentage if not all substantiated cases of psychiatric detentions. Fitzpatrick indicates in a 1987 Helsinki Watch report that for every person discharged in 1987, 1.4 previously unknown incidents came to light. If this ratio (1/1.4) is accurate for the late eighties, it suggests somewhat more than 70 per cent of all cases in that period have probably been found.

15. The transfer data among hospitals and prisons point to a reason that some detainees identified by Mercer and Koppers may have escaped our scrutiny: Many of these detainees were not released until after 1980, sometimes well after, and were in the pipeline at the time of our first investigation. Podrabinek suggests that the main source of information on many lesser known detainees is their cellmates on release. This filtering effect of detainees not becoming known until after their own or a cohort's discharge can hint at the size of the total psychiatric detainee population which is reflected in the well-confirmed cases, and implies a time lag in accuracy of estimates of the total detainee population size perhaps equivalent to average time served in psychoprisons.
16. The information networks developed by extensive travel and work in the USSR make a separate and unique contribution to the study of psychiatric suppression of nonconformity. In the Bloch/Reddaway and Podrabinek lists of detainees, personal contacts clearly tap some subset of information not appearing in our printed sources, since Bloch and Reddaway list 170 cases with which we are not familiar; Podrabinek, 52 (partially overlapping with Bloch and Reddaway).
17. For example, Yu. V. Glukhov, arrested and charged with violating Article 70, a political article, is reported by C. Lubarsky and Moscow monitors to be mentally ill (Mercer, 1991:3). His case is omitted from our analyses.
18. We do consult E.A. Babayan's account of the *structure* of Soviet psychiatry.

3 FOUR EXPLANATIONS OF THE POLITICAL USE OF PSYCHIATRY

1. The American Psychiatric Association's Director of the Office of International Affairs, Ellen Mercer, suggests that psychiatric abuse similar to that practised in the USSR also took place in Eastern European countries such as Czechoslovakia, Romania, and Bulgaria. Bloch and Reddaway note at least some cases in Hungary, Poland, the GDR, and Spain in the 1970s. However, detainees in these countries, apparently lacking the organizational depth of the Soviet dissident movement or comparable structures at local levels, have had less success publicizing their concerns in the West.
2. As discussed in subsequent chapters, we do find that psychiatric measures are targeted on certain types of regime challengers. The nature of differential targeting of Soviet dissidents for psychiatric penalties, and the reasons for it, imply several subsidiary questions. These questions concern the role of psychiatrists in socialist- and capitalist-oriented societies in defining, labelling, and treating or failing to treat criminal behaviour defined as disease.

3. At least a linear decrease is not shown (Bahry, 1987:86); dissent as a parabolic function of age could be hypothesized.
4. For an early discussion of the role of ideology in American psychiatry, consult Anselm Strauss, Leonard Schatzman, Rue Bucher, Danuta Ehrlich and Melvin Sabshin, *Psychiatric Ideologies and Institutions* (London and New York: Collier Macmillan, Free Press Glencoe, 1964).
5. Clinical psychologists or licensed practising psychotherapists were so scarce that Salvendry held that they did not exist in the USSR (Salvendry, 1975:233); certainly no standard certification for licensed psychotherapists has been set. Even in the early nineties only one or two thousand psychologists could be found, and their training appeared unstandardized, sparse, or largely putative.
6. The Ukrainian Psychiatric Association announced to the WPA in 1991 that it intended to increase the term of training in Ukraine to three years.
7. The US Delegation visiting Soviet mental hospitals in 1989 found evidence of physicians deliberately and sympathetically diagnosing as ill healthy people who would otherwise be subject to the standard penalties of prison camp and exile terms (1989:24).
8. Baldessarini (1970) concludes that in the US 1944–68 perhaps 30 per cent or more of the variability in diagnosis of schizophrenia versus affective disorder can be attributed to availability of new drugs and to observer bias.
9. In the US a finding of mental abnormality has functioned as an alternative 'arrest' category for older women and for juveniles who come to the attention of the authorities. Evidently because of societal resistance to their being labelled criminal, older women, perhaps particularly older white women, after arrest are defined as psychotic or psychoneurotic while juveniles – again perhaps particularly white juveniles – have tended to be found suffering from 'transient situational personality disturbance'. See *inter alia* Turk, 1969:143, 148.
10. See Robert van Voren (ed.), *Koryagin: A man struggling for human dignity* (sic) (Amsterdam: Second World Press, 1987); and Dr Semyon Gluzman, *On Soviet Totalitarian Psychiatry* (Amsterdam: International Association on the Political Use of Psychiatry, 1989).

4 WHO ARE THE DISSIDENT DETAINEES? SOME OBSERVATIONS AND DESCRIPTIVE STATISTICS

1. Roy Medvedev (1980) held that dissent largely bypassed the 'middle class' in the former USSR.
2. Our data extend into the late 1920s but are richest for the 1950–91 interval.
3. This is a weak negative correlation between total frequency of detention and occupation as ranked by prestige, where lower numbers reflect higher prestige.
4. Small sample size of the police occupational group means that this finding may not be stable in a larger dataset.
5. N = 172.
6. This number is reduced somewhat by the inclusion of short periods of administrative detention which often amounted to only a few days or a

week and does not imply that court-ordered hospitalizations by themselves resulted in average terms this short.

7. In this chapter all Soviet population estimates are taken from Feshbach, 1982:22.
8. Although our data are most detailed from 1960 onwards, observations from the twenties up to the fifties are in several categories as plentiful as those for the late 1980s and early 1990s, and are included for descriptive purposes. Although we are not confident that our data pre-1960 are completely representative, especially from the Stalin period, enough information is on record to be of interest, especially for purposes of description. Inferential statistics are calculated with and without the pre-1960 data.
9. Here we have included Georgians, Armenians and Azeris in the definition, but not Kazakhs.
10. This interpretation raises subsidiary questions, such as whether in fact women dissidents who commit the same social affronts as men dissidents are charged with violations of the Criminal Code which carry shorter terms if convicted.
11. N=19.

5 TRENDS, CHANGES WITH ADMINISTRATION AND SPATIAL DISPERSION

1. Bloch and Reddaway also see 1971 as showing a real increase in psychiatric repression (1984:73).
2. We include some information dating from the twenties, thirties, forties and fifties because it is available and of descriptive interest. Thus some summary statistics are reported for Stalin's administration, but these must be viewed as illustrative, since the amount of available information is not adequate to presume that stable estimates can be obtained from it.
3. Inevitably our dissident act data are incomplete, if only because we have not included reports of group behaviour such as demonstrations in which participating individuals could not be identified by name. (See Chapter 2.) The dissident act variable represents publicized nonconformist behaviour such as protests, religious processions, unauthorized art exhibits or poetry readings, refusal to be drafted, samizdat production, hunger strikes, flag raising, returning Party cards, etc., which generated a written record.
4. Despite the general tendency for frequency of administrative detentions to decline after 1985, no real reduction in their average length over the Andropov administration took place. Rather Figure 5.8a shows fluctuation. Evidently administrative commitments were an instrument of choice for Andropov, in that they were preferred to criminal commitments.
5. Curve-fitting using a quadratic equation can produce a closer fit. However since no obvious theoretical rationale for specifying the shape of this equation can be found in the literature, and since using more than one form of the dissident acts variable produces statistical estimation problems, interpretation of curve-fitted results is problematical in this case.

   Future research may provide an empirical basis for fitting particular curves. New internments themselves in the Koppers and Mercer data for 1980 through 1991, for example, suggest some possibly cyclical curvature in the process of punitive hospitalization which might be related to Party Congresses. A clear U-shaped curve in frequency of new internments exists in their data (and not in our combined data) after 1981 (26th Party Congress) to 1986 (27th Party Congress), building again after 1986 to 1989, with only one new hospitalization reported in 1990 in these sources. Considering that any given point on a curve might be a relative or absolute maximum, a minimum, or a point on an arc of general increase or of decrease, it is notable that five of the eight Party Congress years from 1956 to 1986 show relative or absolute maxima in new internments in our data. Again a theoretical explanation for such patterns is not forthcoming. It is unclear why policy towards dissidence might be related to internal economic planning or periodic political change, but given the primacy of the Plan in Soviet life, a non-spurious reason for these peaks may be found.

A second methodological issue concerns the inclusion of all our data in these correlations and the regression. It may be argued that data predating 1960 should be omitted from these analyses on the grounds of reduced reliability. Limiting the statistics to 1960–91 data leaves the results essentially the same. Significance levels are not altered, and associations are only slightly reduced. Pearson's r between hospitalization frequency and numbers of dissident acts becomes 0.80 instead of 0.835; r between numbers of dissident acts and frequency of subsequent hospitalization becomes 0.87 instead of 0.89 using all data; and the regression multiple R becomes 0.87 (R squared=0.76) instead of 0.89 and 0.79 respectively. The b coefficient changes to 0.36. These minor reductions in relationships are consistent with loss of information.

6. Apparently having elbowed his way to the head of the line.
7. One caveat, small sample size in the pre-1925 group and the post-1961 age group, limits the confidence we have that all the differences in penalties and dissident activity levels reported here are of necessity stable. As more data are discovered, retesting may allow an increase in sample size at the extremes of the age distribution, and increased confidence in the results obtained at the extremes.
8. We argue that a complete theoretical explanation of this phenomenon, which was not Bahry's objective, also must take even more explicitly into account international events, state response, and change of administration.
9. Small numbers of known dissident acts, which may be a consequence of missing data, give the Stalin administration an annual average frequency of recorded and dated dissident acts of only 1.33, in a tightly packed distribution whose mode and median are both 1, whose maximum is 2 and whose minimum is 1.
10. A subset of persistent dissenters against whom repeated detentions were directed had much higher typical activity levels and in general *increased* their dissident activity after detention, implying both deterrence and compellance failure of repression policies in their specific cases. See Chapter 6.
11. Sample size is 29.
12. Intellectuals in general were at greatest risk of detention in the sense that this occupational category usually provided the most internees in any given year. In his analysis of the data before the Koppers and Mercer additions, Dr Oleszczuk found a number of changes in occupational profile by year

from the sixties onwards. Marginally more students than intellectuals were detained in 1963, and somewhat more white collar employees in 1965 and 1979. The student frequency declines from 1966 through 1970 and 1973–74, and white collar detentions decline from 1968 to 1970, while the frequencies for intellectuals grew rapidly in the same intervals. The 1976–78 interval marks a relative minimum in internments of intellectuals, and relative maxima occur at 1962, 1971–72, 1974, and 1980.

13. We have little information on blue collar nonconformists among the detainees in the Gorbachev years.
14. City of first hospitalization is known for 346/674 or 51.3 per cent, somewhat more than half, of all internees in our data.
15. The missing republic is Kirghizia. Though dissident acts are recorded in Kirghizia, our data do not include dates for the Kirghiz cases.

    We presume that we have a sample of better-known dissident acts which generated a paper record, and that complete records would extend into the tens of thousands. Nevertheless our information has been confirmed in multiple sources and we argue that it is representative.
16. This measure is clearly an underestimate since well-documented dissident behaviour is a subset of all dissent. It does not correct for the size of the dissident population (or the whole Soviet population) in each republic. However, since it is an average per individual of frequency of dissident acts by republic over all years for which data exist within that republic, it can still provide a basis for some meaningful comparisons across republics.
17. Sample size is so small in this case that we would expect subsequent information to generate a different, more stable, and probably smaller estimate.
18. n=286 cases in which republic of residence and year of first dissident act are known.
19. The possibility of diffusion of dissidence by geographical proximity or 'contagion' in some cases suggests that an epidemiological model could be used to explain this phenomenon.
20. The Chernenko interregnum, providing only eight cases, cannot show much dispersion.
21. This number is probably artificially low due to missing data, since detainees are not included in this dataset unless they were forcibly hospitalized. Thus except for missing data, the minimum to which average number of detentions should be able to drop is one per person.
22. This number is also to some extent an artifact of missing residence data, since the calculation omits cases of individuals detained by court order for whom republic of residence is unknown.
23. Results for the two Islamic republics may be artifacts of small sample size.

6 THE RISK OF PSYCHIATRIC DETENTION, DEMOGRAPHIC VARIABLES AND DETERRENCE OF DISSENT

1. All time hospitalized was calculated for each individual in the dataset to include all terms of administrative or criminal detention whose durations are known. Some durations are available even though the corresponding court dates or administrative hearing dates are not known.

2. Priests, nuns, rabbis, ministers, deacons, etc. find that they must describe themselves as 'cult followers' in some Soviet census occupation categories.
3. So too were police, KGB, and invalids, but sample size suggests these observations may not be stable.
4. In Dr Oleszczuk's count during the most active phase of the dissident movement, 1960–81, in most cases of involuntary hospitalization of protesters the trigger event setting off arrest and detention was samizdat activity (printing, distributing, composing, creating, possessing), petitioning, or an offence against the flag.
5. Not surprisingly, the risk of psychiatric detention is well under the group average for those dissenting while already in prison camps (0.125 detentions from 1960–81), though arrests and psychiatric internments – both new and extended – did occur in prisons.
6. These calculations can only be made for individuals for whom we have a record of the nature of the first dissident act, and whose incarceration time and court-ordered and administrative detention durations are known. Maximum subsample size is 71 in these data and can be much smaller.
7. Exceptions are violation of work rules or strikes, characterized by shorter hospitalizations but average incarceration time of 10.5 years, and renunciation of Soviet citizenship, 11 years' average incarceration.
8. Our transfer data include polyclinic placements, ordinary mental hospital commitments, special mental hospital commitments, detentions in Serbsky, and unknown types, as well as information on ordinary labour camp, special regime camp, prison, and exile. Considering only hospitalizations, and calculating the per cent placed first in ordinary hospitals as a proportion of all those placed in both ordinary and special regime psychiatric hospitals for first detentions yields 49.7 per cent in ordinary institutions. Special hospital confinements as a proportion of all ordinary and special hospitalizations then amount to 50.3 per cent. We do not have information on confinements in special wards within ordinary regime hospitals.
9. Our data are consistent with Bonnie's (1990b:334) observation that civil hospitalization is not 'peripheral to the problem of abuse'.
10. Variables recording disposition of victim after each detention or transfer to a new institution do hint at punitive transfers in some respects. Although interpretation is obstructed by missing data and diminishing sample size from first to twelfth transfer (n=319 in the first instance but only 48 by the fifth), it can be argued that deaths in confinement increase over time, as a valid per cent of known cases, from 0.6 at first detention to 5.9 at the eighth transfer. Our data also show a persistent rate of escapes between two and five valid per cent from the first to the seventh transfer.
11. Results are 0.80 as opposed to 0.29 times on average, at $\alpha=0.000$. These frequency of commitment numbers are artificially reduced in this context by the inclusion in the numerator of transfers to prisons, labour camps, and Serbsky Institute, and of exiles.
12. This finding does not imply that political *behaviour* was unaffected by terror.
13. Though perhaps not as alarming to the leadership as the discrepancy between the birthrates in the Islamic and Slavic republics.
14. Future research if more data become available can address the question of

whether some of the observed differences which point to deterrence failure may be attributable instead to an increase in the volume of available information relative to previous years. The findings cannot be solely a function of more years included in the sample after 1971–72, since the data extend 20 years forward to 1991 and 43 years back to 1928. The information for the sixties and later decades is richer, however.

15. For cases in which dates are known, after first administrative detention, 579 show zero recorded additional dissident acts. After first court-ordered hospitalization, 565 show no further dissident acts.
16. As illustration, consider the case of infinitely valued objectives. Suppose deterrence works when the value of an objective times the probability of achieving it via certain means is less than the cost of a penalty times the probability of its being inflicted. Then given the properties of the arithmetic of infinity, no penalty, even an infinite one, will exceed the value of an infinitely desired objective and cause the individual holding it to be dissuaded from seeking it. Even an infinite penalty will only equal the value of the objective, irrespective of the values of the probabilities associated with each, since any quantity times infinity is still infinity. One suspects that deterrence fails for highly valued objectives as well as infinitely valued objectives.
17. Sample size yielding these particular results is small, for two reasons. It includes only those cases in which dates of hospitalizations, or camp terms, and dissident acts are known. Second, for clarity with respect to psychiatric repression method, the groups of dissidents were separated into those who had been hospitalized via the court procedure only, and those hospitalized administratively only, omitting the overlapping group detained via both procedures. Given small sample size (n=64), these findings may not be stable in future research in a larger dataset.
18. That even moderately strong significant findings appear is especially remarkable since the time series data show marked curvilinearity, and the associations have been assessed here preliminarily with linear measures.
19. The Soviet state itself did not maintain heavy penalties across all administrations. Instead the length of administrative hospitalizations tended to decline, and court-ordered detentions declined after 1981.
20. The SIP results show many active nonconformists whose early socializing experiences included the arrest of their fathers, and our data also include father–son records such as those of Vladimir Rybak and his son V.V. Rybak.

7 LEGAL AND POLITICAL DEVELOPMENTS IN THE GORBACHEV AND YELTSIN ADMINISTRATIONS AND AFTER

1. *Vedomosti Verkhovnovo Sovieta SSSR*, 12 Jan., No. 2:22–7, item 19; in *Current Digest of the Soviet Press* 40(6), March: 11–13; see also *Izvestia*.
2. Again, meaningful consent in compulsory hospitalization is unobtainable.
3. The 1992 law directs that insanity shall not be found 'only' because of moral, cultural, political or religious conflicts (article 10(1)).
4. Some analysts might make an exception for the New Economic Plan period.

5. Among dissidents acquitted of some or all charges are K.G. Danilov, R.Ya. Eminov, I.P. Fedotov, L.N. Jagman, M. Makarenko, M.S. Ryshin, V.A. Shavrov, Kh. Teshayev, I.M. Yazydzhieyev and I.D. Zaslavsky (de Boer *et al.* 1982); R. Bairamov, A. Bariev, S. A(kh)metova, R. Gafarov, R.K. Kadiev, I.S. Khairov, M. Khalilova and R. Umerov (Herzen, 1976).
6. One recent exception in 1992 is the Constitutional Court's finding unconstitutional Yeltsin's merger of Russian and formerly All-Union security agencies. Yeltsin had ordered the USSR MVD and the Inter-republic Security Service (MSB) to be combined with the Russian MVD and Russian Federal Security Agency.
7. See for example Special Decree No. 345-209 of 15 May 1969 'On the Means of Preventing Socially Dangerous Acts by Psychiatric Patients', signed by officials of the Ministries of Public Health and Internal Affairs, distributed among police stations and psychiatric hospitals, reportedly, against the terms of the Law of Criminal Procedure of the USSR.
8. See *Izvestia* 18 June 1987, and the Radio Liberty *Research Bulletin* 'USSR This Week', RL 123/87:8, 27 March 1987.
9. See Moscow Television, 14 July 1989, translated in FBIS-USR 17 July 1989:50–1, cited in Gelman, 1990:108 fn.
10. This move is similar to the regime response to pressure to remove corrupt practices from university admissions: periodically some university admissions officers are publicly arrested, presumably for the demonstration effect, since the process of admissions does not seem to have been much altered.
11. Dr Semyon Gluzman asserts (AIPUP, 1990, No. 23:21) that in October 1989 Soviet psychiatrists remained unaware of the provisions of the July 1989 Health Ministry ban on use of electroshock, atropine coma, insulin shock, and sulfazine (except by 'consent' of detainee or family), which had been published in an obscure periodical. Similarly, the printed Soviet response to the findings of the 1989 US Delegation seemed to be regarded by the Ministry of Health as a classified document. In its 1991 visit to the USSR, the World Psychiatric Association found that psychiatrists had become familiar with the 1988 laws and regulations on patients' rights but those detained were not aware of them.
12. Occasional official claims that electroshock has not been used in the USSR/successor states for decades still surface.
13. But again the 1992 law provides for forcible commitment simply for evaluation, mainly done on an outpatient basis in the West (art. 23(4); art. 28(2)).
14. 'Psychiatric Reform Under Way in the Soviet Union?', *CSCE Digest* Jan./Feb. 1988:5; S. Grigoryantz, 'Soviet Psychiatric Prisoners', *New York Times* 23 Feb. 1988.
15. See Deputy Minister of Health A. Koskvichev, 'On Psychiatric Care', in *Izvestia*, 15 Jan. 1988.
16. In March and April 1989 Amnesty International had evidence of at least 25 people still involuntarily hospitalized for political acts, their reports including some long-term hospitalizations. However by August 1990 the IAPUP/Geneva Initiative was confident enough that the systematic political use of mental hospitals in the USSR had abated to cease publication of its information bulletin.

8 SUMMARY OF EMPIRICAL FINDINGS AND CONCLUSIONS

1. See Chapter 2 for a description of data sources. The CPSU Central Committee's Academy of Social Sciences has published a study on 'religious extremism' endorsing one of our sources as follows: 'Catholic extremists have organized the publication of an illegal magazine called "Chronicle of the Lithuanian Catholic Church" [*Khronika katolicheskoi tserkvi Litvy*], which publishes materials of an antisocial nature. Kovalev, who put out this magazine in a clandestine printshop . . . had ties with an anti-Soviet foreign organization and had sent it slanderous materials.' (Filimonov, 1983:abstract).
2. Some denials are irrelevant Cold War point-counterpoint intended only to distract rather than refute. While defenders of Soviet psychiatric practice such as Morozov have countered criticisms by drawing attention to the US Tuskeegee studies (in which black men with syphilis were left untreated to study the course of the disease), when considering the role of the individual v. the state and the power of ideology to submerge good sense, the US plutonium experiments of the 1940s are more nearly analogous, and at least equally immaterial.
3. A standard Soviet rejoinder has been that anyone hospitalized was *ipso facto* truly mentally ill, and that abuses, if any, whether individual errors of 'hyperdiagnosis' or poor judgment, were scattered, unsystematic, certainly not state policy, and confined to the 'period of stagnation' or at least not to recent administrations. Despite some forthright assertions in *Izvestia* and elsewhere, the press coverage identifying psychiatric abuses remained in some respects timid and circumspect into the early 1990s, often implying that the issue concerned only the Khrushchev and Brezhnev periods, or even more narrowly that it was a phenomenon of the sixties and seventies (ex. Kozheurov and Mikhalych, 1992). Alexander Karpov, then chief psychiatrist in the USSR Ministry of Health, as late as 1989 still denied knowing of anyone confined for reasons of conscience, admitting only that psychiatric abuse extended to sheltering in hospitals some draft dodgers or criminals avoiding penalties for their crimes (IAPUP, 1990, No. 23:41 quoting an interview in *Sotsialisticheskaya Industriya* of 31 Oct. 1989). In 1990 Pyotr Morozov still refused to admit political use of hospitalization had taken place; he insisted that the only error had been hospitalizing genuinely ill dissidents in special rather than ordinary psychiatric institutions (*La Croix* interview 21 May 1990, cited in IAPUP, 1990, No. 24:3).
4. Ellen Mercer of the American Psychiatric Association, who was a member of a US Department of State/National Institute of Mental Health/American Psychiatric Association delegation, found, on the basis of interviews with current or former political prisoners conducted in the USSR in 1989 'certainly some . . . were mentally ill' (correspondence, 12 November 1993). Cf. the supplement to the *Schizophrenia Bulletin* of the National Institute of Mental Health. The US Delegation visiting Soviet mental hospitals in 1989 found nine undeniably ill individuals among those presumed political cases still hospitalized, and agreed partially or completely with the Soviet diagnosis in six cases, again indicating a core of agreement on the concept of mental illness.
5. A representative example may be the 1973 Letter from the presidium of the

All Union Society of Neurologists and Psychiatrists (during 1991 the Federation of Societies of Psychiatrists and Neurologists – some sources show 'Narcologists' – of the USSR) printed in the *Guardian*, 29 September of that year. The next year Dr Georgi Vasilievich Morozov of the Serbsky Institute in Moscow, corresponding member of the Academy of Medical Science of the USSR, reports (1974:40) that a group of 13 visiting mental health professionals including World Psychiatric Association Executive Committee members found *one* person detained at Serbsky to be genuinely ill, hence not criminally responsible. Morozov reports that they reached this diagnosis via simultaneous translations of interviews with the individual concerned. They also agreed, on the basis of case histories, that five 'so-called dissidents' were really ill (1974:40). Morozov's account again suggests that some core of agreement exists internationally on what constitutes mental illness. Dr Alfred M. Freedman, president of the American Psychiatric Association in 1973 and apparently one of the outside experts cited by Morozov, also held on the basis of dossiers that six Soviet dissidents had been unnecessarily detained in mental institutions (Sobel, 1978:40).

Essentially the same Soviet response (in *Literaturnaya Gazeta* 4 Feb. 1976, cited in Sobel, 1978:40) argues that Alexis Tummerman and Anatoly Yakovson really were insane and were hospitalized on emigration, in these cases, to Israel; as were Lev Konstantinov, in Vienna, and Viktor Feinberg, in England.

Prof. Marat Yenokhovich Vartanyan, corresponding member of the USSR Academy of Medicine and Deputy Director of the All Union Mental Health Research Centre, in a 1987 domestic Soviet interview, provides another variation of his standard flat denial, asserting that Western visitors shown the Soviet psychiatric wards see 'people who are really mentally ill. Among such people, they were shown so-called dissidents, many of whom later left the USSR . . .'

6. While the Soviet demographic literature shows a concern for low or falling birth rates in Slavic republics in recent decades, these preoccupations did not result in changes in medicine, working or living conditions, transportation, child care, financial support, or household task sharing which would have been required to make feasible a state pro-natalist policy.
7. As opposed to true Communist Party affiliation. Roy Medvedev reports the case of a woman in her 70s in 1980, who despite a number of contributions to the *Chronicle of Current Events* samizdat journal, had not been arrested, prosecuted, hospitalized, or even expelled from the Party, to which she had purportedly belonged for 50 years. Prominent people whose dissident activities are *ignored* raise questions concerning how the discretion to arrest and prosecute is exercised.
8. An exception occurs over the period 1971–76, which shows some increase in average duration for compulsory hospitalizations.
9. Of course a nation-state as vast as the former USSR, correctly mapped as multicultural, might exhibit different cultural norms in different regions, including those norms affecting resort to compulsory hospitalization to cope with radicals or even mere annoyances. The prospect of multiple cultural norms does not imply rapid variability over time either.
10. When military governments in the West are taken adequately into account,

for example, in Latin America, the validity of the casual presumption of greater authoritarianism in Eastern as opposed to Western states disappears. Similarly, it is unclear that Eastern societies are necessarily more conformist than Western societies, though this too is at least in principle an empirical question.

11. Because Leningrad/St Petersburg is more exposed to the West than Moscow, authorities may have been less tolerant of visible dissent there, and may have arrested protesters at higher rates than in Moscow for the same behaviour. However, if true, this explanation of the frequency of detentions in Leningrad would support the instrumental use explanation of punitive psychiatry rather than one of professional socialization.
12. An exception in the Oleszczuk study of Lithuania (1988) shows active dissenters as young as 11.
13. Emilia Grigoryevna Sarantseva was put on the register by her relatives following a dispute over living space.
14. Our data show only a few instances in which a family member requested a psychiatric evaluation, but these can also be explained in non-generational terms. Birute Poskiene's husband, for example, had her committed after she converted to a Protestant group, evidently fearing she would not raise their children to be Catholic.
15. As Podrabinek points out (1980:136), punitive medicine could also be used instrumentally for purposes other than management of the dissident problem, such as to reduce workers' compensation claims, to further factional disputes by dislodging officials from the Central Committee, Council of Ministers, and elsewhere, as well as for other ends and agendas.
16. Substantive accounts do illustrate greater complexity in policy towards dissenters in some administrations than in others. Gorbachev, for example, made selective use of releases such as the large-scale ones in 1988 and crackdowns such as the use of military force against nationalists in 1989 in Baku, Fergana, Tbilisi, and Yerevan.
17. For example, the routine use of abortions for birth control can easily be seen as punitive towards women, expecially as shortages of disinfectants, hot water and anaesthetics made abortion, and in some cases giving birth, brutal.
18. Some hint of leniency is also seen for Belarus in the under-representation of Belarus residents among the detainee population.
19. Alexander Sergeyevich Lyapin, refusing to recant in May of 1979, was interned for six more months.
20. Reddaway has suggested cycles in regime response.
21. Alexeyeff (1986:122) and others have described the available remedies for unjustified detentions – court reviews and psychiatric commission reviews – as resulting in merely pro forma reconsideration of commitments to special regime hospitals taking perhaps two or three minutes per case. This brief and non-substantive reconsideration is probably also partially explainable as a consequence of bureaucratic time-maximization. The appeals process defined in legal reforms of the late 1980s and early 1990s is not functioning, at least in Moscow. In Moscow and environs in 1988, only ten appeals were noted out of tens of thousands of possibly contestable commitments (Barabash, 1989; Shore and Keith, 1989).

    The general failure of the mechanisms of judicial and expert commission re-hearing to result in freeing significant numbers of presumably healthy dissenters can also be interpreted as evidence supporting the argument of deliberate state use of the medical and in this case judicial bureaucracy to deter dissent.

References

Conventions

Citations to the Russian or other Former Soviet Union national press in which no author was provided are listed under the name of the relevant periodical, or, if an interview, the name of the interviewee. Electronic media sources if otherwise unattributed are listed under the name of the appropriate news service or news programme.

Acronyms:

CDSP	*Current Digest of the Soviet Press.*
FBIS	Foreign Broadcast Information Service *Daily Reports*
IAPUP	International Association on the Political Use of Psychiatry (Geneva Initiative)
L/N	from LEXIS/NEXIS services, World Library. Files: SOVNWS (Kremlin News Service), SPD (Russian Press Digest), MOSNWS (*Moscow News*), CDSP (*Current Digest of the Soviet Press*), TASS, and SOVLEG (Soviet/Russian Legislation).

Alexeyeff, Sergei, 'Abuse of Psychiatry as a Tool for Political Repression in the Soviet Union', *Medical Journal of Australia* 31 Jan. 1976 1(5):122–3.

Amalrik, Andrei, *SSSR i Zapad v Odnoi Lodke* (London: Overseas Publishers Interchange, 1978).

American Psychiatric Association, *Diagnostic and Statistical Manual of Mental Disorders DSM-III-R* 3rd Edition Revised (Washington, DC: American Psychiatric Association, 1987).

Amnesty International, *Prisoners of Conscience in the USSR: Their Treatment and Conditions* (New York and London: Amnesty International Publications, 1975, 1980).

Amnesty International, 'Political Abuse of Psychiatry in the USSR: Briefing' (New York: Amnesty International, 1983), EUR 46/01/83, March.

Amnesty International, 'USSR: Human Rights in a Time of Change' (London: Amnesty International, 1989), EUR 46/22/89, Oct.

Andriyanov, V., 'Criminal Diagnosis', *Sotsialisticheskaya Industria* 31 Jan. and 1 Feb.:3, 1987, in *CDSP* XXXIX(9):14. L/N.

Andriyanov, V., 'In the light of day', interview with A. Potapov, RSFSR Minister of Health, *Sotsialisticheskaya Industriya* 1 Sept. 1987.

Antebi, Elizabeth, *Droit d'asiles en Union Soviétique: Document* (Paris: Julliard, 1977).

Arbatov, Georgi A., *The System: An Insider's Life in Soviet Politics* (New York: Random House, 1991). Trans. of Russian manuscript pub. 1991 Moscow: Izdatelstvo Mezhdunarodnye Otnoshenia.

Arbatov, Georgi, and E. Babulin, 'Political Reform and the Evolution of the Soviet State,' in USSR Academy of Sciences *Socialism and Democracy: Topical Aspects of the Present Stage* (Moscow: Nauka Publishers, 1989).

Atay, Joanne E., Michael J. Witkin, and Ronald W. Manderscheid, *Additions and Resident Patients at End of Year: State and County Mental Hospitals, by Age and Diagnosis, by State, United States, 1990* (Rockville, MD: Center for Mental Health Services, US Department of Health and Human Services, 1993), USGPO: 1993–342–356:83633.

Atay, Joanne E., Michael J. Witkin, and Ronald W. Manderscheid, *Additions and Resident Patients at End of Year: State and County Mental Hospitals, by Age and Diagnosis, by State, United States, 1985* (Rockville, MD: US Department of Health and Human Services, Public Health Service, Alcohol, Drug Abuse, and Mental Health Administration, 1988).

Azrael, Jeremy R., 'Varieties of De-Stalinization', in ed. Chalmers Johnson, *Change in Communist Systems* (Stanford: Stanford University Press, 1970), 135–51.

Azrael, J.R. and A.G. Rahr, *The Formation and Development of the Russian KGB, 1991–1994*. RAND MR-355-USDP (Santa Monica, CA: RAND Corporation, 1993).

Babaian (Babayan), Eduard Armeniakovich, with Yu. G. Shashina, *The Structure of Psychiatry in the Soviet Union* (New York: International Universities Press, c.1985).

Bahry, Donna 1987, 'Politics, Generations and Change in the USSR', in James R. Millar (ed.), *Politics, Work, and Daily Life in the USSR: A Survey of Former Soviet Citizens* (Cambridge: Cambridge University Press), pp. 61–99.

Bahry, Donna and Brian D. Silver, 'Intimidation and the Symbolic Uses of Terror in the USSR', *American Political Science Review* 81: Dec. 1987, 1065–98.

Bai, Yevgeny, 'Black Spots on the Human Rights Map: From Castro's Prisons to Pyongyang's Concentration Camps', *Izvestia* 9 Mar.:7 1992, *CDSP* 46(10):14, 8 April 1992.

Baker, Jerry DeWitt, 'Nonimputability in Soviet Criminal Law: The Soviet Approach to the Insanity Plea', *Law and Psychology Review* 11(55)1987:55–102.

Baldessarini, Ross J., M.D., 'Frequency of Diagnoses of Schizophrenia versus Affective Disorders from 1944–1968', *American Journal of Psychiatry* 127(6)1970:59–63.

Barabash, E., 'Psychiatry: Law and Practice', *Pravda* 1 March:3 1989, in *CDSP* XLI(9):23. L/N.

Baranovsky, Igor, 'A Madman Fired at the President', *Moscow News* 36, 4 Sept. 1991.

Barry, Donald B. (ed.), *Soviet Law After Stalin* (Germantown, MD: Sitjthoff and Nordhoff, 1979).

Basaglia, Franco, 'Institutions of Violence' in Nancy Scheper-Hughes and Anne M. Lovel (eds), *Psychiatry Inside Out: Selected Writings of Franco Basaglia* (New York: Columbia University Press, 1987a), 59–86.

Bauer, Raymond, Alex Inkeles and Clyde Kluckhohn, *How the Soviet System Works* (New York: Vintage, 1956).

Bedau, Hugo Adam (ed.), *The Death Penalty in America* (Garden City, NY: Anchor Books, 1964).

Belkin, A., 'Foreign Culture: Jean-Paul Sartre's "Sigmund Freud and the 'Compact with the Devil'"', *Literaturnaya Gazeta* 1 June 1988:15, in *CDSP* XV(29):17. L/N.

Bengelsdorf, Herbert, 'Psychiatric Commitment of Dissenters in Russia: A Myth', *American Journal of Psychiatry* 127(11)1971:1575.

Berman, Harold J., *Soviet Criminal Law and Procedure: The RSFSR Codes*, trans. H.J. Berman and J.W. Spindler (Cambridge: Harvard University Press, 1966).

Bloch, Sidney, 'Soviet Psychiatry and Snezhnevskyism' in Robert van Voren (ed.), *Soviet Psychiatric Abuse in the Gorbachev Era* (Amsterdam: IAPUP, 1989), pp. 55–61.

Bloch, Sidney and Peter Reddaway, *Psychiatric Terror: How Soviet Psychiatry Is Used to Suppress Dissent* (New York: Basic Books 1977a). (American edition of *Russia's Political Hospitals.*)

Bloch, Sidney and Peter Reddaway, *Russia's Political Hospitals: The Abuse of Psychiatry in the Soviet Union* (London: Victor Gollancz, 1977b).

Bloch, Sidney and Peter Reddaway, *Soviet Psychiatric Abuse: The Shadow Over World Psychiatry* (London: Victor Gollancz, 1984).

Bloch, Sidney and Peter Reddaway, *Psychiatrists and Dissenters in the Soviet Union* (Boulder, CO: Westview, 1985).

Bonanni, Andrea, 'Interview with A.A. Churkin, Head of Soviet Diagnostic Service', *Corriere della Sera*, 5 April 1988:5.

Bonavia, David, *Fat Sasha and the Urban Guerilla: Protest and Conformism in the Soviet Union* (New York: Atheneum, 1973).

Bonnie, Richard J. (ed.) with commentary, *Psychiatrists and the Legal Process, Diagnosis and Debate: A Collection of Articles Published in Psychiatric Annals 1973–1977* (New York: Psychiatric Annals, 1977).

Bonnie, Richard J., 'Soviet Psychiatry and Human Rights: Reflections on the Report of the U.S. Delegation', *Law, Medicine and Health Care*, 18(1–2)1990a:123–31.

Bonnie, Richard J., 'Coercive Psychiatry and Human Rights: An Assessment of Recent Changes in the Soviet Union', *Criminal Law Forum*, Winter 1(2)1990b: 319–46.

Bonnie, Richard J., 'Mental Health Law Reform in the Post-Soviet World: A Progress Report'. Paper presented at the Annual Meeting of the American Psychiatric Association, Miami, FL. 24 May 1995.

Breggin, Peter R., *Toxic Psychiatry: Why Therapy, Empathy, and Love Must Replace the Drugs, Electroshock and Biochemical Theories of the New Psychiatry* (New York: St Martin's Press, 1991).

Buianov, Mikhail Ivanovich, *Prezidium, ili kto upravlyaet sovetskoi psikhiatriei* (Moskva: Prometei, 1992).

Bukovsky, Vladimir Konstantinovich and Semyon F. Gluzman, *A Manual on Psychiatry for Dissenters* (Arlington, VA: Keuffel and Esser, 1977).

Bukovsky, Vladimir K., *To Build a Castle: My Life as a Dissenter* (New York: Viking, 1978).

Carrère d'Encausse, Hélène, *Decline of an Empire: The Soviet Socialist Republics in Revolt* (New York: Harper & Row, 1979).

Carrère d'Encausse, Hélène, trans. George Holoch, *Confiscated Power: How Soviet Russia Really Works* (New York: Harper and Row, 1982).

Carrère d'Encausse, Hélène, trans. Franklin Philip, *The End of the Soviet Empire: The Triumph of the Nations* (New York: Basic Books, HarperCollins, 1993).

Chalidze, Valery, *To Defend These Rights* (New York: Random House, 1974).

Chodoff, Paul, 'Involuntary Hospitalization of Political Dissenters in the Soviet Union', *Psychiatric Opinion*, Feb., 11(1)1974:5–19.

Churkin, A., Interviewed in 'Psychiatry and Politics', *New Times* 43, Oct. 1988: 41–3.

Ciucura, Theodore B., 'Dissent, Law and psychiatry in the Soviet Union', *Canadian Slavonic Papers* 21(1)1979:98–108.

Commission on Security and Cooperation in Europe, *Human Rights and Democratization in the Newly Independent States of the Former Soviet Union* (Washington, DC: CSCE, Jan. 1993).

Conference on Security and Cooperation in Europe, 'Psychiatric Reform Under Way in the Soviet Union?', Council for Security and Cooperation in Europe *Digest*, Jan.–Feb. 1988:59.

Connor, Walter D., *Deviance in Soviet Society* (New York: Columbia University Press, 1972).

Conquest, Robert, *Kolyma: The Arctic Death Camps* (London: Macmillan, 1978).

Cook, Warnilla A., *Characteristics of Discharges from Non-Federal General Hospitals with Separate Psychiatric Inpatient Units, United States, 1980* (Rockville, MD: US Department of Health and Human Services, Public Health Service, Alcohol, Drug Abuse, and Mental Health Administration, National Institute of Mental Health, Division of Biometry and Epidemiology, Clinical Services Research Branch, 1985).

Corson, Samuel A. and Elizabeth O'Leary Corson (eds), *Psychiatry and Psychology in the USSR* (New York and London: Plenum Press, 1976).

Cullen, F.T., Jr. and J.B. Cullen, 'The Soviet Model of Social Deviance', *Pacific Sociological Review* 20(3)1977:389–410.

Current Digest of the Soviet Press (see Institute of Man), 'Soviet Psychiatry: a Self-appraisal', 39:6–7 May 1987 13.

Dardykin, S. and B. Ivanov, '"Third Basket": Notes from the First Soviet-American Seminar on Human Rights', *Izvestia* 26 Nov. 1988:6 *CDSP* XL(47): 15, 21 Dec.

De Boer, S.P., E.J. Driessen, and H.L. Verhaar, *Biographical Dictionary of Dissidents in the Soviet Union, 1956–1975* (Boston, the Hague, and London: Martinus Nijhoff, 1982).

Denber, Rachel (ed.), *The Soviet Nationality Reader: The Disintegration in Context* (Boulder: Westview, 1992).

Druzhinin, N.M. and Mitskevich, E.S., 'Sergei Ivanovich Mitskevich', *Istoriia SSSR* 2, 1967:111–18.

Ellman, Michael, 'A Note on the Distribution of Income in the USSR under Gorbachev', *Soviet Studies* 42(1), Jan. 1990:147–8.

Etkind, Efim Grigorevich, trans. Peter France, *Notes of a Nonconspirator* (New York: Oxford University Press, 1978).

Faraone, Stephen, 'Psychiatry and Political Repression in the Soviet Union', *American Psychologist* 37(10):1105–12, Oct. 1982.

Feldbrugge, F.J.M., '"Does Soviet Law Make Sense?"' Rationality and Functionality in Soviet Law: An Epilogue', in Donald B. Barry, F.J.M. Feldbrugge, George Ginsburgs, and Peter B. Maggs (eds), *Soviet Law After Stalin* (Alphen aan den Rijn, Netherlands and Germantown, MD: Sijthoff and Noordhoff, 1979).

Feshbach, Murray, *The Soviet Union: Population Trends and Dilemmas*, Population Bulletin, 37(3)1982 (Population Reference Bureau, Inc., Washington, DC).

Feshbach, Murray and Alfred Friendly, Jr., *Ecocide in the USSR: Health and Nature Under Siege* (New York: Basic Books (HarperCollins), 1992).

Filimonov, E.G., 'The Social and Ideological Essence of Religious Extremism', *Nauchny ateizm* 8, August 1983, in *CDSP* XXXV(39):9, 26 Oct. 1983. L/N.

Fireside, Harvey, *Soviet Psychoprisons* (New York: Norton, 1979).

Flanagan, Tim J. and Katherine M. Jamieson (eds), *Sourcebook of Criminal Justice Statistics 1987* (Bureau of Justice Statistics. Washington, DC: US Government Printing Office, 1988).

Gelman, Harry, *Gorbachev's First Five Years in the Soviet Leadership: The Clash of Personalities and the Remaking of Institutions.* R-3951-A (Santa Monica, CA: RAND, 1990).

Gershman, Carl, 'Psychiatric Abuse in the Soviet Union', *Society: Transaction Social Science and Modern Society* 21(5)1984:54–9.

Gevorkyan, Natalya, 'In the Madhouse', *Moscow News* 49, 4 Dec. 1991. (Grigorenko Materials released by Military Procurator's Office.)

Glebov, Oleg and John Crowfoot, *The Soviet Empire: Its Nations Speak Out: The First Congress of Peoples Deputies, Moscow, 25 May to 10 June 1989* (Chur, London, Paris, New York, Melbourne: Harwood Academic Publishers, 1989).

Gluzman, Semyon, *On Soviet Totalitarian Psychiatry* (Amsterdam: IAPUP, 1989).

Goffman, Erving, *Asylums: Essays on the Social Situation of Mental Patients and Other Inmates* (Garden City, NJ: Anchor Books, 1961).

Golyakhovsky (Zak), Vladimir, *Russian Doctor* (New York: St Martin's Marek, 1984).

Gorbanevskaya, Natalya, *Red Square at Noon* (New York: Holt Rinehart & Winston, 1972).

Gorbunova, E., 'In the Shadow of Semiknowledge: Russian Republic Minister of Public Health A.I. Potapov on the Problems of Soviet Psychiatry, Real and Imaginary', *Sovietskaya Rossia* 20 Nov. 1987:4, *CDSP* 16 Dec. 1987 XXXIX (46):5–7.

Gordeyeva, A. and Ya. Chernyayev, 'People's Control: The Drug-Treatment Service is Called Upon to Operate Efficiently and Energetically, But Does It?', *Meditsinskaya Gazeta* 12 July 1985:12, in *CDSP* XXXVII(29):17. L/N.

Gorman, Mike, 'Soviet Psychiatry and the Russian Citizen', *International Journal of Psychiatry* 8(5)1969:841–54.

Grigorenko, Pyotr, *The Grigorenko Papers* (Boulder: Westview Press, 1976).

Grigoryents, S., 'Soviet Psychiatric Prisoners', *New York Times* 23 Feb. 1988; cf. 22 Nov. I9:1.

Gupta, Dipak K., Harinder Singh and Tom Sprague, 'Government Coercion of Dissidents: Deterrence or Provocation?' *Journal of Conflict Resolution* 37(2)1993: 301–39.

Gurr, T.R., 'Persisting Patterns of Repression and Rebellion: Foundations for a General Theory of Political Coercion' in M.P. Karns (ed.), *Persistent Patterns and Emergent Structures in a Waning Century* (New York: Praeger, 1986).

Helsinki Watch Group, *Documents of the Helsinki Watch Group in the USSR: Sbornik Dokumentov* (New York: Khronika Press, 1977).

Helsinki Watch Group, *Soviet Abuse of Psychiatry for Political Purposes* (New York and Washington, DC: Helsinki Watch Committee, 1987).

Henderson, C.W., 'Conditions Affecting the Use of Repression', *Journal of Conflict Resolution* 35 1991:120–42.

Herzen Foundation, *Tashkentskii Protsess* (Amsterdam: Alexander Herzen Foundation Press, 1976).

Holden, Constance, 'Politics and Soviet Psychiatry', *Science* 239 5 Feb. 1988:551–3.

Holden, Constance, 'Psychiatrists Examine the Soviet System', *Science*, March 24 1989, 243(4898):1547.

Holden, Constance, 'Soviet Psychiatry: Real Progress or Just PR?', *Science* 28 July 1989, 245(4916):348.

Holland, J. and I.V. Shakhmatova-Pavlova, 'Concept and Classification of Schizophrenia in the Soviet Union', *Schizophrenia Bulletin* 3(2)1977:277–87.

Hopkins, Kenneth D. and Gene V. Glass, *Basic Statistics for the Behavioral Sciences* (Englewood Cliffs, NJ: Prentice-Hall, 1978).

Horelick, A.L., 'The Political Character of Soviet Anti-Semitism', P-2945 Santa Monica, CA: RAND, 1964.

Hubner, Peter, 'The Political and Social Relations of the Dissidents', in Wolfgang Berner (ed.), *The Soviet Union 1978–1979: Domestic Policy, the Economy, and Foreign Policy Vol. 5*. Trans. of *Sowjetunion, 1978–79* (New York and London: Holmes and Meier, 1980).

IAPUP Working Group on Internment of Dissidents, *Soviet Political Psychology: The Story of the Opposition* (London: UK Publications Ltd., 1983).

IAPUP, *Information Bulletin*, Nos. 18–24 (ed.), Dr C.M. Shaw (Cambridgeshire and Amsterdam, 1988–90).

Illich, Ivan, *Medical Nemesis* (New York: Pantheon, 1976).

Inkeles, Alex and Raymond A. Bauer, *The Soviet Citizen: Daily Life in a Totalitarian Society* (New York: Atheneum, 1968).

Institute of Man, 'Speaking Frankly about Something Important: The Institute Interviews Prof. M. Ye. Vartanyan: Soviet Psychiatry: A Self-Appraisal', *Argumenty i fakty*, 14–20 March 1987:5 and 21–27 March 1987:5–6; *CDSP* 39(15)1987:6–7.

ITAR-TASS Moscow English service.

Ivanov, F., 'Details for *Izvestia*: The USSR and World Psychiatry' (Interview with A. Karpov, Chief Psychiatrist USSR Ministry of Health), *Izvestia* morning ed. 27 Oct. 1989:6, FBIS SOV-89-210, 1 Nov. 1989:99.

Izvestia unattributed, 'Decision Adopted on Conditions and Procedures for Administering Psychiatric Assistance', *Izvestia* morning ed., 6 Jan. 1988:27, FBIS SOV-88-003, 6 Jan. 1988:27.

Izvestia unattributed, 'The Congress of USSR People's Deputies – Verbatim Report', *Izvestia* 3 June 1989:1–7, *CDSP* 41(27):12, 2 August 1989.

Izvestia unattributed, 'The Second Congress of USSR People's Deputies: Verbatim Report', *Izvestia* 21 Dec. 1990:2–5, *CDSP* 42(4)1990:17.

Jacobson, Bobbie, 'Sinister Psychiatry: The Position of British Psychiatrists at the World Psychiatric Association Symposium of Schizophrenia, Russia, 1973', *World Medicine* 9(1)1973:15–23.

Kassis, V. and L. Kolosov, 'Behind the Scenes of Subversion: Concealed by a Flowering Lotus' (Moscow Krishna Circle Broken Up, Activities Traced to CIA Agent), *Nedelya* (22) 30 May–5 June 1983:10, in *CDSP* XXXV(33):15. L/N.

Kazanetz, E.P., 'Differentiating Exogenous Psychiatric Illness from Schizophrenia', *Archives of General Psychiatry* 36 1979:740–45.

Kerblay, Basile H., *Modern Soviet Society* (New York and Toronto: Methuen and Co. Ltd. and Random House, Inc., 1983. Trans. 1977 'La société soviétique contemporaine', Librairie Armand Colin).

Khamriv, Viktor, 'Fellow Countrymen: For Now, Kazakhstan Political Prisoner is Free – Boris Suprunyuk Has a Grievance against the Moscow Press', *Sevodnya* 31 May 1994:2, *CDSP* 46(22):20, 29 June 1994.

Knight, Amy W., 'The Future of the KGB', *Problems of Communism* 39(6)1990: 20–33.

Konchakov, A., G. Kozhevnikov, A. Meisner and V. Raikov, 'Health Service – Experience and Problems: Let Words Heal', *Izvestia* 27 Nov. 1984:3, in *CDSP* XXXVI(49):25, 2 Jan. 1985. L/N.

Koppers, Andre, *A Biographical Dictionary on the Political Abuse of Psychiatry in the USSR* (Amsterdam: IAPUP, 1990).

Korneev, V., 'Indefinite Stay in Lunatic Asylum', *Izvestia* Union edition 23 Dec. 1990:6, FBIS SOV-91-002, 3 Jan. 1991:36–7; also trans. 'An Insane Asylum with No Set Term', *CDSP* 42(51):27, 23 Jan. 1991.

Korolkov, Igor, 'Torture Has Been Used in Russia and Will Continue To Be Used . . .', *Izvestia* 16 Mar. 1994:1, 4, *CDSP* 46(12):15, 20 April 1994.

Koryagin, Anatoly, 'Unwilling Patients', *Lancet* 11 April 1981:821–4.

Koryagin, Anatoly, 'Soviet Psychiatrist Describes Abuse', *Science News* 131:328(1), 23 May 1987.

Koryagin, Anatoly, 'World Psychiatry: Readmitting the Soviet Union', *The Lancet* 2, 30 July 1988:268–9.

Koryagin, Anatoly, 'A Green Light for Injustice', in Robert van Voren (ed.), *Soviet Psychiatric Abuse in the Gorbachev Era* (Amsterdam: IAPUP, 1989), pp. 86–92.

Kozheurov, Ya. and S. Mikhalych, 'KP Investigation: What Children and Dissidents Have in Common – Unknown Pages from Present-Day Psychiatry', *Komsomolskaya Pravda* 1 Feb. 1992:5, *CDSP* 44(5):30, 4 March 1992.

Kozlov, Sergei, 'Kazakhstan: Boris Suprunyuk Gets Two-Year Suspended Sentence', *Nezavisimaya Gazeta* 8 Sept. 1994:3, *CDSP* 46(36):20, 5 Oct. 1994.

Kreindler, Isabelle, 'The Soviet Deported Nationalities: A Summary and an Update', *Soviet Studies* XXXVIII(3), July 1986:37–405.

Kremlin International News Broadcast 15 Nov. 1993. *Draft Constitution of the Russian Federation.* Broadcast in English. L/N.

Kuropayeva, Tatyana, 'Psychiatry and Politics – What Has Changed?' (Interview with Roy Alexandrovich Medvedev), Moscow domestic news services 1745 GMT, 5 April 1990, FBIS SOV-90-068, 9 April 1990:45.

Lane, David, *The End of Social Inequality: Class, Status and Power under State Socialism* (London: George Allen and Unwin, 1982).

Lebedev, Anatoly, 'Human Rights: Human Rights Defenders Count Each Other – There Were Significantly More Dissidents in the USSR Than Is Generally Believed', *Nezavisimaya Gazeta* 28 Aug. 1992:2, *CDSP* 44(35):23.

Leonhard, Karl, *The Classification of Endogenous Psychoses* (New York: Irington Publishers, 1979: dist. Halsted Press. 5th ed. Trans. *Aufteilung der endogenen Psychosen.*

Lichbach, I.L., 'Deterrence or Escalation? The Puzzle of Aggregate Studies of Repression and Dissent', *Journal of Conflict Resolution* 31 1987:266–97.

Literaturnaya Gazeta, 'Plenary Session of the Board of the Writers' Union: Speech by Lyudmila Shchipakhina' (Moscow) (Call to Rehabilitate Turkmenian Poet who Died in Psychiatric Hospital) 10, 9 Mar. 1988:7, *CDSP* 40(11):28, 13 April 1988.

Lopez, George A. and Michael Stohl (eds), *Dependence, Development and State Repression* (New York: Greenwood Press, 1989).

Lukacher, G., 'Humanization of Psychiatric Assistance', *Meditsinskaya Gazeta* 14 June 1991, in World Psychiatric Association Report (unpublished), Appendix 9:44.

McInerny, Peggy, 'Russian Legal Reform and the Case of *Izvestia*', *Meeting Report* XI(17) (Washington DC: Kennan Institute for Advanced Russian Studies, 1994).

Maguire, Kathleen, Ann L. Pastore and Timothy J. Flanagan (eds), *Bureau of Justice Statistics Sourcebook of Criminal Justice Statistics–1992* (Washington, DC: US Department of Justice, 1993).

Maier, Mark, *The Data Game: Controversies in Social Science Statistics* (Armonk, NY: M.E. Sharpe, 1991).

Maksimova, E., 'On Psychiatric Assistance' Interview with I. Samoshchenko and A. Moskvichev, *Izvestia* 15 Jan. 1988:6, *CDSP* 40(6):13–14.

Maksimova, E., 'In the Work of the Psychiatric Service' (Interview with A. Churkin, Chief Psychiatrist USSR Ministry of Health), *Izvestia* 27 April 1988:6, *CDSP* 40(17):22, 25 May 1988.

Maksimova, E. and I. Markovich, 'Defenseless', *Izvestia* 11 July 1987:3, *CDSP* 39(29):1, 19 Aug. 1987.

Manucharova, Ye., 'Psychiatry without Zones of Silence', *Izvestia* 18 April 1989:3, in *CDSP* XLI(16):24. L/N.

Marchenko, Anatoly, *My Testimony* (New York: E.P. Dutton and Co., 1969).

Marchenko, Anatoly, *From Tarusa to Siberia* (Royal Oak, MI: Strathcona Publications, 1980).

Mason, T. David and Dale A. Krane, 'The Political Economy of Death Squads: Toward a Theory of the Impact of State-Sanctioned Terror', *International Studies Quarterly* 33(2), June 1989:175–98.

Meditsinskaya Gazeta, 'In Memory of A.V. Snezhnevsky' (Obituary), 17 July 1987:3.

Medvedev, Roy, *On Soviet Dissent: Interviews with Piero Ostellino*. Trans. William A. Packer, (ed.) George Saunders (London: Constable, 1980).

Medvedev, Zhores A. and Roy A., *A Question of Madness* (New York: Alfred A. Knopf, 1971).

Mercer, Ellen, *Internments* (Washington, DC: American Psychiatric Association Office of International Affairs, unpublished, 1991a).

Mercer, Ellen, *Releases* (Washington, DC: American Psychiatric Association Office of International Affairs, unpublished, 1991b).

Mercer, Ellen, *Summary of American Psychiatric Association Activities Related to the Use of Psychiatry for Political Purposes in the Soviet Union* (report) (Washington, DC: American Psychiatric Association, 4 March 1992).

Merskey, Harold and Bronislava Shafran, 'Political Hazards in the Diagnosis of "Sluggish Schizophrenia"', *British Journal of Psychiatry* 148 1986:247–56.

Millar, James R. (ed.), *Politics, Work and Daily Life in the USSR: A Survey of Former Soviet Citizens* (Cambridge, New York, New Rochelle, Melbourne and Sydney: Cambridge University Press, 1987).

Miller, Martin A., 'The Theory and Practice of Psychiatry in the Soviet Union', *Psychiatry: The Journal for the Study of Interpersonal Processes* 48(1)1985: 13–24.

Ministry of Health of the USSR, 'On Measures for Further Improvement of Psychiatric Assistance', No. 225, 21 March 1988.

Moroz, I.B., 'Slowly Progressive Schizophrenia with Signs of Chronic Hypomania during Its Course', *Korsakoff Journal of Neuropathology and Psychiatry* I 1983:79–85.

Moroz, Oleg, 'Diagnosed Insane', *Literaturnaya Gazeta* (International) 1(18):20–21, Dec. 1990.

Morozov, Georgi, 'Psychiatry in the Soviet Union', *British Medical Journal* 2(922)1974:40.

Morozov, G.V. and I.M. Kalashnik (eds), *Forensic Psychiatry* (New York: International Arts and Sciences Press, 1970).

Morozov, Pyotr, 'Statement by P. Morozov on Behalf of the All Union Society of Neurologists and Psychiatrists at the World Psychiatric Association General Assembly' (1989), Record of Motion and Vote, in *Report by the WPA Team of the Visit to the Soviet Union*, 1991, Appendix 1:34. WPA Unpublished report.

Moskvichev, A., 'After *Izvestia* Has Spoken: Expert Commissions Will Be High Quality', *Izvestia* 16 Sept. 1987:3, *CDSP* 39(37):22, 14 Oct. 1987.

Motyl, Alexander J., *Sovietology, Rationality, Nationality: Coming to Grips with Nationalism in the USSR* (New York: Columbia University Press, 1990).

Motyl, Alexander J. (ed.), *The Post-Soviet Nations: Perspectives on the Demise of the USSR* (New York: Columbia University Press, 1992).

Nekipelov, Viktor (ed.) and trans. Marco Carynnyk and Marta Horban, *Institute of Fools: Notes from the Serbsky Institute* (New York: Farrar Straus Giroux, 1980).

Nezavisimaya Gazeta (eds.), 'Medicine' (Interview with Dr James Berley), *Nezavisimaya Gazeta* English edition, Jan. 1991:20–21.

Nie, Norman H., Sidney Verga and Jae-on Kim, 'Political Participation and the Life Cycle', *Comparative Politics* 6, 1974:319–40.

Novikov, A., 'Let's Examine It: A Sore Point – Or, Who Needs "Psychiatric Terror in the USSR"?', *Komsomolskaya Pravda* 15 July 1987:3, *CDSP* 39(29):4.

Novikov, A., S. Razin and M. Mishin, 'A Closed Subject', *Komsomolkaya Pravda* 11 Nov. 1987:11, *CDSP* 39(46):1–3, and 'Assignment in Response to a Disturbing Letter: A Closed Subject . . .' FBIS SOV-87-224, 20 Nov. 1987:45–51.

Olcott, Martha B. (ed.), with Lubomyr Hajda and Anthony Olcott, *The Soviet Multinational State: Readings and Documents* (Armonk, NY: M.E. Sharpe, 1990).

Oleszczuk, Thomas A., 'Soviet Repression: An Empirical Examination', paper presented to American Association for the Advancement of Slavic Studies, Washington, DC, 16 Oct. 1982.

Oleszczuk, Thomas A., 'An Analysis of Bias in Samizdat Sources: A Lithuanian Case Study', *Soviet Studies* XXXVII(1), Jan. 1985:131–7.

Oleszczuk, Thomas A., *Political Justice in the USSR: Dissent and Repression in Lithuania, 1969–1987* (Boulder, CO: East European Monographs and New York: Columbia University Press, 1988a).

Oleszczuk, Thomas A., 'The Human Rights Offensive in the USSR: The Fourth Side of Liberalization', paper presented to Annual Meeting of the American Political Science Association, Washington, DC, Sept. 1988b.

Oleynik, Igor, Natalia Alexeyeva and Tracey A. Ryan (eds), *Russian Government Today* (Reference) (Washington, DC: Carroll Publishing, 1994).

Patyulin, Valentin *et al.*, *Human Rights in Socialist Society* (Moscow: Novosti Press Agency Publishing House, 1981). (Russian ed. 1980).

Peterson, D.J., *Troubled Lands: The Legacy of Soviet Environmental Destruction* (Boulder: Westview, 1992).

Petras, James and Morris Morley, *Latin America in the Time of Cholera: Electoral Politics, Market Economics and Permanent Crisis* (New York and London: Routledge, 1992).

Plyushch, Leonid Ivanovich, trans. and ed. Marco Carynnyk, *History's Carnival: A Dissident's Autobiography* (New York and London: Harcourt Brace Jovanovich, 1977).

Podolsky, Edward, *Red Miracle: The Story of Soviet Medicine* (Freeport, NY: Beechhurst Press Inc., 1947).

Podrabinek, Alexandr Pinkhosovich, *Psychotherapy in the Soviet Union.* Citation and year unclear, perhaps Paris: Poiski Press.

Podrabinek, Alexandr Pinkhosovich, *Punitive Medicine* (Ann Arbor MI: Karoma, 1980). Alexander Lehrman trans. of A.P. Podrabinek, *Karatelnaia meditsina* (New York: Khronika Press, 1979).

Podrabinek, Alexander Pinkhosovich, 'Punitive Psychiatry during the Period of Perestroika' in Robert van Voren (ed.), *Soviet Psychiatric Abuse in the Gorbachev Era* (Amsterdam: IAPUP: 1989), 93–106.

Popov, Yu., 'A Troubling Topic: Is Everything All Right at Psychiatric Hospitals?', *Pravda* 21 June 1991:3, *CDSP* 43(25):17, 24 July 1991.

Presidium of the Supreme Soviet of the USSR, 'On the Confirmation of the Regulation of Conditions and Procedures Governing the Provision of Psychiatric Assistance' 5 Jan. 1988, Moscow.

Prokoshenko, S., 'Sent for Examination', *Pravda* Moscow ed., second ed. 28 Sept. 1990:2, FBIS SOV-90-192, 3 Oct. 1990:50.

Rainbolt, William R., *A History of Underground Communication in Russia Since the 17th Century* (Palo Alto: R&E Research Associates, 1979).

Razboynikov, V., 'Instructions to Put Him Away', *Izvestia* morning ed. 29 June 1989:3, FBIS, SOV-89-133, 13 July 1989:83–4.

Razboynikov, V., 'Follow-Up', *Izvestia* morning ed., 9 Jan. 1990:6, FBIS SOV-90-004 12 Jan. 1990:101–2.

Reddaway, Peter (compositor and editor), *Uncensored Russia: Protest and Dissent in the Soviet Union* (New York: McGraw Hill American Heritage Press, 1972).

Reddaway, Peter, *The Forced Labour Camps in the USSR Today: An Unrecognized Example of Modern Inhumanity* (Brussels: International Committee for the Defence of Human Rights in the USSR, 1973).

Reddaway, Peter, 'The Development of Dissent in the USSR' in William E. Griffith (ed.), *The Soviet Empire: Expansion and Detente* (Lexington, MA: D.C. Heath, 1976), pp. 57–85.

Reddaway, Peter (ed.) with Archie Brown and T.H. Rigby, *Authority, Power, and Policy in the USSR* (New York: St Martin's; London: Macmillan, 1980).

Reddaway, Peter, *Soviet Policy Towards Dissent since Khrushchev* (Munich: Radio Liberty Research Paper 297/80, 21 August, 1980).

Reddaway, Peter, 'Dissent in the Soviet Union', *Problems of Communism* 6, 1983.

Reddaway, Peter, 'Soviet Politics on Dissent and Emigration: The Radical Change of Course since 1979: Colloquium Paper' (Washington, DC: Kennan Institute for Advanced Russian Studies, Woodrow Wilson International Center for Scholars, 1984).

Reddaway, Peter, 'The Case of Dr Koryagin', *New York Review of Books* 31:10(1), 10 October 1985.

Reddaway, Peter, 'Does Moscow's Purge of Corrupt Psychiatrists Threaten the Psychiatric Gulag?', *IAPUP Information Bulletin* July (15–16)1987:7–14.

Reddaway, Peter, 'Will Perestroika End Political Abuse in Soviet Psychiatry?', 3 July 1988 draft, published as 'Soviet Psychiatry: an end to political abuse?', *Survey,* Autumn (O):25–38.

Reddaway, Peter, 'The WPA and Soviet Psychiatry, 1983–1989', in Robert van Voren (ed.), *Soviet Psychiatric Abuse in the Gorbachev Era* (Amsterdam: IAPUP, 1989), pp. 73–85.

Reddaway, Peter, 'The Current Situation in Soviet Psychiatry Regarding Political Abuses', *IAPUP Information Bulletin* Sept. 1989, No. 22:1–8.

Reddaway, Peter, 'Should World Psychiatry Readmit the Soviets?' *New York Review of Books*, 12 October 1989, 36(15):54.

Reddaway, Peter, 'Are You Ready for the Next Russian Revolution?', *Washington Post National Weekly Edition*, Dec. 4–10 1989:23.

Reddaway, Peter, 'Reform of Soviet Psychiatry: Is the Establishment Beginning to Panic?', *Radio Liberty Research Bulletin Report on the USSR: All-Union Topics*, 2(44), 2 Nov. 1990:1–13.

Reddaway, Peter, 'Civil Society and Soviet Psychiatry', *Problems of Communism* July–Aug. 1991, 40(4):41–48.

Redick, Richard W., *Trends in Number of Additions to Mental Health Organizations, United States, 1971, 1975, and 1981* (Rockville, MD: US Department of Health and Human Services, Public Health Service, National Institute of Mental Health, Division of Biometry and Epidemiology, Survey and Reports Branch, 1985).

Reich, Walter, 'Diagnosing Soviet Dissidents', *Harpers* Aug. 1978:31–7.

Reich, W., 'Psychiatric Diagnosis as an Ethical Problem', in S. Bloch and P. Chodoff (eds), *Psychiatric Ethics* (New York: Oxford University Press, 1981).

Rich, Vera, 'USSR: Doubts about Psychiatric Reform', *The Lancet*, 8 September 1990, 336(8715):616–17.

Rich, Vera, 'Soviet Union Admits to Abuses of Psychiatry', *New Scientist* 16 Nov. 1991 132(1795):13.

Rollins, Nancy, *Child Psychiatry in the Soviet Union: Preliminary Observations* (Cambridge: Harvard University Press, 1972).

Romanenko, V., 'Institute of Man: Speaking Frankly About Something Important – What Tasks is Psychiatry in the USSR Tackling Today?', *Argumenty i fakty* 14–20 Mar. 1987:5, in *CDSP* XXXIX (15):6. L/N. (Interview with M. Ye. Vartanyan).

Romanenko, V., 'Institute of Man: Speaking Frankly About Something Important – Soviet Psychiatry Favors an Open Dialogue with Our Western Colleagues', *Argumenty i fakty* 21–27 Mar. 1987:5–6, in *CDSP* XXXIX(15):6. L/N.

Rosenstein, Marilyn J., *Characteristics of Admissions to the Inpatient Services of State and County Mental Hospitals, United States, 1980* (Rockville, MD: US Department of Health and Human Services, Public Health Service, National Institute of Mental Health, Division of Biometry and Applied Sciences, Survey and Reports Branch, 1986).

Roth, Loren H., Yuri Reshetov, Darrel A. Regier, and Samuel J. Keith (issue eds) (cf. Shore and Keith), *Schizophrenia Bulletin: National Institute of Mental Health:*

Issue Theme: Report of the US Delegation/Soviet Response. Supplement to 15(4) (Rockville, MD: US Department of Health and Human Services, Public Health Service, Alcohol, Drug Abuse and Mental Health Administration, 1989). (English and Russian texts.)

Rubenstein, Joshua, *Soviet Dissidents: Their Struggle for Human Rights* (Boston: Beacon Press, 1985).

Rubin, Sol, *Psychiatry and Criminal Law: Illusions, Fictions, and Myths* (Dobbs Ferry, NY: Oceana Pubs, 1965).

Rueschemeyer, Marilyn, Igor Golomshtok and Janet Kennedy, *Soviet Emigré Artists: Life and Work in the USSR and the United States* (Armonk, NY and London: M.E. Sharpe, 1985).

Rush, Myron, *The Fate of the Party Apparatus Under Gorbachev.* R-4001-A (Santa Monica: RAND, 1991).

Ryan, Michael (comp. and trans.), *Social Trends in Contemporary Russia: A Contemporary Source-Book* (New York: St Martins, 1993).

Safronova, N., 'Is the Iceberg Melting? A Law of Psychiatric Care is Being Drafted', *Izvestia* 29 March 1990:3, *CDSP* 42(13):5.

Salvendry, John T., M.D., 'Psychiatry in the Soviet Union Today', *Canadian Psychiatric Association Journal* 20 1975:229–36.

Samatan, Marie, *Droits de l'Homme et Repression en URSS: L'appareil et les Victimes* (Paris: Editions du Seuil, 1980).

Sapiets, Marite, Peter Reddaway and Caryl Emerson (translators), *The Case of Leonid Plyushch* (Boulder, CO: Westview, 1976).

Savenko, Yuri, 'Law: A Cunning Move to Join the World Psychiatric Community: Russia's Punitive Psychiatry Upholds its Right to Existence', *Moscow New Times International,* in English 50, Dec. 1992:32, FBIS-USR (not FBIS-SOV)-93-006.

Scarnati, R., 'The Prostitution of Forensic Psychiatry in the Soviet Union', *Bulletin of the American Academy of Psychiatry and Law* 8(1):1980:111–13.

Scheflen, Albert E., *Levels of Schizophrenia* (New York: Brunner Mazel, 1981).

Scheper-Hughes, Nancy, *Saints, Scholars and Schizophrenics: Mental Illness in Rural Ireland* (Berkeley and Los Angeles: University of California Press, 1979).

Scheper-Hughes, Nancy, *Death Without Weeping: The Violence of Everyday Life in Brazil* (Berkeley, Los Angeles and Oxford: University of California Press, 1992).

Scheper-Hughes, Nancy and Anne M. Lovell (eds), *Psychiatry Inside Out: Selected Writings of Franco Basaglia* (New York: Columbia University Press, 1987).

Schmidt, Y., G. Morozov and L. Badalyan *et al.*, 'A. Letter from the Presidium of the All-Union Society of Neurologists and Psychiatrists' to *The Guardian* 1973, in Bloch and Reddaway, *Russia's Political Hospitals* (London: Victor Gollancz, 1977).

Segal, Boris, M., 'Involuntary Hospitalization in the USSR' in Corsons (eds), *Psychiatry and Psychology in the USSR* (New York and London: Plenum Press, 1976).

Sharlet, Robert, 'Soviet Institutions and the Administration of Law', Part III in Donald B. Barry, F.J.M. Feldbrugge, George Ginsburgs, and Peter B. Maggs (eds), *Soviet Law After Stalin* (Germantown, MD and Alphen aan den Rijn, Netherlands: Sijthoff and Noordhoff, 1979).

Shatz, Marshall, *Soviet Dissent in Historical Perspective* (New York: Cambridge University Press, 1980).

Shaw, Christine, 'The World Psychiatric Association and Soviet Psychiatry' in Robert van Voren (ed.), *Soviet Psychiatric Abuse in the Gorbachev Era* (Amsterdam: IAPUP: 1989), pp. 36–54.

Shchipakhina, Lyudmila, 'Writers Debate National Culture: Call to Rehabilitate Persecuted Turkmenian Poetess Who Dies in Psychiatric Hospital' (Speech by L. Shchipakhina at Board of Writers' Union), *Literaturnaya Gazeta* 10(9)1988:7, *CDSP* 40(11):28, 13 April.

Sheley, Joseph F., *Criminology: A Contemporary Handbook.* Second edition (Belmont, Albany, Bonn: Wadsworth Publishing, 1995).

Shifrin, Avraham, *The First Guide to Prisons and Concentration Camps of the Soviet Union* (New York: Bantam, Stephanus Edition Verlags GmbH, 1982).

Shore, David and Samuel J. Keith (eds); (issue eds) Loren H. Roth, Yuri Reshetov, Darrel A. Regier, and Samuel J. Keith, *Assessment of Recent Changes in Soviet Psychiatry: Report of the US Delegation, Soviet Response*. Supplement to *Schizophrenia Bulletin* 15(4) (Schizophrenia Research Branch, National Institute of Mental Health, Alcohol, Drug Abuse, and Mental Health Administration. Washington, DC: US Government Printing Office, 1989).

Shtromas, Alexander, *Political Change and Society: The Case of the Soviet Union* (Frankfurt: Peter Lang, c.1981).

Smith, T.C. with T.A. Oleszczuk, 'Trade and Arrests (for dissent): Soviet-American Linkages in the 1970's', *Coexistence* 23(3)1986:209–25.

Smith, T.C. with T.A. Oleszczuk, 'Soviet Domestic Political Behavior: Patterns in Psychiatric Detention for Political and Religious Dissent in the USSR', paper presented at March Joint Annual Meetings of the British and US International Studies Associations, London, 1989.

Smith, T.C. with T.A. Oleszczuk, 'The Brezhnev Legacy: Nationalities and Gorbachev' in Zvi Gitelman (ed.), *The Politics of Nationality in the Contemporary USSR* (New York: St Martin's and London: Macmillan, 1992).

Snezhnevsky, A.V., 'The symptomatology, clinical forms and nosology of schizophrenia', in J.G. Howells (ed.) *Modern perspectives in World Psychiatry* (New York: Brunner/Mazel, 1971).

Snezhnevsky, A.V. and Marat Vartanyan, 'The Forms of Schizophrenia and Their Biological Correlates', in H.E. Himwich (ed.), *Biochemistry, Schizophrenias and Affective Illnesses* (Baltimore: Williams and Wilkins, 1970).

Sobel, Lester A. (ed.), *et al.*, *Political Prisoners: A World Report* (New York: Facts on File, 1978).

Sokolov, Valentin, 'Conversion Table Showing Numbers of Some Articles of the Criminal Codes of the Union Republics and Their Equivalents in the Russian Criminal Code', in Cronid Lubarsky (ed.), *Vesti iz SSSR: Prava Cheloveka/ USSR News Brief List of Political Prisoners in the USSR* 1 May 1983:9–13.

Solomon, Peter H., 'The Case of the Vanishing Acquittal: Informal Norms and the Practice of Soviet Criminal Justice', *Soviet Studies* XXXIX(4), Oct. 1987:531–55.

(Soviet Supreme Court), *Statute on Conditions and Procedure for the Provision of Psychiatric Assistance.* 5 Jan. 1988 *Vedomosti Verkhovnovo Sovieta SSR* No. 2, [2440], 13 Jan. 1988, item 19:22–7, *CDSP* 40(8), March:11–13: also via L/N.

Sparre, Victor, (trans.) Alwyn and Dermot McKay, *Flame in Darkness: The Russian Human Rights Struggle, as I Have Seen It* (London: L. Grosvenor, 1979).

Spechler, Dina R., *Permitted Dissent in the USSR: Novy Mir and the Soviet Regime* (New York: Praeger, 1982).

Staroselskaya, S., 'A Special Case: Look Before You Leap' (Patients' Aggressiveness Linked to Incompetent Articles in Press), *Meditskinskaya Gazeta* 13 Jan. 1988:4, *CDSP* 40(6):14, 9 March 1988.

Stepanov, L., 'Psychiatry or Psychosis?', *Izvestia* 16 July:4, in *CDSP* XXXV(28):12. L/N.

Stohl, Michael and George A. Lopez, *The State as Terrorist: The Dynamics of Governmental Violence and Repression* (Westport, CT: Greenwood Press, 1984).

Stone, Irving F., 'Betrayal by Psychiatry', *New York Review of Books* 10 Feb. 1972:7–14.

Stover, Eric and Elena O. Nightingale (eds), *The Breaking of Bodies and Minds: Torture, Psychiatric Abuse, and the Health Professions* (American Association for the Advancement of Science, New York: W.H. Freeman, 1985).

Strauss, Anselm, Leonard Schatzman, Rue Bucher, Danuta Ehrlich, and Melvin Sabshin, *Psychiatric Ideologies and Institutions* (London: Collier Macmillan, 1964).

Sukhareva, Grunia Efimovna, *Clinical Schizophrenia Among Children and Adolescents* (Kharkov, 1937).

Sukhareva, Grunia Efimovna, *Klinicheskie lektsii po psikhiatrii detskogo vozrasta* (Moskva: Gosudarstvennoe izdatelstvo med. literatury, 1940, 1955, 1959).

Szasz, Thomas, *Psychiatric Justice* (New York: Macmillan, 1965).

Tabakov, George A., *Medicine in the United States and the Soviet Union: A Comparative and Critical Study* (Boston: Christopher Publishing House, 1962).

Tappan, Paul W., *Crime, Justice and Correction* (New York: McGraw-Hill, 1960).

Taranov, Sergei, 'A Medical Diagnosis Still Has the Force of a Court Sentence', *Izvestia* 6 June 1992:6, *CDSP* 44(23):27, 8 July 1992.

Tarsis, Valery Ya., *Ward 7: An Autobiographical Novel.* Trans. Katya Brown (London: Collins and Harvill Press, 1965).

Tarsis, Valery Ya., *Testimony, Executions by Madness* (Frankfurt: Possev-Verlag, 1971).

Tausig, Michael, 'Terror as Usual', *Social Text*, Fall-Winter 1989:3–20.

Tempest, Richard, 'Madman or Criminal: Government Attitudes to Petr Chaadaev in 1836', *Slavic Review*, 1986.

Thorne, Ludmilla 'Prisons of Madness', *Journal of Current Social Issues* 15:55–60 Summer, 1978.

Ticktin, Hillel, 'Political Economy of the Soviet Intellectual', *Critique* 2 1973:5–22.

Timerman, Jacobo, *Preso sin Nombre, Celda sin Numero* (Caracas, Venezuela: Editorial Ateneo de Caracas, 1981).

Tkachenko, Ye., 'People Are Profitting from Illness' (Interview with N. Movchan), *Sovetskaya rossiya* 1st edition, 26 Jan. 1988:3, FBIS SOV-88-023, 4 Feb. 1988:35.

Tolz, Vera, with Melanie Newton (ed.), *USSR in 1990: A Record of Events* (Boulder: Westview, 1992).

Turk, Austin T., *Criminality and Legal Order* (Chicago: Rand McNally, 1969).

Turk, Austin T., *Political Criminality: The Defiance and Defense of Authority.* Volume 136 (Sage Library of Social Research. Beverly Hills, London and New Delhi: Sage, 1982).

US Congress: Senate Committee on the Judiciary, Subcommittee to Investigate the Administration of the Internal Security Act and other Internal Security Laws, *Abuse of Psychiatry for Political Repression in the Soviet Union* (New York: Arno Press (New York Times Company), 1973).

US Department of Health, Education and Welfare Public Health Service, *Patients in Mental Institutions 1960* (Washington, DC: National Institutes of Health, 1963).

USSR Supreme Soviet Presidium, *Statute on the Conditions and Procedures Governing the Provision of Psychiatric Assistance.* 5 January 1988, No. 8282-XI. See above, Soviet Supreme Court.

Van Voren, Robert (ed.), *Koryagin: A Man Struggling for Human Dignity* (Vladimir Bukovsky Foundation, Amsterdam: Second World Press, 1987).

Van Voren, Robert, 'Soviet Psychiatry Criticized in the Soviet Press' in Robert van Voren (ed.), *Soviet Psychiatric Abuse in the Gorbachev Era* (Amsterdam: IAPUP, 1989), 62–72.

Van Voren, Robert (ed.), *Soviet Psychiatric Abuse in the Gorbachev Era* (Amsterdam: IAPUP, 1989).

Vedeneyeva, Irina, 'At the Devil's Door: *Ogonyok* Visits Moscow's Drug-Treatment Hospitals', *Ogonyok* 8 Feb. 1988:19–23, *CDSP* 40(13):10, 27 April 1988.

Vigon, A.G., 'Information About the Work of the Ethical Medical Examination Commission of the All-Union Society' (Dr Vigon's report on the work of the Belov Commission), in World Psychiatric Association 1991, Appendix 6:41–2.

Vilensky, O., 'Psychiatry and Politics', *Argumenty i fakty* 14, 7–13 April 1990:7, FBIS SOV-90-073, 16 April 1990:68–9.

Vinitskaya, Galina, 'Parliament Adopts Law on Psychiatric Aid', ITAR-TASS English service, Moscow 2 July 1992 17:58 GMT, FBIS-SOV-92-132, 9 July 1992:59.

Waller, J. Michael, *Secret Empire: The KGB in Russia Today* (Boulder, San Francisco and Oxford: Westview Press, 1994).

Weinstein, Edwin A., *Cultural Aspects of Delusion: A Psychiatric Study* (New York: Free Press, 1962).

White, Stephen, '"Democratisation" in the USSR'. *Soviet Studies* 42(1), Jan. 1990:3–24.

Wimbush, S.E. and A.R. Alexiev, 'Is the Soviet Union Islam's Best Friend? Not Exactly' (Santa Monica, CA: RAND, Aug. 1980).

Windholz, George, 'Psychiatric Commitments of Religious Dissenters in Tsarist and Soviet Russia: Two Case Studies', *Psychiatry* Nov. 1985, 48(4):329–40.

Winn, Ralph B. (trans. and ed.), *Psychotherapy in the Soviet Union*, trans. of *Vsesoiuznaia Konferentsia po Voprosam Psikhoterapii* (Conference Proceedings, 1956: Moscow) (New York: Greenwood Press, c.1961, 1969).

Wishnevsky, Julia, 'Revelations of Corruption among Soviet Psychiatrists', *Radio Liberty Research Bulletin* 61, 12 Feb. 1989:1–4.

World Health Organization, *Report on The International Pilot Study of Schizophrenia. Vol. 1: Results of the Initial Evaluation Phase* (Geneva: World Health Organization, 1973).

World Psychiatric Association, *Report by the World Psychiatric Association Team of the Visit to the Soviet Union 9–29 June 1991*. Unpublished report copy.

Wynn, A., 'The Soviet Union and the World Psychiatric Association', *Lancet* 19 February 1983, 1(8321):406–8.

Yanowitch, Murray, *Social and Economic Inequality in the Soviet Union: Six Studies* (White Plains, NY: M.E. Sharpe, Inc., 1977).

Yastrebov, V.S., 'The Organization of Addiction-Treatment Services', *Feldsher i akusherka* 8: August:3–9 1985, in *CDSP* XXXVII(44):15. L/N.

Yelin, Lev, 'Psychiatry and Politics', interview with A.A. Churkin, Moscow *New Times* 43, Oct. 1988:41–3.

Yelin, Lev, 'A Split and Personalities', Moscow *New Times* 37, 11–17 Sept. 1990: 38–9, FBIS SOV-90-183, 20 Sept. 1990:33–5.

Yergin, Daniel and Thane Gustafson, *Russia 2010 and What It Means for the World* (New York: Vintage Random House, 1995).

Young, John W., *The Longman Companion to Cold War and Detente 1941–1991* (London and New York: Longman, 1993).

Zheludkov, Arkady, 'Who Will Now Be Treated for Alcoholism, How and Where', *Izvestia* 20 Jan. 1994:3, *CDSP* 46(3):14, 16 Feb. 1994.

Ziferstein, Isadore, 'A Critical Evaluation of Gorman's "Soviet Psychiatry and the Russian Citizen,"' *International Journal of Psychiatry* 8(5)1969:858–61.

General Index

Entries are arranged alphabetically, letter-by-letter. Laws, decrees and administrative instructions are listed separately, following the General Index.

Conventions: SPH special psychiatric hospital (maximum security forensic hospital)
OPH ordinary or standard psychiatric hospital

Index of Laws, Decrees, Administrative Instructions